Contracts, Benefits, and Practice Management for the Veterinary Profession

CONTRACTS, BENEFITS, AND PRACTICE MANAGEMENT FOR THE VETERINARY PROFESSION

JAMES F. WILSON, DVM, JD

JEFFREY D. NEMOY, DVM, JD

ALAN J. FISHMAN, CLU, CFP®

Managing Editor: Elise P. Wilson
Editor-in-Chief: Suzanne Neilson
Production: The Thornhill Group, Los Angeles, CA

James F. Wilson, DVM, JD
  Visiting Lecturer, University of Pennsylvania, Colorado, and North Carolina
  State University Schools of Veterinary Medicine
  Veterinary Pet Insurance Company sponsored speaker at 17 other veterinary
  schools per year
  Proprietor, Priority Veterinary Management Consultants, Yardley, PA

Jeffrey D. Nemoy, DVM, JD

Alan J. Fishman, CLU, CFP

Priority Press, Ltd., 2111 Yardley Rd., Yardley, PA 19067

Library of Congress Cataloging in Publication Data:

Wilson, James, 1943 -
  Contracts, Benefits, and Practice Management of the Veterinary Profession

ISBN: 0-9621007-3-0

Printed in the United States of America

10 9

In memory of Christina Hynoski,
animal lover, pre-veterinary student, leader, and mentee
who died before she could fulfill her dream of
becoming a member of the veterinary profession and

Thomas G. Prior, athlete, avid reader, rugged individualist,
beloved brother-in-law, who treasured books
and the knowledge buried within them

James F. Wilson

To my beautiful wife, Kim

Jeffrey D. Nemoy

To the three women in my life,
my wife Karen and two daughters, Danielle and Lauren,
and in memory of my parents

Alan J. Fishman

ACKNOWLEDGMENTS

Having researched and written the *Law and Ethics of the Veterinary Profession* book 11 years ago, I knew it would be difficult to write this book while working full-time without some major help from many people. It also was obvious that unless my family was willing to put up with my hours at the office working on this project, it would create more disharmony than it could ever be worth. Thus, the first thanks go to my wife, Elise, for understanding and tolerating my ridiculously long hours staring into a computer screen instead of spending time with her. What made it bearable for both of us was that her father, Thomas J. Prior, was such good company during those empty evenings that she never felt like she had been abandoned.

The next two people in line for some recognition are patriarch, Thomas J. Prior, who along with Elise edited most of these chapters, and our son Mike, who gave up some ski weekends, camping trips, and time at the pitch and putt course with his dad who was forever working on "the book." Tom's editing consistently forced me to plug all the holes when it appeared I didn't really know what I was talking about. Unfortunately, he was always right, even when it took several hours of additional work to correct the defects. As for Mike, here's hoping that this book creates enough supplemental income so I can meet him in the Rockies twice each year while he's in college to catch up on our skiing. Fortunately, his sister, Amy, was in college throughout most of this effort and thus, didn't know what she was missing.

Another key person is Jeffrey Nemoy, DVM, JD. Jeffrey is the UC Davis graduate who decided he wanted to work on this project with me after finishing veterinary school even if it meant uprooting himself from his native California and moving cross country. Jeffrey became the office and computer systems manager, Power Point instructor, big brother and teacher for Mike, and researcher and initial draftsman of the chapters covering restrictive covenants, employment benefits, and independent contractors. Jeffrey read nearly 200 employment contracts, gleaning the pertinent statistical data referenced throughout the chapters. He has now received his JD degree from Loyola Law School in Los Angeles and is licensed in California, following up on the dream he had when we first had dinner in Davis, CA. As we initiated this project, his hope was (1) to help practice owners and managers understand the value of a wide array of employee benefits and learn how to offer them and (2) to help new graduates entering the profession grasp the intricacies of veterinary practice finances well enough to be able to negotiate contracts where both sides come out winners.

Next up is Chris Johnson, selected by Jeffrey to manage our office after he left, approved by me, and a true jack of all trades. Chris created all the figures and tables found in this book, double checked all the citations to be sure they matched the text, and proofed and formatted much of the book. Best of all, she did this while playing mother to a family with two teenagers, wife to a working husband, caregiver to two parents who died in her home during the writing of this book, and student in accounting at Temple University.

Another major contributor with a most understanding spouse is Alan Fishman, CLU, CFP, the author of the chapters on life insurance, disability income coverages, and retirement plans. Alan cut his writer's teeth with the materials in this book. One of the side effects was an increased knowledge of how to teach people about his material, an understanding of the financial shortcomings of the veterinary profession, and preparation for his growing role as a financial planner and advisor for practitioners, residents, interns, and new graduates. Alan, too, lost a parent during the unending gestation of this book. He encouraged me to get it published soon because the changes in the retirement plan industry were occurring so fast and furiously he'd have to rewrite his materials yet one more time if we didn't get it to the market.

As with the *Law and Ethics* book, our editor, Suzanne Neilson, played an important role. Although some of the gaps in delivering text to her were so big she had to call and ask what the name of this book was, Suzanne once again was the literary surgeon who dissected out the "diseased" text Jeffrey, Alan, and I submitted to her and sutured it back together like a vascular surgeon - reestablishing flow and continuity without destroying our thoughts. And, when I was so burned out and needed to leave for a three-week vacation just as this book was being completed, Suzanne and Chris finished the details. Thanks, you two, because that will make it easier for me to deny responsibility for any of the errors that are bound to occur.

Having lost our production manager from the *Law and Ethics* book to retirement, we desperately needed someone to take our text from Word Perfect and Word to the page-proof stage. One of the great fortunes of hiring Jeffrey was that we inherited his father, Sheldon Nemoy, and his production company entitled The Thornhill Group. Always the gentleman, always happy to achieve perfection, Sheldon and his crew designed the presentation and layout of our text in the contemporary manner in which you see it. It's a tedious task but an incredibly important one, done by a real professional.

Many other people played key roles, too: Charlotte Lacroix, DVM, JD of Priority Veterinary Legal Consultants, and my partner in the Priority Veterinary Management Consultants business, who edited and critiqued portions of this book; Larry McCormick, DVM, MBA, CBA who did the same. Barry Stupine, the hospital administrator for the Veterinary Hospital of the University of Pennsylvania; and University of Penn Deans Edward Andrews and Alan Kelly who had the desire to help Penn's new graduates, interns, and residents improve their success negotiating educational debt- and life-sustaining employment contracts and agreed to fund my assistance for them for the past eight years. Without that opportunity this book would be based largely on personal opinions instead of the hands-on, in the trenches, real world experience gained from reviewing hundreds of employment offers.

Other people with smaller but important roles include: Frances S. Shofer, Adjunct Assistant Professor of Epidemiology and Biostatistics from the University of Pennsylvania School of Veterinary Medicine, who helped Jeffrey harvest all the data about percentages of contracts containing important clauses discussed throughout this book. Also Laura Leasburg, DVM who read and analyzed some of the contracts and researched and wrote much of the text about health insurance, and AVMA New York Life insurance agent, Lesley Snider, who assisted with those materials.

Thanks are in order to Alex Baccini, University of Pennsylvania law student who researched and drafted a difficult section on restrictive covenants; large animal practitioners Jeff Ott, VMD, and Ron Stuber, DVM and his wife, Sue, who because of their first-hand experiences with veterinarians who destroyed vehicles or were lousy drivers helped create the section covering the use of business-owned autos; William Fegley, CPA and Lou Gatto, CPA, who answered key questions and provided material about independent contractors and tax-deductible employee benefit programs; and Tom Kendall, DVM for his insights and experience with a highly successful cafeteria plan. Not to be forgotten are Lloyd Meisels, DVM, for his help defining income production by veterinarians; Rich Blose, DVM and Nick Holland, VMD for their creativity tying compensation to performance appraisals; Dennis Cloud, DVM for sharing his unique veterinary compensation and performance criteria with the rest of the profession; Ms. Marty Bezner, CVPM for helping show that compensation based on 20% of production plus benefits is virtually identical to 25% with all benefits deducted; and my sister-in-law Mary Prior for her comments about managing a successful day care program for children. Thanks also are in order for Bernard Rollin, ethicist from Colorado State University, whose friendship, encouragement, and huge contributions to veterinary ethical decision making over his career have helped mold my thoughts about this ethereal but crucial component of core business values and contractual issues.

All veterinarians, and especially I, owe unending thanks to Harold (Hank) Hannah whose *JAVMA* Legal Briefs pushed veterinarians out of the legal Dark Ages and into the twentieth century. Several of the algorithms depicting legal principles and procedures were provided by Hank.

Last and not least, thanks are in order to my parents, Jim and Helen Wilson, who taught me that with enough perseverance and effort, I could accomplish anything I set out to do. This text and the events surrounding it taxed my abilities and stamina to the limit, but in the end their example was golden and here, at last is the completed book. Happy reading.

PREFACE

During the Christmas season of 1988 my wife, Elise, and I attended our first SCAVMA Auction at the University of Pennsylvania. At that fun-filled event we donated a copy of our newly published textbook, *Law and Ethics of the Veterinary Profession*, for auction along with three hours of assistance coaching the purchaser with his or her initial employment contract negotiations. Little did I know that the seeds for this book had been sown.

By the spring of 1991, because of what they were learning in the University of Pennsylvania's two-credit law and ethics course, so many of Penn's graduating students were asking for contract negotiating assistance that I approached Barry Stupine, Hospital Administrator for the teaching hospital and then Dean, Ed Andrews, to see if the school would be willing to pay me for my time. In spite of a tight budget, the answer was, "We think this is a great idea, Jim. Yes, we'll find the funds for your time, just don't anger any of our alumni who may have to pay more to hire these new grads as a result of your coaching." Fortunately, Dean Alan Kelly has continued his support of this effort during his tenure—an incredibly valuable service I wish all veterinary schools would offer their new grads.

I have heeded Barry Stupine's and Dean Andrews' words of warning carefully and, although a tiny group of alums have expressed concern about paying higher salaries and benefits than they had planned, very few feel my suggestions for more appropriate compensation and benefits have created adversarial relationships between them and their new doctors. And in the process, we have raised average salaries in the Mid-Atlantic states to levels well beyond the AVMA's published yearly norms.

Since 1991, over 250 individual students, interns, and residents at Penn have had an opportunity to listen to my evaluation of the salary, benefits, and restrictive covenant offers they were receiving. Utilizing local legal counsel for the final review of contract terms, by press time an additional 300 practice owners, office managers, and students from other schools have presented contract offers for me to evaluate. In the process, I continue to learn about new compensation and benefit ideas, absorb the language from creative contract clauses, and gain access to the salary, benefit, and restrictive covenant norms being offered across the country. Those observations and that knowledge are shared with readers in the text and sample contract clauses scattered throughout this book.

Those who have sought my business consultation services know that my review of their offers often has involved a heavy dose of "parental" advice coupled with ideas for negotiating better agreements and, in some cases, rejecting the offers and pursuing better opportunities elsewhere. One thing they have learned consistently is that negotiating a good contract is a two-way street. If new hires expect to be paid the salaries they want and think they deserve, they had better produce sufficient income for the practices at which they work to pay them accordingly. If potential employers expect to attract and retain good employees, they had better pay adequately, include a reasonable array of benefits, provide some training, coaching, and mentoring, and treat their new doctors with respect.

While teaching at UC Davis in 1995, a junior student named Jeffrey Nemoy approached me and told me that as a result of the law and ethics course and my passion for the subject, he wanted to attend law school. During January of his senior year he asked whether he might come to Pennsylvania in June of '96 and work in my office. The idea struck me that this might be just what was required to prompt me to put all that I was learning about employment contracts into print and, hopefully, influence the way practice owners and associates view their employment relationships. In addition to the research and writing, Jeffrey proved to be instrumental in bringing my office computer system and me into the 21st century of networked computers, email, and web-based research and teaching. He also was instrumental in training our son Mike to build animated, graphics-illustrated Power Point teaching programs for me to use in the 10 veterinary schools at which I teach this subject each year.

The arduous task of writing this text began in the fall of 1996 and was, perhaps, half finished by the time Jeffrey decided to move back to Los Angeles in July of 1997. My goal was to finish the project by the summer of 1998. Well, as fate would have it, my role in helping to start two new businesses in 1998 slowed the research and writing pace considerably.

During the winter of 1997-1998 another UC Davis student I have mentored for many years, Charlotte Lacroix, DVM graduated from the University of Pennsylvania's law school and became licensed to practice law in Pennsylvania and New Jersey. Working in tandem with Dr. McCormick and me, she started Priority Veterinary Legal Consultants, a sole proprietorship that assists veterinarians with their business-related legal matters. During the same time period, veterinary school classmate, practice owner, and friend, Larry McCormick, DVM, MBA, CBA (certified business appraiser), partnered with me to form Priority Veterinary Management Consultants. That business offers practice management advice, veterinary practice appraisals, and operational audits of practices. By the summer of 1998, I was back in the saddle supplementing Jeffrey's research on employee benefits and drafting the materials gleaned from many years of teaching experience.

Perhaps the death of Christina Hynoski, our daughter's high school classmate, family friend, and my mentee, in May of 1998 might have been an omen for what was in store for the rest of the year. Bright, charismatic Christina stopped in to see me and report on her academic pre-vet progress during every college break. She had completed her junior year of pre-veterinary studies at Clemson when she died suddenly while traveling in Tasmania. Her family lost a vibrant, endearing person and beloved child; the veterinary profession lost a fantastic future colleague. Without a doubt, her death was an inspiration to me to finish this project and help other enthusiastic young veterinary career professionals find employment opportunities that allow them to repay their educational debts, enjoy their jobs, and have some money left over for a vacation. Thus, Christina is the first person to whom this book is dedicated.

In mid August, my wonderful critic, editor, cheerleader, and wife of 29 years, Elise, had an ovariohysterectomy. During her post-op recovery, I recall very clearly sitting by her bedside plunking away on my lap top, trying to finish Chapter 3. Because there were no phone calls, I made some major progress while serving as her private duty nurse. However, in the middle of finishing the 15th draft of the "Five Tiers of Owner Compensation" section of Chapter 1, we learned that Elise's follow-up care would involve eight months of an aggressive combination of radiation-chemotherapy for metastatic uterine cancer. In September our daughter, Amy, put her life on hold and came home from the first semester of her senior year at the University of Colorado, Boulder to take care of her mom, her dad, and her grandfather, Thomas J. Prior. The book was relegated to the back burner.

One thing I have learned in 16 years of private veterinary practice is that troublesome cases always come in threes. It was in December of 1998 that number three struck. Elise's brother, Thomas G. Prior, the other party to whom this book is dedicated, had exploratory abdominal surgery during which the surgeon determined that he had metastatic pancreatic cancer. All fall he and our sister-in-law had been central to our support system and we hadn't even known he was sick!

The winter and spring of 1999 were fully occupied caring for Elise through her last three months of therapy; pursuing the latest in medical care for my canoeing and skiing buddy, Tom; providing business consultations for former students and colleagues around the country who were almost afraid to ask how things were going; and teaching business management, law and ethics, and personal, professional, and financial development at veterinary schools. Well, as fate has it for people with pancreatic cancer, Tom died at the end of June. I lost a dear friend; we all lost a scholar and family and community activist.

So more than a year later than planned, most of the knowledge I have gained over the past nine years about veterinary employment contracts, employee benefits, and the need for new graduates to create their post-graduation debt-repaying budgets now is in print. My hope is that by covering the gamut of topics tied to employment relationships, those of you who read this book can avoid many of the pitfalls your predecessors have endured. Read it with a probing mind. Search for ways to make the employment relationships of your future more harmonious and financially, personally, and professionally rewarding. Whenever possible, improve upon the concepts and ideas included here. The greatest profession on earth, veterinary medicine, needs to become even better and you can make it happen. Let Christina's enthusiasm for veterinary medicine serve as an inspiration to all of us to learn to negotiate contracts where both parties become winners; and for my dear friend Thomas G. Prior, lover of books, the perpetual free spirit, the best-read man I have ever known, here's one for you.

TABLE OF CONTENTS

Chapter 2

THE BASICS OF CONTRACT LAW

Chapter 3

COMPENSATION

Chapter 4

BASIC EMPLOYMENT BENEFITS

Chapter 5

HEALTH AND DISABILITY INSURANCE

Chapter 6

Life Insurance

Chapter 7

ANCILLARY EMPLOYMENT BENEFITS

Chapter 8
RETIREMENT BENEFITS

Chapter 9

RESTRICTIVE COVENANTS

Chapter 10

INDEPENDENT CONTRACTORS

Appendix I

PRINCIPLES OF VETERINARY MEDICAL ETHICS

Appendix II

MANDATORY CONTINUING EDUCATION FOR VETERINARIANS

Chapter 1

VETERINARY ETHICS AND THE BASICS OF AMERICAN LAW

By James F. Wilson, DVM, JD

The practice of veterinary medicine is based on a wide variety of legal concepts and precedents. The laws and regulations affecting veterinary medicine are innumerable. Some laws define the rights and duties of veterinarians as owners and managers of veterinary practices or providers of medical care. Others focus on the legal use of FDA and controlled veterinary drugs, biologicals, and pesticides as well as animals and their relationship with the law.

For coverage of these subjects, the complaint process and its link to professional liability, antitrust law and its effect on restraints of trade, credit management and collection of bad debt; medical records for business value and legal defense, equine purchase examinations, and wildlife law, readers are encouraged to contact the publisher and obtain a copy of the *Law and Ethics of the Veterinary Profession* textbook, first published in 1988 and reprinted nine times since then.[1]

animal welfare issues and stewardship for the animal kingdom than were graduates of the 1960s, '70s, and '80s. This changing ethical milieu requires more careful moral-ethical-legal decision making by veterinary practice owners and their staff than ever before. Otherwise employers find themselves compensating associates highly and providing quality benefits but experiencing continuous turnover because their practice philosophy and ethical standards are far afield from that of the recent graduates they have hired.

Because of a need for discussion of ethical determination in all phases of veterinary practice, including the formation of successful employment contracts, this first chapter reviews and explains contemporary moral-ethical-legal resolution as well as how the American legal system works. The subsequent nine chapters focus on employment contracts, employee benefits, and financial planning.

A NEW AGE DAWNING

Twenty years of teaching experience has led the author and veterinary school administrators to conclude that today's veterinary school graduates are much more attuned to

ORIGINS OF LAW

The laws regulating business relationships are a part of a comprehensive legal system that has evolved over centuries. Various cultures have had an effect on our current law, the first being those civilizations associated with the creation of the Bible. The Greek and Roman cultures also contributed to present-day legal concepts. Trials by judges, the assistance of lawyers for those involved in the trial process, and the creation of written laws available for all people to inspect comprise some of the contributions these earlier societies made to today's legal system.

The English Common Law System has had the biggest impact on American law. Unlike some other legal systems, the English common law does not rely solely on statutory law (laws created by legislatures or dictatorships). Instead, under the common-law system, judges have the discretion to establish binding legal precedents by interpreting the customs and beliefs of the people as they pertain to a set of facts presented. As in all systems, the court is also charged with interpreting the language and intent of legislatively enacted laws.

Judicially created law, or *case law*, as it is called, is law derived from judicial decisions and interpretations. The customs and beliefs of the times gradually become law as judges rely upon the doctrine of *stare decisis* ("the decision stands"). This legal principle means that decisions made in prior cases are to be followed in current cases and will be followed in future cases when the same set of facts exists.

Because of this principle, lawyers can anticipate how courts will decide cases, and they can advise people regarding ways to avoid future legal conflicts. Nonetheless, variations in the facts associated with similar cases make predicting case outcomes somewhat tenuous. Depending on these variations, courts will always have some leeway to alter their decisions. The result is that since very few sets of facts are identical, even with exceptional legal research, it is still difficult to predict the outcomes of cases. Much to the chagrin of science-oriented veterinary practitioners and staff, this means that the law is frequently gray rather than black or white, as most would like to see it.

It must also be kept in mind that prior decisions are binding only in courts of the same *jurisdiction*. There are various legal jurisdictions including the federal, state, municipal, tax, and several other court systems. Because of jurisdictional variations, what is law in Florida may not be the same as the law on a given issue in Pennsylvania. For example, money damages for the emotional distress associated with the loss of a pet are judicially allowed in Florida,[2] Hawaii,[3] Louisiana,[4] and Texas[5] but have either (1) not been considered, (2) been allowed by trial courts but not yet heard or decided by appellate courts, or (3) not been allowed by appellate courts in the remaining 46 states.

Morals, Codes of Ethics, and Laws

Morals

Moral and ethical constraints, although less well defined than the law, are as important as the legal constraints imposed upon the veterinary profession. In fact, the basis of all constraints on the practice of veterinary medicine is the underlying morality of each person. An individual's moral perception of right and wrong will consistently affect how that person responds to or obeys the ethical and legal constraints of society and the profession.

Moral constraints constitute the first limitations on the practice of veterinary medicine. *Webster's* offers the following definition of morals: "of or relating to principles of right and wrong behavior, sanctioned by or operating on one's conscience or ethical judgment." Specifically, this means that moral constraints on the practice of veterinary medicine have to do with practitioners' personal views of right and wrong and the guilt they feel when they do not comply with these very personal feelings.

A person's moral standards are determined largely by family influences and to some degree by religious upbringing or philosophical principles. Other factors influencing moral judgment emanate from schools, peers, clients, girlfriends, boyfriends, spouses, staff members, the public, and, ultimately, the press.

When analyzing people's conduct, the famous newspaper columnist, Ann Landers, said it best in a column where she set forth some guidelines for "telling the difference between right and wrong."[6] These consist of advice from a retired pastor, Dr. Preston Bradley, of the Peoples Church of Chicago, and contain the following caveats:

1. Does the course of action you plan to follow seem logical and reasonable?

2. Does it pass the test of sportsmanship? In other words, if everyone followed this same course of action, would the results be beneficial for all?

3. Where will your plan of action lead? How will it affect others? How will it affect you?

4. What will you think of yourself when you look back at what you did?

5. Separate yourself from the problem; pretend the problem is that of a person you admire. How would you expect them to solve it?

6. Hold up your final decision to the glaring light of publicity. Would you want family and friends to know what you have done?

One cannot help wonder how much influence the veterinary educational process has on a professional person's morality. Traditionally, there has been little mention of this subject in veterinary school. The international animal rights movement of the 1980s and '90s has changed this, though, in that veterinarians more than ever before find themselves in the mainstream of issues concerning people's interactions with and responsibilities for the treatment of animals. In the past decade many veterinary schools have added or expanded courses on law and ethics in their curricula. Thus, it appears that as Nixon's Watergate affair of the '70s upgraded the ethics curricula in the nation's law schools, advances in the animal rights movement and the human animal bond have done the same for the nation's veterinary schools in the '90s.

TEACHING AND UNDERSTANDING ETHICS

Many science-oriented veterinary school professors and administrators, research-oriented clinicians, and private practitioners have questioned whether it is possible to teach ethics to veterinary students who range from 23 to 43 years of age. After all, hasn't the moral and ethical fiber of students who have reached these ages already been decided?

The best answer to this question is that yes, people's personal moral code has formed by the time they are adults, but they still can be taught to identify ethical issues and think things through methodically according to certain ethical mores.[7] A recent text on the subject of veterinary ethics, by Bernie Rollin, ethicist from Colorado State University's College of Veterinary Medicine, speaks to this issue:

Detecting ethical questions is, in some ways, like detecting lamenesses. Prima facie, ordinary people not particularly knowledgeable about veterinary medicine would think that anyone can tell when a horse is lame and which leg is affected. After all, we can do so easily with humans. In fact, when actually confronted with a lame horse, inexperienced lay people, and even veterinary students, can at best detect that something is wrong (and sometimes not even that), but can rarely pinpoint the problems. This is exactly analogous to the activity of identifying ethical problems. People (sometimes) know something is problematic, but they have trouble saying exactly what the problem is.[8]

Codes of Ethics

Ethical constraints or guidelines come from a body of principles or ideals developed by a group of people to encourage high standards of conduct and to regulate the conduct of members belonging to that group. In veterinary medicine it usually is a professional association such as the AVMA, AAEP, AABP, or other specialty group that develops these guidelines. Ethical guidelines differ from morals in that they reflect the views of groups of people as opposed to individual opinions of right and wrong.

The basic code of ethics for veterinarians in the United States is the American Veterinary Medical Association (AVMA) *Principles of Veterinary Medical Ethics.*[9] Individual state and local veterinary associations usually adopt the AVMA code to fulfill their own needs for a script on the topic of ethics.

Etiquette is often confused with ethics when considering standards of conduct in the veterinary profession. This may be because of the focus the *Principles of Ethics* traditionally had on testimonials, advertising, marketing of products and services, and solicitation of clients. Etiquette consists of the accepted forms, manner, and ceremonies established by convention that are expected for someone to be a member of a group or professional association. Historically, etiquette is more procedural in nature, whereas ethics relates to standards of conduct promoted by and demanded of members of veterinary associations.

One author helped clarify the difference between ethics and etiquette in veterinary practice as follows: ...etiquette is the set of rules of decorous behavior, whereas ethics are the moral principles of the veterinary profession or its associations.[10] Historically the profession classified many rules of etiquette as principles of ethics, but this has changed. For example, current rules on advertising and client solicitation that can be ethically disseminated to the public have become local rules of etiquette. Whereas

older versions of the *Principles* have focused considerable attention on accepted standards of advertising, the 1998 revisions to the *Principles* have simplified them. What once was several paragraphs limiting the volume and type of information that could be disseminated to the public now reads as follows:

> Advertising by veterinarians is ethical when there are no false, deceptive, or misleading statements or claims. A false, deceptive, or misleading statement or claim is one which communicates false information or is intended, through a material omission, to leave a false impression.[9]

The new *Principles* go on to explain and simplify the ethical requirements regarding testimonials and endorsements by members of the profession. In doing so, they say,

> Testimonials or endorsements are advertising, and they should comply with the guidelines for advertising. In addition, testimonials and endorsements of professional products or services by veterinarians are considered unethical unless they comply with the following:
>
> 1. The endorser must be a bonafide user of the product or service.
> 2. There must be adequate substantiation that the results obtained by the endorser are representative of what veterinarians may expect in actual conditions of use.
> 3. Any financial, business, or other relationship between the endorser and the seller of a product or service must be fully disclosed.
> 4. When reprints of scientific articles are used with advertising, the reprints must remain unchanged, and be presented in their entirety.[9]

Since this is virtually all the current *Principles of Ethics* say regarding etiquette, it is clear that the new principles have become more tightly linked to ethical decisions than to etiquette.

VETERINARY ETHICS AND ANIMAL ETHICS

As a branch of ethics, veterinary ethics lacks a single accepted usage, which sometimes results in confusion. Some people consider that the term *veterinary ethics* relates to animals, and animal use by society, just as veterinary medicine relates to the care and use of animals. If this is the case, any ethical issue concerning animals, whether or not it is related to veterinarians, is considered an issue of veterinary ethics. As one author said,

> In this sense, whether people have a moral obligation to protect endangered wildlife, or whether it is morally proper to wear animal fur, are questions of veterinary ethics, because these are questions concerning what is morally right to do with or to animals.[11]

Other people, however, believe that "veterinary ethics" means ethics as it relates to veterinarians and their relationships with others within the profession who are involved in providing veterinary care. Most veterinarians have this understanding of the term. Thus, the AVMA's *Principles of Veterinary Medical Ethics*" is a document about ethical issues in veterinary practice, focusing more on the relationships one has with colleagues than on the broader range of moral or ethical issues relating directly to animals.[11]

THE FOUR BRANCHES OF VETERINARY ETHICS

Even when one conceives of veterinary ethics as the study of ethical issues relating to the practice of veterinary medicine, Tannenbaum says there are four different things one might have in mind.[12] The first of these relates to what members of the profession think is right and wrong regarding professional behavior and attitudes. In this sense, understanding the "ethics" of a profession is a matter of describing its actual values and does not involve making value judgments about what is moral or immoral in a professional person's behavior. Tannenbaum calls the study of the actual ethical views of veterinarians and veterinary students regarding professional behavior and attitudes *descriptive veterinary ethics.*[12]

The second branch of veterinary ethics according to Tannenbaum involves the creation of the official ethical standards adopted by organizations comprised of professionals and imposed upon their members. With this interpretation of ethics, one can understand or appeal to a part of a profession's ethical standards without personally believing those standards are morally correct. Thus, the process of articulating and applying ethical standards to and by organized veterinary medicine is called *official veterinary ethics.*

Another source of moral and ethical standards for veterinarians involves action by administrative government bodies that regulates veterinary practice and activities in which veterinarians engage. In many cases, these administrative bodies adopt sections of the AVMA's *Principles of Ethics* into their statutes or regulations. When that is the case, violations of these ethical standards can result in criminal or civil penalties, up through and including license revocations. It is this branch of ethics to which Tannenbaum applies the term *administrative veterinary ethics.*

Lastly, one can focus on attempts to discover or determine the correct moral standards for veterinarians and other veterinary caregivers to pursue. According to Tannenbaum, the philosophical literature uses the term *normative ethics* to refer to the search for correct principles of good and bad, right and wrong, justice and injustice. Thus, he titles the activity of looking for correct norms to define veterinary professional behavior and attitudes *normative veterinary ethics.*

This multitude of definitions seems to complicate matters more than necessary. Nonetheless, because of Tannenbaum's stature as a well-known veterinary ethicist, a discussion is included here in hopes that readers will pursue this excellent reference as a resource to help solve many of the daily ethical puzzles that occur in veterinary practice.

LAWS

Laws are bodies of rules developed and enforced by government to regulate peoples' conduct. The powerful influence of the law in veterinary medicine emanates from court rulings, statutes, or governmental regulations that affect animal care and the practice of veterinary medicine. Many of these laws stem from the public's moral and ethical concerns about life, death, and how people should conduct themselves in society.

The main difference between ethical principles and laws lies in their enforcement. While laws are enforced by governments, ethical principles are enforced solely by the professional associations that developed them. Since there is no government involvement in the enforcement of veterinary ethics, the sanctions are limited to suspensions and expulsions from veterinary associations. Professional associations may reprimand, suspend, or expel members for failure to adhere to their ethical codes, but they must rely on their own organizational rules, not those of the court system, to effect the expulsion. The benefit to society or an association from such action is questionable, because members can continue to behave unethically even after they have been expelled. It is because of this fact that action taken against unethical veterinarians by associations rarely has the impact that court or state boards of examiners decisions do.

Although ethical guidelines are extremely important in encouraging cooperation and respect within a profession, their value goes beyond that limited effect. This is because courts and governments can and do look to the ethical principles established by the various professional associations for guidance when legal precedents need to be updated to fit today's professional and societal expectations.

The legal ramifications of wrongdoing are clearly greater than a professional association reprimand. The enforcement of laws can lead to civil lawsuits, state board hearings, or criminal prosecutions. Such actions can result in monetary damages awarded plaintiffs in civil court actions against veterinarians for the negligent practice of veterinary medicine; license suspensions or revocations or fines assessed by state boards for unprofessional conduct; and even imprisonment, as in cases involving violations of anticruelty, FDA, or DEA laws.

Whatever the case, though, morality and ethics always must be considered in conjunction with the law. The attitudes and perceptions of young veterinarians must evolve from those of ordinary citizens to those of medical professionals. How this is accomplished and whether it is successful will greatly affect the professional behavior patterns and standards by which they conduct their practices in the years to come.

THE EVOLUTION OF MORAL PRINCIPLES TO ETHICAL AND LEGAL PRECEDENTS

As moral attitudes change and evolve, some of the principles espoused by individuals are adopted by groups of individuals or professionals and become embodied in their principles of ethics. Over time, some of those ethical principles are integrated into laws adopted by government or legal precedents developed by courts (Figure 1.1). In other cases, the moral attitudes of certain segments of the public bypass the consensus ethical principles of society stage and are churned directly into laws, e.g., laws dealing with pornography or abortion.

Rollin redefines the terminology of the process when he explains that there are three subcategories under the umbrella of ethics: (1) social ethics, (2) personal ethics, and (3) professional ethics.[8] Of these, social ethics is the most basic and objective even

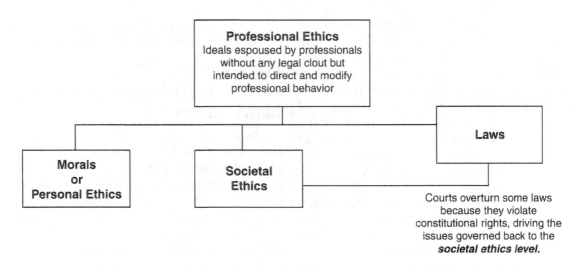

Figure 1.1. The formation of laws

if, to many, the words *objectivity* and *ethics* do not fit in the same sentence. Rollins' category called *personal ethics* equates to what has been presented herein as moral judgment. Professional ethics obviously applies to decisions by professionals and is explained in more detail later.

SUBJECTIVITY AND OBJECTIVITY

People who consider themselves scientists sometimes are tempted to assert that, unlike scientific judgments, which by definition are objective, ethical judgments are subjective opinion and not fact and, thus, not subject to rational discussion or adjudication. It is true that conducting experiments to gather data to decide what is right or wrong and, therefore, what is "ethical" is difficult. However, ethically correct decisions are not based simply on personal whim and caprice.

If people doubt this principle, they should simply go out and rob a bank in front of witnesses. Subsequently, they can argue in court that such conduct was in their opinion ethically and morally acceptable because they needed the money to avoid starvation for a failing parent, themselves, or their children. However, from a societal perspective, what was good for them will not be good for society as a whole and, therefore, is unacceptable conduct. Furthermore, the fact that such ethical judgments are not validated by gathering data or doing experiments to determine what is right vs. wrong behavior does not mean that these judgments are simply a matter of individual subjective opinion. Instead, consensus rules about rightness and wrongness of actions that have an impact on others need to be and are articulated into clear social principles, which in turn are encoded into laws and policies.[8]

SOCIETAL, PERSONAL, AND PROFESSIONAL ETHICS

According to Rollin, the ethical rules that people believe to be universally binding on all members of society are called the *social consensus* ethic.[7] Without consensus ethics, society would deteriorate into chaos and anarchy. Rules can vary somewhat for different societies around the globe as long as there is a common core in all of these ethics.

The social consensus ethic, though, does not regulate all areas of life; certain areas of behavior are left to the discretion of individuals who apply their moral judgment, or their *personal ethic*.[7] An excellent example of a matter that has recently moved from the concern of the social ethic and the laws that mirror it to the purview of one's personal ethic is the area of sexual behavior.

Whereas once laws constrained activities like homosexual behavior, adultery, and cohabitation, in western democracies these things now are left to one's personal ethic. In many states or locales, homosexual couples can receive medical benefits as if they were married dependants and can adopt children as couples, while heterosexuals who cohabit out of wedlock no longer face actions for criminal behavior, nor is such activity frowned upon socially as it once was.

On the other hand, certain areas of personal ethics have been converted by laws to social consensus ethics. An example entails one's personal choice of renting or selling one's property or hiring or firing on a whim. Historically, the prevailing attitude was that such decisions were one's own damn business and no one else's.[8] This is no longer the case, because federal law has interceded to impart what it finds to be a more socially acceptable consensus ethic that governs such decisions and mandates equality irrespective of age, race, religion, and national origin.

The third component of ethics is *professional ethics*. Because of the special education and training of professionals, society generally leaves it to these groups to set up their own rules of conduct. This allows them to deal with situations pertinent to their work. For example, psychiatrists may not have sex with their patients, and veterinarians have a responsibility to provide essential medical services for animals when it is necessary to save life or relieve suffering. The social ethic offers general rules with which all people are to comply, while subclasses of professionals develop their own more specific ethical codes to cover their special circumstances; hence, the codes of ethics for lawyers, physicians, veterinarians, farriers, ministers, and others. Professional ethics thus occupies a position midway between social consensus ethics and personal ethics.

ETHICAL CHANGES

FROM ANIMAL WELFARE ACTIVISM TO ANIMAL WELFARE LEGISLATION

In recent years, a wider recognition of the value of the human-animal bond, coupled with the activities of animal right's activists, has tended to advance man's moral concerns about animals. Generally, this activism has changed the moral feelings society has about animals. This has led to considerable animal welfare legislation and, more recently, the teaching of animals and the law in at least six law schools in the United States.[13] This reform movement has also impacted the veterinary community, whose members have changed their moral and ethical feelings regarding their professional responsibility for the welfare of their patients. The changes are reflected by the following societal examples:

1. The whales caught in the Bering Sea over a decade ago which could be saved only by a thawing of relations between the then Soviet Union and the United States. This was a major worldwide animal rights/animal welfare situation dealing with the fate of two animals. This increased interest in the welfare of specific animals continued in 1998 with the freeing of Willie the killer whale, the star of several movies using his name, from his wonderful home in Newport, Oregon to his ancestral habitat off the coast of Newfoundland.

2. Sweden's 1982 legislative action granting cattle in its country the "right to graze."

3. Great Britain's 1988 ban on dehorning and castration of livestock older than eight weeks of age without anesthesia.

4. The 1985 amendment to the U.S. Animal Welfare Act affirming the rights of laboratory animals to be free of pain and suffering not essential to a piece of research; providing that nonhuman pri-

mates have the right to be housed under conditions which enhance their psychological well-being; and requiring that research dogs be granted the "right to exercise." The adoption by the state of Minnesota of many laws similar to this federal legislation into its state animal welfare statutes in 1983 (dogs, cats, horses, rodents, and pet birds).

5. The unwillingness of today's veterinary graduates to euthanize pets solely because owners ask them to do so. This moral precept has gained enough importance that it was included in the employment contract of a recent Colorado State University graduate.[14]

This focus on the moral and ethical consequences of our daily activities is not exclusive to the animal welfare movement. In recent years, Wall Street and Washington, D.C. have been faced with multiple moral, ethical, and legal nightmares. For example, the Michael Milken-Ivan Boesky junk bonds case in the early 1990s sent multimillionaire financial dealers on Wall Street to prison, only to be joined by Charles H. Keating, Jr. and others from the Savings and Loan industry a few years later.

Government leaders are now forced to place their assets into blind trusts so that their decisions in office do not directly benefit their financial holdings in business. And if cabinet members fly around the country excessively in private jets paid for by taxpayer dollars, they will be out of a job, not because they violated the law but because they used poor moral and ethical judgment.

The animal welfare/animal rights movement is constantly pushing man's moral concerns for animals into new laws. These include activities such as the

- active enforcement of the Endangered Species Act, responsible for saving virgin forests in the Pacific Northwest in order to conserve the spotted owl and preventing removal of the bald eagle from the endangered species list in 1999;

- passage of laws allowing pets in public housing;

- passage of consumer protection bills called *dog and cat lemon laws*, providing purchasers of pets with legal rights to return unhealthy pets to dealers and obtain replacement animals or refunds for veterinary expenses incurred treating their sick pets; and

- the Proctor and Gamble company's decision to stop most animal testing of many of its household products except for pharmaceuticals, foods, and new products.[15]

A front-page business section feature article in the *Philadelphia Inquirer* stated that, in some cases, animal testing is required by law, and only in those cases will Proctor & Gamble continue testing on animals.[15] The company's policy against the use of animal testing now covers 80% of its total product portfolio, including color cosmetics, shampoos and hair styling products, skin care products, tissue and towel products, laundry and dishwashing detergents, and household cleaners. P & G has spent more than $100 million over the last 15 years to study alternatives to animal testing.

As a result of pressures from animal advocacy groups and research into nonanimal testing, science has advanced to the point that nonanimal testing methods now can be relied on to ensure that those products are safe for people. Three other consumer product manufacturers including Dial, Gillette, and Mary Kay cosmetics have already agreed to end animal testing. However, the FDA still requires animal testing on pharmaceuticals.[15]

It seems clear that as long as the world is free of economically draining world wars or military conflicts and societies continue to become more affluent, moral concerns for animals will increasingly be converted into legal rights. Although it may sound preposterous, the following quote explains the nature of the changing times.

There is this thick legal wall with humans on one side and all nonhuman animals on the other side...While the law currently protects pets from abuse and endangered species from extinction, animals do not actually have rights—an age-old position of the legal system. But over the last 50 years, science has shown that some animals—chimps in particular—have extraordinary mental capacities beyond what the ancient Greeks, Romans, and Hebrews ever imagined....If they have human-like intelligence, shouldn't that entitle them to human-type rights?

While the concept may sound far fetched, it wasn't too long ago that women and blacks were denied rights because they were considered, to some degree, less than human. It took a 13th Amendment to the Constitution for us to outlaw slavery at a time when people were treated as property because of the color of their skin. There are occasions in the law for taking a very fundamental look at the treatment of other living things.[13]

FROM ETHICAL TO ILLEGAL

Occasionally what goes up the flagpole from a moral attitude to an ethical principle to a law also comes down. A classic example of a law superseding an ethical principle is found in the anticompetition, restraint of trade context. Prior to 1975, it was common for professional associations to develop minimum fee schedules to which their members were expected to comply, and for courts to accept the propriety of such fee schedules. This principle changed in 1975, with a landmark decision by the United States Supreme Court,[16] which held that it was a violation of the Sherman Antitrust Act for professional associations to suspend or expel members for refusing to follow minimum fees set by the association. Where it had heretofore been unethical conduct *not* to comply with association fee schedules, it now was *an illegal restraint of trade to agree* in any way with colleagues to establish fees or for members of associations to even discuss them.

As if that weren't enough to force major change upon the learned professions, in 1977 the Supreme Court again broke new ground. In this case it held that ethical principles prohibiting the advertising of routine professional services were unconstitutional limitations of free speech.[17]

Before these landmark decisions, both of these professional-association-adopted ethical principles were free from governmental review. Since that time, however, the Federal Trade Commission (FTC) has demanded upon at least two occasions that the AVMA remove numerous anticompetitive ethical principles embodied in its guidelines. The FTC also has required that several state boards of examiners repeal board regulations that restrained trade and competition.

The ethical principles that were removed corresponded with what members of the profession felt constituted morally and ethically appropriate conduct and etiquette among colleagues. However, the FTC felt that some of those rules of conduct restrained trade and enhanced unfair competition, causing harm to the consumers of veterinary services. Thus, one can see that the moral, ethical, and legal constraints on veterinary practice are in a constant state of flux. What is deemed morally, ethically, and legally appropriate today may no longer be the case in the future.

THE VETERINARIAN'S ROLE IN DECIDING MORAL AND ETHICAL ISSUES

It is important that veterinarians consider what impact, if any, moral, ethical, and legal constraints have when they are applied to day-to-day business decisions. From a moral point of view, practitioners must consider their roles as

- protectors of animals' interests;

- professionals applying their own standards to issues of right and wrong treatment of animals based on their upbringing, education, and religious beliefs; and

- educators of owners regarding responsible animal ownership.

Ethically, veterinarians have been forced to become

- representatives of the veterinary profession looking to the *AVMA Principles of Veterinary Medical Ethics* for guidance;

- highly visible professionals trying to retain the public's trust that we care more about animals' well-being than we do about maintaining the status quo of animals as property or making money; and

- reformers of the veterinary profession's ethical standards and advocates for animals and society's relationships with them.

When considering the veterinarian's role from a legal point of view, members of the profession must consider themselves as

- servants of animal owners carrying out their contractual wishes and demands (after all, animals are still regarded as property under the law);

- assistants in the enforcement of state or federal laws, as may be required by a state, to report suspected staged animal fights,[18] acts of animal cruelty,[19] or the chemical impairment of colleagues;[20]

- professionals required to know something about and understand laws regarding the care of animals and the practice of veterinary medicine; and

- authors and reformers of laws and rules relating to contemporary and controversial issues such as ownership of veterinary practices by nonveterinarians, minimum standards of veterinary practice, registration of veterinary facilities by state boards independent of one's li-

cense to practice veterinary medicine, the adoption of state puppy and kitten lemon laws, and new FDA laws and regulations maintaining food safety.

THE VETERINARIAN'S DILEMMA

Fulfilling one's moral duties toward animal patients can put veterinarians at odds with their clients. Let's look at a couple of examples.

EXAMPLE 1

An owner brings in "Maggie," a severely neglected, maggot-infested mongrel, and requests or can afford only "Class D" medicine. The doctor considers the owner's prior neglect of the animal to be cruelty to animals and knows that the patient needs at least "Class B" and maybe "Class A" medicine to recover. Her choices include the following:

1. refuse to lower her standards to the point she delivers Class D medicine and, instead, send Maggie and her owner down the street to find another veterinarian willing to provide this type of care.

2. recommend euthanasia because Class D medicine will bring with it a poor prognosis for Maggie's recovery, the probability of an unpaid bill and, perhaps, additional cruelty or abuse of the patient.

3. provide Class C treatment, saying nothing to the owner about the neglect. The doctor does not get involved, but allows her desire to receive some income from the case and the owner's wishes to take precedence over Maggie's interests.

4. agree to provide care but be determined to educate the owner about the anticruelty laws and how they apply to the owner's apparent neglect of Maggie.

If traditional property law principles are applied in situations like this, veterinarians are merely servants of owners, disregarding the interests of animals. If veterinarians consider their moral views of right and wrong, however, they will or should feel guilty that this animal will receive inferior care and, in all likelihood, suffer additional neglect at the hands of its owner. In fact, it is reasonable to consider that Maggie probably should either be placed in another home or euthanized.

When practitioners look to the AVMA's *Principles of Ethics* under the section entitled *Professional Behavior*, the messages regarding the issue are unclear. Two different sections addressing this type of situation say

Veterinarians should first consider the needs of the patient: to relieve disease, suffering, or disability while minimizing pain or fear.

The choice of treatments or animal care should not be influenced by considerations other than the needs of the patient, the welfare of the client, and the safety of the public.[9]

The *Principles* fail to address what one should do when the interests of a badly neglected patient are in direct conflict with the intentions, abilities, or actions of the owner. For example, it may be in the patient's best interest to proceed with high-quality veterinary care to save its life or restore it to normal function. However, the owners may lack a strong bond with this particular pet, be unhappy with its undesirable aggressive behavior, be concerned about the spread of a zoonotic disease to an immunocompromised family member, or lack the funds to pay for veterinary services.

Since the *AVMA Principles* fail to provide clear direction to deal with this conflict, it is in this type of confusing ethical dilemma where a practitioner's knowledge of the law can be most helpful. Attempting to deal with the problem from a strictly moral perspective by heaping moral indignation on a neglectful or abusive animal owner probably will not win the owner's respect nor produce better care for the animal. Yet saying nothing won't help the poor animal, either.

Knowledge of state or local animal cruelty laws that define cruelty to include "the deprivation of necessary sustenance, food, drink or veterinary care from an animal" can provide veterinarians with a hefty club with which to convince owners it is time to mend their ways or be reported to the local SPCA. In other words, using a legal argument in the above example to alter a client's attitude about owner responsibility probably will be much more effective than the judgmental impact of a purely moral one. With that in mind, practitioners could present the following blend of moral and legal arguments to such an owner:

Mr. and Mrs. Badowner, my staff and I are absolutely appalled that you could allow Maggie here to become so horribly neglected. You may have all kinds of excuses for what has happened, but in my judgment the facts presented here make things look like this may be a case of cruelty to animals, which is a crime, you know. I realize you cannot do anything today about what has happened in the past, but I want you to know that you are on trial. If you follow our directions and show us that you can take care of Maggie like a responsible owner, you will regain our respect and you'll be off the hook. However, if you do not come back for the follow-up appointments that we will schedule for you today, and if you do not show us that you can provide proper care for Maggie, I will be compelled to report you to my good friend Vickie at the SPCA. (Veterinarians who would like to make an even stronger impression, will take pictures of Maggie to document the severity of the neglect.)

This is what is called an *armtwister*, and it is amazing how powerful the effect of such a constructive reprimand can be. When there is serious doubt about the intentions of the client, the following dialogue can be added:

You know Mr. and Mrs. Badowner, your irresponsible care of and attitude towards Maggie upsets me so much that I am going to call my friend Vickie at the SPCA today and tell her about what my staff and I have seen. As of this time your name will be kept confidential. The SPCA will be on notice not to take any action until we determine whether you can satisfactorily care for Maggie and follow our directions, but you are definitely on trial.

The example involving a neglected dog with maggots used a practitioner's knowledge of the law to help bring about a morally beneficial result for the animal. However, in other cases the anger induced in an animal's owner or the reluctance to return and endure further admonishment brought about by a veterinarian's knowledge and application of the law could place a damper on what otherwise appears to be a morally correct course of action. In some circles, veterinarians elect not to employ this type of threat but, instead, automatically report such neglect or abuse to the proper authorities for them to ascertain whether other animals, children, or spouses in the family also are affected.

EXAMPLE 2

This example involves a cat, "Missy," that was spayed while 55 days pregnant and is now lying in a postsurgery recovery cage. It is a few minutes before closing time in a metropolitan practice, and rush hour traffic has begun. Because Dr. Slasher was unable to complete all of his diagnostic procedures on another client's feline urological syndrome-suspect cat, that client elected to leave "Blackie" overnight rather than take him home and fight the traffic to bring him back tomorrow.

Blackie's owner leaves, and Dr. S walks back into the treatment room where he is confronted by his technician who excitedly says, "Dr. Slasher, that pregnant cat you just spayed? She's in shock and she and the cage are soaked in blood."

Dr. S responds with furor, "Oh my God." He quickly restarts the IV fluids and then discovers that the patient's PCV is a mere 18. After an additional 15 minutes, the patient looks worse and Dr. S decides the only alternative is to reopen the abdomen and find the bleeder.

Dr. S's recently opened veterinary practice does not have a feline blood donor and, thus, his only source of blood for an immediate transfusion is Blackie, whose owner just departed. He could perform the additional surgery without giving the transfusion, but due to the rapid drop in the PCV, he feels his patient's chances for survival will be greatly enhanced if he can give some fresh blood during the additional surgery. Stressed by the excitement of the moment, he decides to draw 50 to 60 cc of blood from Blackie if he can do so without the need for any sedation. After all, this poses no apparent threat to Blackie but great benefit to the bleeding patient. Blackie is a great patient and donates his blood like a hero.

Dr. S's moral principles, or in Rollin's words his *personal ethic*, tell him that the survival of the hemorrhaging cat (and his professional reputation) are more important at this moment than any medical risks to Blackie. He does not have time to peruse his AVMA *Principles of Ethics* for advice, but had he done so he might well have been comforted by the section which says, "Veterinarians should first consider the needs of the patient: to relieve disease, suffering, or disability while minimizing pain or fear."

Under traditional property law principles, the taking of blood from Blackie without the consent of the owner is an illegal act. Still, Dr. S's medical (and moral) standards tell him to draw blood from Blackie regardless of his failure to obtain the owner's consent because he knows that the hemorrhaging cat will have a much better chance of survival if she receives fresh blood.

In other words, from a moral (and medical) perspective he feels totally justified in drawing blood without permission, while from a legal point of view he realizes that his actions violate the owner's lawful rights of ownership. Had he read his copy of the *Principles of Ethics*, he would have felt even better about his decision to draw blood from Blackie.

Because of the crisis nature of the moment, Dr. S fails to consider the medical alternatives that might help him solve this moral-ethical-legal dilemma such as the following:

1. calling a colleague and attempting to borrow some blood from another practitioner (this implies being on good terms with one's colleagues)

2. sending an employee home to retrieve his or her cat to use as a donor (unfortunately, it's rush hour)

3. calling a good client who lives nearby and who is already on the practice's "willing blood-donor list" (This "Marketing 101" concept requires advance planning for avoiding dilemmas like this.)

4. trying to call Blackie's owner to get permission first, documenting such attempts in the medical record, and trying again 15 minutes later (He failed to do this.)

5. opening the abdomen, suctioning the free blood into a syringe and autotransfusing the patient (Up-to-date continuing education would have made it more likely that he would think of this alternative.)

6. applying a pressure body bandage to the patient to slow or stop the internal hemorrhaging until blood could be acquired for a transfusion

7. administering plasma expanders or one of the new oxygen-carrying blood replacement products entering the marketplace

8. drawing blood from Blackie without shaving the jugular furrow and simply not telling the owner: In this approach, he might have avoided the entire conflict with Blackie's owner but would have violated the ethical guideline calling for veterinarians to be "honest, fair, courteous, considerate, and compassionate."

Additionally, he probably would be violating his own moral principles of honesty and integrity.

Blackie's owners return the following evening, and Dr. Slasher saunters into the room announcing that "You should be proud of your 'son' because shortly after you departed yesterday, Blackie became a hero. He donated 60 cc of blood to a beautiful calico in need of his assistance and, consequently, saved her life."

Unfortunately, Blackie's owners do not see things that way. They file a three-page letter to the California State Board of Veterinary Examiners asking, "How dare they allow a morally deficient practitioner like Dr. S to retain his veterinary license."

The clinician who actually experienced this nightmare had never thought about this moral-ethical-legal dilemma in the above terms before it happened. Have you? Which course of action would you have pursued? What do you think the outcome of this case was once it was reviewed by the State Board?

Answer: After 16 hours of discussion and $800 of legal counsel assisting with a response that analyzed the moral, ethical, and legal ramifications of Dr. Slasher's actions, the State Board reviewed his letter and dismissed the complaint with a reprimand. One lucky, but wiser veterinarian.

MORAL-ETHICAL-LEGAL ISSUES IN EMPLOYMENT CONTRACTS

In that veterinary students are more attuned to animal rights and welfare issues and personal safety concerns than at any time in the history of the veterinary profession, many new applicants for veterinary employment value appropriate animal welfare policies and ethical decision-making by their employers as much as or more than they do compensation and employee benefits. For employment relationships between veterinary employees and employers to be successful and long lasting, some discussion and an understanding and acceptance of many moral, ethical, legal, and other practice philosophy issues should occur before applicants accept jobs or employers hire veterinary nurses or associates. Among the most problematic issues and, thus, those requiring discussion prior to signing any contract, are the practice's and applicant's views regarding:

- convenience euthanasia.

- credit management policies for after-hours and daytime emergencies examined by doctors with or without the assistance of other staff members.

- the need for individual sterile surgery packs for each sterile surgery procedure.

- positions and policies on cosmetic surgeries and whether agreement can be reached by the parties on the amputation of puppies' tails and dew claws, declawing of cats, the cropping of ears, and the debarking of dogs.

- other personal animal rights issues and the willingness of the employer to support some form of pro bono work by associates for the indigent.

- overnight hospitalization of emergency and critical care patients without appropriate medical supervision and without apprising owners of the availability of 24-hour care for patients that need it when it is within 20 minutes of the practice.

- the use of heavy-handed, brutal restraint (sometimes referred to sarcastically as "brutesthesia") or excessive disciplinary actions by staff members when contemporary chemical restraint constitutes a more humane and efficacious method (also called "technesia," i.e., technician-induced anesthesia).

- the use of chemical restraint when taking radiographs to reduce human exposure to x-rays.

- the handling of off-hour emergencies without backup veterinary nursing assistance or adequate experienced veterinary supervision.

- the presence (or absence) of anesthetic gas scavenging and radiation safety systems, and compliance with other OSHA safety requirements for employees.

- the safety and contemporaneity of the (1) intubation procedures; (2) IV catheter use; (3) cardiac, respiratory, body temperature, and blood pressure monitoring systems; and (4) anesthetic protocols associated with anesthetic, surgical, and dental procedures.

- the prevention of sexual harassment in the workplace.

- the willingness of the practice to refer patients in need of more competent and complete medical care to specialists, in spite of any negative effect on the practice's income.

- staff pregnancies in general and establishing a safe work environment to accommodate pregnant employees in the workplace.

- the creation of an environment for learning and professional growth with opportunities to discuss cases with colleagues.

Some job applicants and practice owners feel so strongly about certain ethical concerns that they have incorporated clauses in their employment contracts to assure compliance with their ethical standards. Two such examples include clauses addressing a job applicant's views on convenience euthanasia and a practice owners's views on animal restraint and abuse.

Euthanasia: *The responsibility for carrying out convenience euthanasia of client-owned and abandoned healthy animals will be performed in equal numbers by Employee and Employer and Employer agrees to provide Employee with reasonable financial* *and management support required to institute programs to decrease the numbers of healthy animals euthanized by Employer's practice.* (Revised from a Colorado State University student's proposed employment contract with a Wisconsin mixed animal practice employer—December, 1997.)

Animal Cruelty: *No professional person will strike, kick or whatsoever lay any abuse on any animal at any time for any reason. All personnel are expected to show complete emotional control both in examination rooms and all hospital and ward areas. Hospital policy will be to control unruly animals with muzzles, sedation, tranquilizers or anesthesia. If this is not possible, then requesting that either another staff doctor handle the case or that it be referred to another hospital is the preferred course of action rather than physical violence. Remember, even the most vicious dog or cat is part of someone's family. The persistent question always is, "Can you handle the case professionally as a compassionate veterinarian?"* (Revised and reprinted from a 1999 New Jersey small animal practice contract with a University of Pennsylvania graduate.)

In dealing with the many moral, ethical and legal issues on a daily basis, veterinarians and their staff are encouraged to read the AVMA *Principles of Veterinary Medical Ethics*, know more about their state and. local laws, and purchase some references to help them reach defensible moral-ethical-legal decisions. Many state boards of examiners now make tests on state laws and ethical principles their entire written state board examination.[21] State VMAs will be doing their members a great favor if they will have their association's legal counsel (or a local law librarian) help them assemble the most important laws relating to animals and veterinarians. These would include abandoned animal laws, lien laws, anticruelty laws, livestock protection laws, standard leash laws, dangerous dog laws, rabies vac-

cine and quarantine laws, and pet shop lemon laws.

It is well accepted that veterinarians are not expected to solve medical and surgical problems without using many of the basic continuing education references readily available in the profession. Similarly, they should not expect to be able to solve moral-ethical-legal dilemmas without devoting a little time to reviewing the laws of their states and the excellent references that have become available in the past few years.[1,7,10-12,22] The Florida Animal Control Officers Association, Minnesota Federated Humane Societies, and the State Humane Association of California have assembled publications covering all of the laws related to animals in their states. Animal control associations and humane associations in other states probably have done the same.

CLASSIFICATION OF LAWS

Many different types of laws exist in this country, with most having specific procedures for enforcement and an established set of remedies. Figure 1.2 illustrates various types of American law, while Figure 1.3 charts the general types of American law. Figure 1.4 illustrates the origins of animal law.

CRIMINAL LAW VERSUS CIVIL LAW

One of the traditional methods for classifying law has been on the basis of the type of activity that is being regulated. Criminal law defines the boundaries of the relationship between the individual and society. Acts that are harmful to people and to the fabric of an orderly society are crimes. In conjunction with the creation of criminal laws, society has developed a set of procedures and laws allowing for the investigation of a crime, the arrest of a suspected criminal, the prosecution of such an individual, and the determination of punishment. Most criminal laws

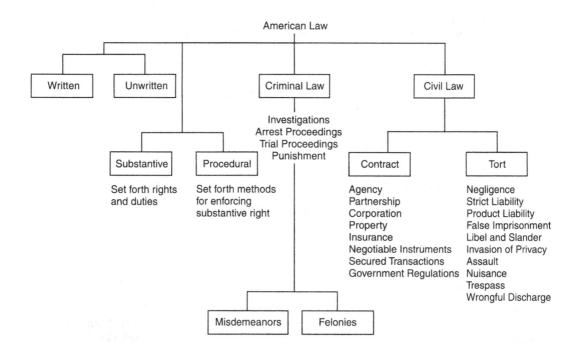

Figure 1.2. General types of American law

focus on acts that can injure people, go against the public interest, or offend public morality. When legal action is initiated, it is brought by society acting through a district attorney at the local level or the U.S. Attorney General on a national level.

Civil law pertains to the relationships among individuals within a society. A contract dispute between a veterinarian and an employee is an example of a civil law action. In some cases both civil and criminal suits occur. A horse thief, for example, could be charged in a criminal action for committing a wrong against society. In addition, the horse owner could file a civil lawsuit against the thief in an attempt to attain compensation for damages that occurred to the animal at the time of the theft.

Contract Law versus Tort Law

Civil law has two major subdivisions—contract law and tort law. Contract law deals with duties established by individ-

uals as a result of a contractual agreement. This area of law developed because merchants needed a means to assure that promises between persons would be fulfilled. A failure to respect or fulfill the duties set forth in the contract creates the potential of a lawsuit for breaching that duty. Within contract law are laws regulating specific types of business contracts, negotiable instruments (like checks), insurance (including worker's compensation), bankruptcy proceedings, securities (stocks and bonds), etc.

Conversely, tort law deals not with duties created by the parties through a contract, but with duties toward other people that are established by law. For example, the law of negligence, a subdivision of tort law, imposes a duty upon business people to maintain the premises in a manner that will prevent injuries to any people invited to enter those premises.

Courts and legislatures have expanded tort law, creating standards to which every person in our society must adhere. Under

Law is the body of authorized pronouncements made by duly established public entities and binding on all those within the jurisdiction of the particular entity.

Primitive Customs

Force and combat gradually replaced by rules and penalties except that force is still sanctioned for:

- Disputes between nations - wars
- Control of illegal mob action
- Taking custody of a suspected criminal
- Self-defense
- Terminating a trespass
- Defending home and family

Primitive customs gave way to formalized statements of the law.

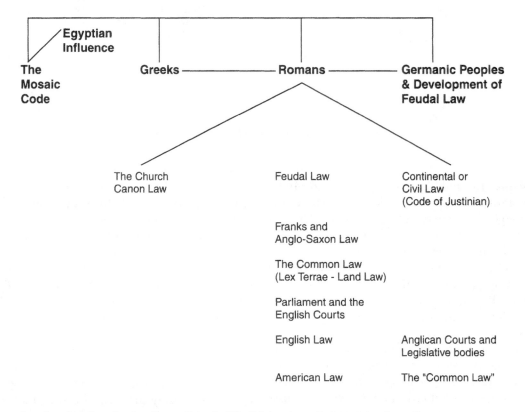

American law, though primarily an offshoot of English law, nevertheless draws from other systems. The state of Louisiana, for example, is a European-style "civil law" state.

Figure 1.3. The origin of American law

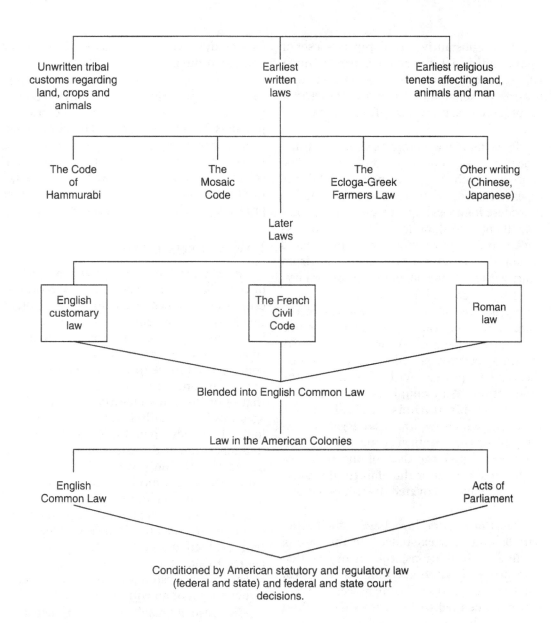

Figure 1.4. The origins of "animal" law

tort law, standards of care exist for the protection of one's body, business interests, personal property, and reputation. Tort law permits people to sue for relief of an injury that occurred as a result of damages inflicted on their bodies, family, or property due to a wrongful act. In general, a legal action of this type seeks not to punish the wrongdoer, but only to obtain monetary compensation for the injury that occurred. If the action was intentional, occurred with malice, or involved gross negligence, large monetary awards may be allowed by the court in order to punish the individual financially.

SUBSTANTIVE VERSUS PROCEDURAL LAW

References to *substantive law* or *procedural law* are frequent. Each has its own function. Substantive law comprises a set of rights and duties to which a person must adhere in today's society. Tort law, encompassing personal injuries and a concurrent set of remedies, is an example of substantive law.

Procedural law comprises the rules and procedures for conducting a lawsuit. The court in which an action must be filed, the types of evidence that are admissible, and the procedure for appealing a verdict are all components of procedural law. Errors in following the proper procedures can allow a valid substantive lawsuit to be dismissed from court without being heard by a judge or jury.

The procedural laws that most commonly pose problems for attorneys are the statutes of limitations. Such laws provide that unless people commence lawsuits within a specified period of time, they lose the right to proceed with or maintain the legal action. An example is the California Statute of Limitations on Malpractice Actions,[23] which requires that legal actions for professional negligence be filed within three years after the date of the injury or within one year after the plaintiff discovers or should have discovered the injury, whichever occurs first.

Most procedural laws have a good rationale behind their existence. In the case of statutes of limitations, the theory is that evidence and witnesses tend to disappear and lose recollection as time passes. Thus, a suit must be filed within a reasonably short time after the injury occurred or was discovered. In addition, speedy resolution is important because it is not fair for defendants to be subjected to the threat of a lawsuit indefinitely.

WRITTEN VERSUS UNWRITTEN LAWS

Written laws are rules and regulations that have been enacted by a legislative arm of government and codified (placed in a code of laws). This body of law is comprised of federal and state statutes as well as county and city ordinances.

Unwritten law, or *common law*, refers to the interpretation by our court system of written laws as well as the interpretation of previous court decisions. Therefore, even though it may appear that a particular action is not covered by a given statute, legal counsel must research the unwritten law (legal interpretations) of all pertinent cases before providing a client with a legal opinion.

LAW VERSUS EQUITY

As the legal system evolved, a rigid set of *remedies at law* was created for various crimes or breaches of conduct. These often involved the payment of monetary damages for an injury caused by such conduct. It soon became apparent, however, that the court needed more flexibility than this provided. In some situations, a remedy at law that only allowed a plaintiff to collect damages would be totally inadequate. Instead, a judicial remedy that, for example, prohibited repetition of the crime or the undesired action was the only way to prevent future damages. Furthermore, since very few sets of facts were ever the same, judges needed the opportunity to customize a punishment or a remedy. As a result, a second legal system evolved under English law allowing courts to develop *remedies in equity*. In today's court system, a judge can dispense either a legal or an equitable remedy.

In a case of breach of contract, instead of merely determining a dollar value for the damages, the court can order one of the parties to perform the contract in certain limited situations. This is titled *specific performance* and is an equitable remedy rather than a rigid legal remedy. For example, the court could specifically require a defendant to transfer title of a unique piece of property to the plaintiff if simply requiring the defendant to pay damages would result in an inequitable and unjust remedy.

Another example of a remedy in equity is the issuance of an *injunction*, prohibiting specific conduct or activity. If any action is taken in violation of the injunction, the defendant can be found to be in contempt of court and sent to jail.

THE JUDICIAL SYSTEM

The court system plays a major role in the administration of justice in the United States. It is through the orderly, although sometimes painstakingly slow, judicial branch of government that individuals have a means to settle personal conflicts peacefully. These same courts also function to preserve the fabric of society by trying and punishing disruptive people who commit crimes against other people or society itself. Lastly, the courts seek to maintain the public's social values and traditions by interpreting the Constitution, laws, and interpersonal relations in a manner that improves society while still respecting the ever-changing customs and mores of its people.

CLASSIFICATION OF COURTS

Courts of Original Jurisdiction

There are basically two types of courts within the judicial branch of government. The first is the *court of original jurisdiction*, which has the authority to hear a case when it is first brought before the court system. One of the key elements in determining which court can hear a case involves the extent of that court's jurisdiction. Each court has a designated area of authority, granted by the Constitution or the legislature, to hear and decide cases.

The court's jurisdiction is sometimes determined by the type of legal activity involved in the suit. For example, traffic courts decide only traffic cases, while tax courts deal only with interpretations of the United States tax codes. The court's jurisdiction can also be governed by the dollar value of the suit. Small claims courts, for example, only deal with suits in which the

damages sought are less than a certain amount, depending upon the state, and in some states, in which legal counsel is not permitted in the courtroom. The next higher court system (sometimes called the *court of common pleas, municipal court*, or *superior court*) may encourage or require the parties to retain legal counsel. Courts in this group have the authority to hear civil cases when the dispute does not exceed, e.g., $15,000 or, in criminal cases, when the fine does not exceed, e.g., $5,000 and the prison term is less than five years. In addition, there are territorial boundaries within which one or both parties to the lawsuit must reside which establish the jurisdiction of a court to hear and decide the case.

These courts of original jurisdiction are where the trials are held and where evidence and testimony are considered. They have a wide variety of designated titles from state to state, as indicated in Figure 1.5. The federal courts of original jurisdiction are entirely separate from the state courts and have their own titles. The jurisdiction in the federal ladder of courts is limited to such areas as disputes between states, conflicts between residents of various states, matters governed by federal law, patent law, and other areas as shown in Figure 1.6.

Courts of Appellate Jurisdiction

The second type of court is called a *court of appellate jurisdiction*. Appeals from courts of original jurisdiction go first to an intermediate court of appeal. Some of the various titles for these state courts are the *court of appeals, appellate session of superior court*, and *supreme court, appellate division*. These appellate courts have the power to review cases for errors in the admission of evidence, errors in legal interpretations by the trial court judge, and errors in instructions to juries. Appellate courts only consider transcripts of evidence presented at the trial and arguments presented by legal counsel about the law applied to the case. They do not rehear any of the evidence

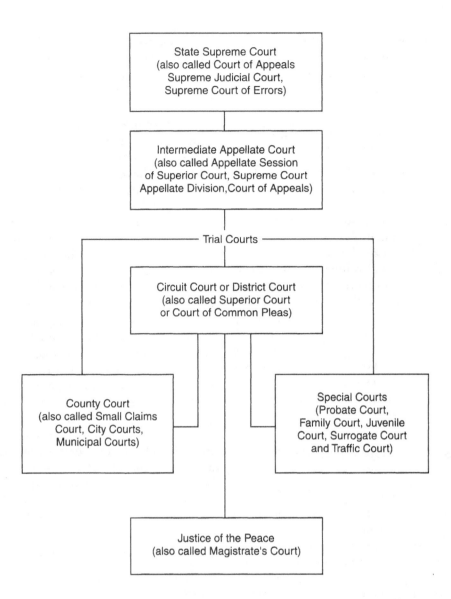

Figure 1.5. State courts of original jurisdiction

presented by witnesses at the trial. They can, however, *remand* the case (send it back) to the trial court for it to hear additional evidence if their review shows that legal procedures were improperly followed and some evidence was therefore incorrectly admitted or omitted.

The rights of appeal do not end at this appellate system. There are still the state supreme courts, also called *supreme judicial courts* or *supreme courts of errors* and, ultimately, there is the *United States Supreme Court*. In general, because of the significant costs incurred in the appeals process, only cases involving a considerable amount of money or critical legal principles are appealed all the way to the state or United States Supreme Court level. Fortunately, most cases against veterinarians do not contain either of these ingredients. As a result, excessive trial and appellate legal expenditures are uncommon in veterinary medicine.

For most general business law disputes involving veterinarians, ample precedents are

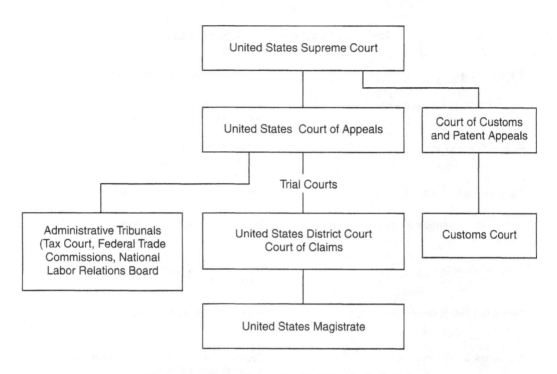

Figure 1.6. Federal courts of original jurisdiction

available so that counsel can offer sound advice. When it comes to veterinary negligence and malpractice disputes, however, relatively few cases have been tried and appealed. Since case law and precedents are only created by the writing of legal opinions at one of the appellate levels, this paucity of case law makes it difficult for attorneys to predict outcomes of veterinary malpractice cases.

THE LEGAL CODIFICATION, CITATION, AND LIBRARY SYSTEMS

Legal references and citations are scattered profusely throughout most legal writings. To follow up on these, people with even the most basic legal knowledge can use a law library. Most law libraries have a reference librarian available to assist the novice. County and city courthouses, law schools, large- and medium-sized law firms, and many public libraries all have an array of legal references for anyone who wishes to use them. For a table illustrating where various types of law can be found, see Table 1.1.

LEGAL CASE HEADINGS

Case titles are generally defined by the names of the parties to the lawsuit. A small "v." separates the names and stands for versus, e.g., *Brown* v. *The Board of Education*. At the trial court level, the plaintiff's name, the person bringing the lawsuit, appears first. The defendant's name, the person defending the legal actions, appears last.

If a suit is appealed after a verdict at the trial court level, the name of the party who is appealing the case appears first. If a case appears as *People* v. *Atchison*, it is most likely a criminal case brought by the local district attorney or state attorney general on behalf of "the people" in that jurisdiction.

Whenever a case is cited, the place where it can be found follows the name of the case. For example, 250 U.S. 620 (1916) means that the written report of this case can be found in volume 250 of the *United States Reports*

Table 1.1. Locating Various Kinds of Law

Kinds of Law	Where the Law May be Found
International treaties and agreements	"Treaties, conventions, international acts, protocols and agreements," treaty series
Federal Constitution	United States Code; most history or political science texts and state statutes
Congress (federal statutes)	United States Code; statutes at large
Federal administrative agencies (rules and regulations)	Federal Register; Code of Federal Regulations
State constitutions	Revised or compiled statutes; pamphlets issued by secretary of state
State legislature (state statutes)	Revised or compiled statutes; annotated statutes; session laws
State administrative agencies	Separate publications by departments and divisions; administrative codes
Political subdivisions of the state, local and special units of government (ordinance)	Minutes of the governing body may be codified.
Municipal corporations (ordinances)	Printed copy of ordinances — book or pamphlet. There may be printed municipal or county codes.
Public corporations (rules, regulations, ordinances)	Printed copies; minutes; proclamations
Quasi-public corporations (rules, regulations, rates)	Letters, minutes, published records and schedules
Courts (common law)	Court records and case reports — digests and encyclopedias
Contracts (enforceable private rights)	Written or oral agreements

(reporting cases decided by the United States Supreme Court) on page 620. The (1916) means that the case was decided in 1916. The year that the case was decided is virtually always a part of the citation.

Citation of a case heard by a state supreme court is slightly different. An example is *Burke* v. *Fine*, 51 NW 2d 818 (Sup Ct Minn. 1952). Although this case would most likely be reported in a book of cases solely pertaining to Minnesota, the United States has also been sectioned into groups of states. This is done for ease, so that all the cases decided by the supreme courts in each group of states can be placed in one volume to save law libraries and law offices the need for stocking books from all 50 states.

In the example, the case cited could be found in Volume 51 of the second series of the *North Western Reporter* on page 818. Table 1 lists the courts included in each of the most commonly abbreviated citations.

A citation like 287 F Supp. 840 (W.D. Va. 1968), for instance, means that the decision came from the United States district court in the western district of Virginia.

Statutes are also found frequently as components of legal citations. They follow a similar basic style. These too are easy to locate in a law library by looking at the title and the section, §, citations. An example appearing as Calif. Evidence Code §1230 would be found by locating the books of state statutory codes within a library. These are often stacked alphabetically around the perimeter of the library, while the books reporting appellate court decisions are alphabetical by state or region within the central part of the library. Common abbreviations for case reports are shown in Table 1.2.

THE ADVERSARY SYSTEM OF JUSTICE

Several components are necessary in order for the American legal system, also called the *adversary system of justice*, to function effectively. These are an unresolvable issue, an impartial tribunal, equality in competence, and equality in adversariness.

Table 1.2. Common Abbreviations for Case Reports

Abbreviation	Title	Courts Included
U.S.	United States Reports	United States Supreme Court
F.	Federal Reporter	Federal circuit courts of appeals
F.Supp.	Federal Supplement	United States district court decisions
A. a.2d**	Atlantic Reporter*	PA, MD, DE, NJ, CT, VT, NH, ME, RI
N.E. N.E.2d	North Eastern Reporter*	MA, NY, OH, IL
N.W. N.W.2d	North Western Reporter*	MI, WI, MN, IA, ND, SD, NE
P. OR, WA, AK, HI	Pacific Reporter*	KS, OK, NM, CO, WY, MT, ID, UT, NV, AZ, CA,
So. So.2d	Southern Reporter*	LA, MS, AL, FL
S.E. S.E.2d	South Eastern Reporter*	WV, VA, NC, SC, GA
S.W.	South Western Reporter*	TX, AR, MO, TN, KY

* These regional reporters include decisions of all appellate courts in these states.
** The abbreviation 2d means the second series of volumes collecting specific reports (e.g. F2d means Federal Reporter, second series.)

An Unresolvable Issue

The first item is that of identifying an unresolvable issue. Almost any situation can become controversial, so finding enough substance for a lawsuit is not difficult. Examples of issues which may be unresolvable without court intervention can include whether or not the facts of a case support a plaintiff's contention that the medical care provided for their animal was below the standard for their community, their state, or for the country as a whole. In another case, the primary issue may involve a determination of the magnitude of the damages incurred. In still others, the major unresolvable issue could be one of determining which states' laws apply to the case.

An Impartial Tribunal

The second key element needed to allow for the American legal system to function is that of an impartial tribunal. Our forefathers chose the judge and jury system to fulfill this need. Although some judgeships are elective positions, the majority of judges are appointed. Some, as in the United States Supreme Court, are appointed for life. They are therefore unlikely to be beholden to any person or business interest. Historically, the judicial system seems to have met the test of impartiality well.

To assure the maximum potential for impartiality, however, the Constitution also established trial by a jury of one's peers. Not all legal actions are open to this option, but most serious offenses for large-dollar suits may have a jury trial. Courts such as traffic court and small-claims court do not have the full protection of a jury trial.

Equality in Competence

The third component for a fair and effective legal system is reasonable equality in the competence of legal counsel on each side of the case. It is in this area that the system is most likely to break down. Overburdened counsel working for the public defender's office of a county or city court system may not have resources sufficient to defend individuals against well-directed police evidence or aggressive district attorneys. On the other hand, the district attorney's office may be underbudgeted and undermanned to compete with the wealthy defendants who can hire top attorneys and private investigators.

The old adage "you get what you pay for" is as apropos in the legal world as in any other area of the free-enterprise marketplace. Veterinarians in need of legal counsel should anticipate spending $125 to $300 per hour for an attorney's services depending upon the complexity of the legal problem, the need for experienced senior counsel versus less-seasoned junior counsel, and whether they live in a metropolitan or rural area. It should be kept in mind that good legal care is as important as good medical care, depending on the seriousness of the legal issue.

Equality in Adversariness

The fourth essential ingredient for the effective application of justice is equality in adversariness. The English system of justice is based on what is termed *the adversary system of justice.* The continental system, used generally throughout Europe, is not an adversary system.

The English and American systems allow the attorneys for each side of the case to ask nearly all the questions of the witnesses and to select expert witnesses. In the continental system, the judge is the primary interrogator, with attorneys presenting written questions and arguments on behalf of their clients to the judges. As the action proceeds in the continental system, the judge may interject new theories and new legal and factual issues, thus reducing the disadvantage of the party with the less competent lawyer.[24] In addition, the court may obtain evidence from expert witnesses on its own initiative. Neither of these is likely to occur in the American system.

It is because of the adversary element in our system that law students are taught to represent their sides of cases to the maximum of their abilities. They are instructed not to determine or assume anything regarding the guilt or liability of their clients; that job is up to the tribunal, i.e., the judge or jury. The attorneys' duty is to present the facts and arguments in the case as effectively as they can regardless of what their clients said or did.

One cannot help but wonder what effect some of the procedures inherent in the continental system might have on the issues of adversariness. In that system costs of litigation are taxed in such a way as to discourage hopeless or frivolous cases and, as a rule, the defeated party bears the cost of litigation including attorney's fees.[24]

Although the adversary system has worked satisfactorily for years, it is because of the adversary element that many legal controversies which start out as molehills ultimately become mountains. The parties to the lawsuit often become enemies engaging in war instead of individuals seeking to negotiate amicable solutions that are satisfactory to each. Too often both parties end up losing and, because of the legal fees incurred, the attorneys are the biggest winners.

ATTORNEYS

Lawyers are considered "officers of the court" and must be licensed by the state in which they are practicing. Figure 1.7 illustrates some of the key issues surrounding the licensing and services provided by legal counsel.

SELECTION OF LEGAL COUNSEL

Selecting an attorney is as difficult a task as choosing an auto mechanic, physician or, for the animal owner, a veterinarian. Because many veterinarians think that they cannot afford attorneys, they are often undercounseled regarding the law. Practitio-

ners who seek legal counsel should consider the following in making their choice:

1. The candidate's reputation in the community. Due to the huge number of attorneys in practice, this may be difficult to ascertain. If questioning a few other attorneys familiar with the lawyer being considered is not feasible, it may help to ask the candidate for a reference of someone with a legal problem similar to the one at hand.

2. Determine the candidate's record for punctuality. Time is very important in certain veterinary activities such as a proposed partnership or corporate buy in or buy out, and an inordinate delay can kill a deal.

3. Determine the candidate's reputation for returning phone calls. The frustration of being unable to contact one's legal counsel within a reasonable time after the need arises can also create ill will. It may be best to casually ask a secretary in the attorney's office this question as well as questioning the attorneys themselves.

4. Establish, as well as possible, how adversary minded the attorney is. Questions that focus on the attorney's flexibility regarding solutions to a given legal problem can help one estimate this characteristic. Sometimes practitioners need a very adversary-minded attorney who will dogmatically look after their best interests. Other times they will merely want counsel to assemble the papers for a business deal as expeditiously as possible. It helps to find out if candidates are willing to meet with both of the parties to a proposed business deal or if they wish only to work with the opposing counsel. If the case is, for example, a contract negotiation that definitely requires independent legal representation for each side, a call to the opposing attorney to see how well the two attorneys can work together may also be worthwhile.

5. Assay competence by posing questions to references provided by the attorney.

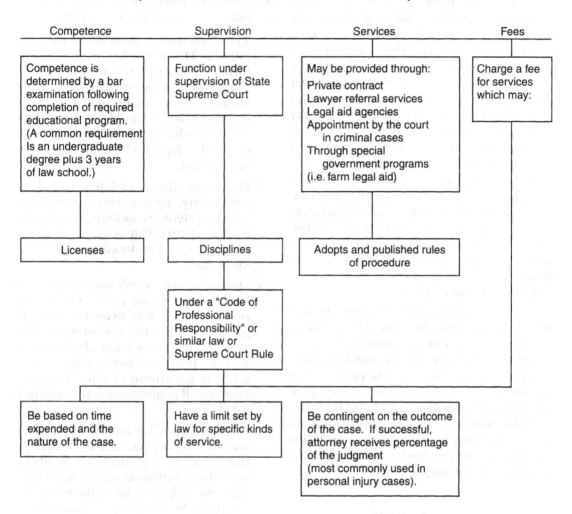

Figure 1.7. Legal licensing and services

When very little background information about an attorney exists, it is worthwhile to ask for the names of clients with similar legal problems who could provide some references. In addition, asking questions which determine how much experience the candidate has with legal issues like the ones under consideration allows at least some measure of competence to be determined.

6. Locate more than one candidate. Most veterinarians would be as leery about choosing an attorney by perusing the yellow pages as they would be about picking a physician that way. It is far better to assemble a list of potential candidates and then narrow the list to two or three choices.

Traditionally, word of mouth has been the best approach in this type of search. However, in recent years an association of lawyers and veterinarians focusing on veterinary-related legal issues has come into existence. The American Veterinary Medical Law Association, founded in 1993 and incorporated in 1994, is a national association consisting of over 100 attorneys, veterinarians, and other individuals and organizations with an interest in veterinary medical law and its pertinence to the veterinary profession and allied fields. Veterinarians seeking legal counsel familiar with the profession are encouraged to contact the AVMLA for references to speakers on veterinary legal subjects or for legal counsel with an interest and knowledge of veterinary medicine.[25]

An alternative way to locate competent legal counsel is to ask friends who manage small businesses, local dentists and physicians, accountants, or bankers for names. Often legal counsel employed by a local corporation, a government agency, or a local law school can provide good, unbiased referrals. Sometimes these references may be able to advise which attorneys not to hire as well as which to consider. If no other sources are available, veterinarians can contact the local bar association. Most associations provide a referral service to members who will offer an initial 15-minute consultation free of charge.

Should specialists in veterinary law be unavailable, seeking attorneys who specialize in the type of legal counsel that is needed is worth some extra effort. The usual areas of attorney expertise are bankruptcy, probate and estate planning, criminal, patent, corporate, commercial, worker's compensation, property, litigation, and trade. As reported in several regional newspapers, an emerging group of attorneys, Linda Cawley in Denver and Michael Rotsten in Encino, CA, now exists who even specialize in laws focusing on animal ownership.[26,27] Attorneys who specialize in commercial or trade law are generally best suited for business-related advice.

THE ISSUE OF FEES

The adversary training that lawyers undergo during their legal education encourages them to "dot every i and cross every t without regard for economic realities."[28] In addition, attorneys are traditionally accustomed to taking on legal assignments without explaining to their clients what each, or

for that matter, any component of the legal representation is likely to cost.

Part of the rationale for vague fees evolves from the difficulty in ascertaining how much time it might take to research all the current legal precedents, tax ramifications, or witness testimony pertaining to the case in question. Determining the best course of action can require considerable homework, depending on the complexity of the facts. Of course, the same can be said for difficult veterinary cases, but most veterinarians were not taught to charge for medical research in the manner that attorneys and accountants have been taught to charge for legal and tax research.

Negotiations about fees are as important when choosing attorneys as many of the previous items are. The following are some points to consider in this area.

1. Discuss and negotiate fees well before deciding to hire legal counsel. Request an itemized estimate which includes, for example, the lawyer's hourly fee, charges for photocopying documents, costs for filing legal documents, and fees for secretarial services. Flat fees for some particular services can be negotiated, but occasionally this reduces the attorney's incentive to do a thorough job on more difficult cases.

Determine whether the attorney has a minimum billing time for work performed. If the minimum billing time is 15 minutes, plan phone calls to take full advantage of the 15-minute time span that will be charged, using a clock or stopwatch to stay within the minimum billing time increments. Have a notepad available to write down information gathered during the conversation. Since much of the discussion will be about unfamiliar concepts, written notes are essential if one expects to be able to remember and explain what has been learned during the conversation.

Fees may be lower in smaller firms where fewer people are involved in the case and there often is more contact between the lawyer assigned to the case and the client. Find out whether junior associates are able to resolve the case or whether more expensive senior partners will be needed.

2. Determine the type of billing. An itemized monthly bill is essential. A breakdown of the components of the legal services rendered and the time each took can help define what progress is being made in resolving the case.

3. Insist on monthly status reports in order to ascertain what type of progress is being made. If costs are escalating or progress seems too slow, remember that the person who hired the attorney is the one who should retain control of the case.

4. Do not become obsessed with economics. Veterinarians should always remember that the main objective in seeking legal counsel is the creation of an ideal document or providing the best possible representation for their particular interest. Penny pinching on legal fees can sometimes save money in the short run but cost dearly in terms of emotional aggravation and monetary losses in the long run.

5. Do some homework. Perhaps the best way for practitioners to control expenditures on legal fees is for them to prepare as many of their own materials as they possibly can themselves and then pay counsel to apply the legalese. Providing attorneys with some sample language for a partnership agreement, for an employment contract, or for a buy-sell agreement that has been hashed over by the involved parties can greatly reduce essential legal time. Although attorneys should be able to create an agreement that establishes what the parties have agreed to, it is often helpful for those parties to thoroughly discuss and write down what they have in mind before their attorneys draft the document. If they do not do this, they may discover that what they have just paid well for does not reflect what they wanted at all.

This book will provide a discussion of contract issues and language to address them so that veterinarians can discuss and attempt to resolve many of their concerns about employment contracts before they seek legal counsel. Those people willing to devote personal time to home preparation before seeking competent legal counsel will earn dramatic reductions in legal costs.

The Course of Events in a Legal Action

The course of events in civil cases is different from the course in criminal cases, so each is covered separately. For an illustration of how the system works, see Figure 1.8.

The Initiation of a Civil Case

A Complaining Party

The first notice that a veterinarian usually has regarding a potential legal problem is in the form of a complaining or angry client, staff member, or supplier. Although this may seem to be nothing more than an irritant, be thankful for the notice. It is much more difficult if the first notice arrives in the form of a summons rather than in the form of an upset individual. A summons is a legal document that states that the plaintiff (complaining party) has been injured because of certain acts or omissions for which the defendant is liable.

The reason that it is preferable to face a complaining person rather than a summons is because it is possible to reason and negotiate with an individual on a personal basis outside of the confines of the legal system. Once a legal summons appears, this option is usually gone. Instead, the reality of attorneys' fees and the judicial system are part of the future.

If the complaining parties are clients with injuries to themselves personally or to

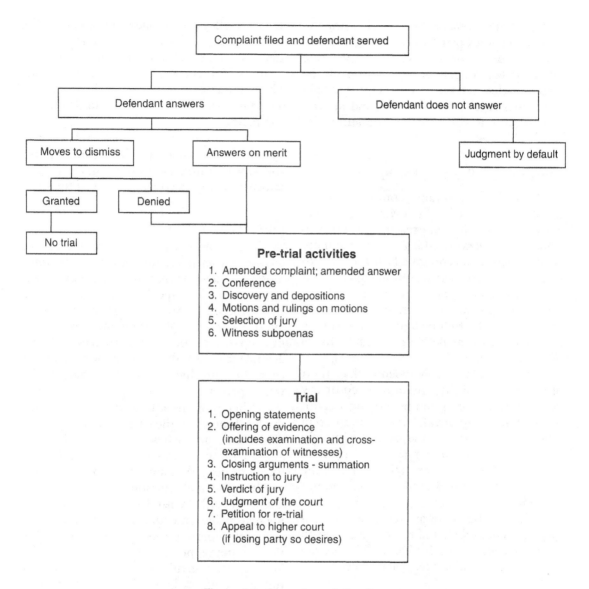

Figure 1.8. Steps in a civil action

their animals, the appropriate first response for a veterinarian before doing anything besides listening quietly to the complaint is to call one's insurance agent. Only veterinarians who have good professional liability insurance will have this option, though.

Do not admit any liability or offer any type of settlement options without first notifying and consulting with a spokesperson from the insurance company. It is at this stage that good insurance representatives have the best opportunity to resolve grievances. Any comments made by the insured party that might compromise the insurer's ability to defend or settle the case must be avoided or the insurer may have the option of refusing to defend the insured party.

When the complaint is in the form of a civil lawsuit, legal counsel is generally required. Where insurance is involved, the insurance carrier will choose and pay for such counsel. If no insurance coverage is in force, e.g., a criminal action for violating the Food Drug and Cosmetic Act, allegations of animal cruelty, or an action by the State Board of Examiners for a violation of the state Practice Act, practitioners must supply their own legal representation and answer the allegations contained in the summons within 30 days.

Options for Early Settlement

Experienced insurance company personnel can often settle a grievance relatively easily because they are reasonably unemotional bystanders. In addition, it is normally within their own economic best interests to settle cases instead of sustaining major legal fees. Insurance companies have been known to procrastinate in paying claims, though, in order to forego paying for as long a period of time as possible. In fact, this is not uncommon.

Practitioners should ensure that their professional liability insurance company does not have the option of settling a claim without their approval. Any veterinarian who thinks a lawsuit or grievance is merely a nuisance action rather than a legitimate case should reserve the right to have the insurance company defend the case and not settle it.

When settlements are deemed impossible, legal counsel should be selected as soon as possible after a suit is filed, well before the *discovery phase* of the legal action begins.

PLEADINGS

Once a plaintiff has decided to file a lawsuit, the defendant and the court need to know what alleged wrong needs to be righted. The *complaint* filed by the plaintiff, which sets forth the alleged facts along with a request for a remedy, is the first component of the *pleadings*. The defendant is required to answer all allegations in that document, which is why any *summons* ordering the veterinarian to appear before the court is a serious matter. In the answer to a civil suit, the defendant may admit or deny the allegations made in the complaint or claim any defenses to the charges. In addition, the defendant may file a *counterclaim*, which is a request for action to remedy a wrong caused by the plaintiff arising out of the same set of facts contained in the complaint.

The complaint, any counterclaim, the answer, any answer to the counterclaim, and any preliminary motions made by the attorneys comprise the pleadings of the case.

Preliminary Motions

To test the strength of a complaint or an answer, either party may file a *preliminary motion* requesting that the judge make a ruling or take some specific action before the case proceeds. Some motions are procedural. For example, they may attack an improper method in notification of the defendant about the legal action or allege that the suit has been filed against the wrong person.

Other motions attack the substance or the legal theory of the case. An example is a defendant who wishes to admit to the facts alleged in the complaint but nevertheless wants to deny that any injury occurred as a result. In such a situation, a motion called a *demurrer* is filed with the court. After allowing reasonable time for either side to respond to a preliminary motion and after reviewing the arguments presented by the parties, the judge either overrules the motion and orders the case to proceed, upholds the motion filed and orders corrections in the documents filed with the court, or dismisses the case.

Subpoenas and Summons

A subpoena is a court-ordered command to provide testimony or to turn over particular items of evidence for examination by the opposing party.

SERVICE OF PROCESS

The procedure for delivering a summons, a complaint, or a subpoena to the defendant is called *service of process*. This may be performed by the plaintiff, by a court marshall, or by someone from the office of the plaintiff's attorney. The summons, complaint, or subpeona may be delivered in person, by leaving it with someone at the defendant's residence or business, or, sometimes, by publishing it in a newspaper. Each court has procedural rules specifying who may deliver the service of process and how it must be done. Improper service of process, sometimes referred to as *sewer service*, can result in a case being dismissed.

THE INITIAL STAGES OF A CRIMINAL CASE

The types of criminal activities that veterinarians most commonly would become involved in are assault and battery because of a failure to control one's temper, abuse of alcohol or controlled substances, allegations of animal cruelty, or driving under the influence of alcohol or a drug. Although these abuses could involve a state law enforcement agency, procedures vary from state to state, so only federal procedures will be discussed here.

Crimes are generally classified as misdemeanors and felonies. Misdemeanors are offenses lower than felonies, usually punishable by fines or imprisonment for less than one year. Felonies are offenses punishable by death or imprisonment for terms exceeding one year.

Complaints to the U.S. Attorney

The procedures in the federal court system for misdemeanor crimes can unfold in one of two ways. Most cases begin with a law enforcement agent complaint to the office of the United States Attorney. That office then has a choice of proceeding either by issuing a complaint based on testimony under oath before a United States magistrate or by requesting or requiring that the evidence be submitted to a grand jury.

Grand Jury Indictments

If the grand jury decides that there is enough evidence to support a finding of *probable cause*, it will return an indictment. Probable cause exists when facts and circumstances would warrant a person of reasonable caution to believe that an unlawful offense was or is being committed. An *indictment* is a formal written accusation originating with a prosecutor and issued by a grand jury charging that the person named has done some act or been guilty of some omission that by law is classified as a crime.

In some cases the complaint or the indictment leads to a summons commanding the appearance of the accused person in court. In other cases an arrest warrant is issued.

If the offense constitutes a felony and the crime was committed in the presence of a government agent or the agent had probable cause to believe that a felony was committed, an arrest can be made immediately without a summons or arrest warrant. More commonly, though, in felony cases the United States Attorney's office convenes a federal grand jury, presents the evidence, and requests that the grand jury return an indictment.

If the crime is a simple misdemeanor, the initial appearance of the defendant is made before the magistrate. For more serious misdemeanors, the magistrate informs the defendants of their rights and adjourns the case until legal counsel can be appointed or retained.

Preliminary Hearings

If the misdemeanor or felony was initiated through the complaint process rather than by the indictment of a grand jury, a preliminary hearing will take place. This is a test of the prosecutor's evidence to see whether there is probable cause that a crime was committed and that the defendant committed it. If a defendant is being prosecuted under a grand jury indictment, there is usually no preliminary hearing. In *United*

States v. *Mase*, 556 F2d 671 (1977), the court ruled that a grand jury indictment constitutes a finding of probable cause and avoids the need for a preliminary hearing.

Pretrial Motions

Just as in civil cases, pretrial motions are important. These raise issues that can be either procedural or substantive in nature. Some of the most common ones involve whether or not the evidence was acquired during an illegal arrest or illegal search which violated the defendant's constitutional rights. Other pretrial motions concern discovery, e.g., providing defense counsel with copies of any statements made by the defendant to government agents, results of chemical or physical tests performed on the defendant, and any information that might aid in the defense effort.

THE MID STAGES OF LEGAL ACTION

Discovery

The discovery phase of a case is that portion of time after a suit has been filed and after any preliminary motions have been decided. During this stage, attorneys for both sides assemble all materials that are relevant to the case. Subpoenas are used to obtain otherwise inaccessible evidence. The first items to be subpoenaed in cases involving the practice of veterinary medicine are generally the medical and business records related to the case; any laboratory or pathology reports, radiographs, or other images or photographs; the appointment book; and any relevant portions of the laboratory, surgery, anesthesia, or radiology log books.

In an effort to expedite a dispute when veterinarians are certain they have a strong defense to any action, it may be beneficial to provide these items to the plaintiff or plaintiff's counsel before the issuance of a subpoena. This should never be done without authorization from an agent for the insurance company or from legal counsel assigned to the case. However, such a demonstration of cooperation and openness is sometimes quite valuable.

After the provision of this type of information, the next step is to subpoena witnesses who have information about the incident that provoked the suit. "Interrogatories" (formal written questions) are prepared by opposing counsel for questioning during a deposition. The "deposition" stage of the case involves an informal hearing with counsel for the plaintiff, counsel for the defendant, the witness who will be questioned, and a court reporter. Questions about the witness's educational background, how the case was handled, and anything else that seems relevant are posed. Carefully thought out answers to these interrogations are essential, because when the deposition ends, the witnesses are required to sign a statement that all testimony is true. If the case goes to trial, testimony at the trial is compared with that from the deposition. Discrepancies will be clearly pointed out to the judge or jury in an attempt to impugn the credibility of the witness.

Settlement Conferences

Settlement conferences are part of civil actions and can occur at any time. If the case has not been settled within two weeks prior to the trial date, however, a mandatory settlement conference generally takes place. This includes the attorney for the plaintiff, the attorney employed by the insurance company or the defendant, and the judge.

Plea Bargaining

While the mid stages of civil actions are marked by settlement conferences, the mid stages of criminal cases involve attempts to settle using the plea bargaining process. To understand plea bargaining, one must first know the various pleas. A guilty plea means just what it says, i.e., the defendant admits that a violation of the law has transpired. The only thing left to determine, then, is the sentence. Most defendants are advised by counsel to plead not guilty because it gives counsel time to evaluate the evidence and pursue the best course of action.

Another plea that can be used is that of *nolo contendere*, or *no contest*. Such a plea may be made only with the consent of the court. It is different from a guilty plea in that a plea of no contest may not be used against the defendant in a civil action based upon the same facts, whereas a guilty plea can. No contest pleas might be used, for example, in antitrust cases in which there is a likelihood of a civil action for damages following a criminal charge of an antitrust conviction.

The only other pleas allowed are not guilty or not guilty by reason of insanity. A not guilty plea in a criminal case means that the prosecution must proceed to trial and attempt to prove *beyond a reasonable doubt* that the defendant committed a criminal act. Fulfilling this burden of proof is considerably more difficult than the burden applied to civil cases, where the requirement is to show that a *preponderance of the evidence*, i.e., more than half, supports one side of the case or the other.

In many states, a conviction of a crime pertaining to the abuse of or dispensing of a controlled drug is sufficient grounds for the state board to seek a license revocation or suspension. Since a no contest plea is the equivalent of a conviction of the controlled drug violation, and that conviction is sufficient for the state board to initiate action,[29] a no contest plea provides no value to veterinarians who find themselves in this situation.

Plea bargaining is an integral component of the criminal justice system. Counsel for the defendant negotiates with the prosecutor to reduce the magnitude of the offense or the sentence depending upon the strengths and weaknesses of each side's case. Unlike civil cases, where judges are involved in settlements, judges are forbidden from participating in these negotiations. The bargain can involve the defendant pleading guilty in exchange for either dropping some charges in a multiple-charge prosecution, or allowing the defendant to plead guilty to a lesser crime instead of going to trial for the more serious crime. It can also involve recommendations satisfactory to both sides regarding the length of the sentence for the guilty plea.

THE TRIAL

If no settlement occurs and the case goes to trial, the first item to be determined is whether the trial is to held only before the judge or in front of a jury. If the choice is for a jury trial, jury selection becomes the first item of business.

Jury Selection

Potential jurors are drawn by chance from a drum containing names of people called for jury duty. From this group, a jury is selected consisting of 12 people in criminal cases and 6 or 12 people in civil cases plus 1 or 2 alternates. The size of the jury varies, depending upon the court and jurisdiction from which the case originates. The selection process is called *voir dire*.

In federal courts, the judge asks questions of prospective jurors. These questions generally are meant to reveal any prejudices relevant to the type of case or the defendant personally. In state courts, the judge and the attorneys for each side may ask questions. Prospective jurors are then either selected or eliminated based upon their answers to these questions.

The judge or either attorney may have grounds to remove a prospective juror because of a prejudice, in which case the request to remove a juror is called *removal for cause*. Each side also has the right to reject three potential jurors for no apparent reason at all, in which case it is called a *peremptory strike*.

Opening Statements

In the event of a jury trial, once the jury has been chosen, opening statements are usually presented by both sides to describe the facts of the case to the jury. In addition, the attorneys for each side have the opportunity to summarize the evidence in the case. The plaintiff always starts out with an opening statement, but differences can occur as to when in the trial the opening statement is made on behalf of the defendant. The delivery of the defendant's opening statement depends upon the wisdom of counsel and the type of case involved, i.e., criminal or civil.

Evidence

After opening statements are completed, the actual trial with the presentation of evidence commences. The plaintiff must present evidence first. When counsel for the plaintiff has completed questioning a witness, counsel for the defense has the right to cross-examine the witness. If some issues need additional review, the plaintiff's counsel may engage in re-direct examination of the witness. Counsel for the defendant then has another opportunity to cross-examine the witness concerning the specific questions raised during the re-direct exam. At this point, witnesses may be dismissed or, with sufficient justification, requested to remain available in case they need to be recalled for further testimony.

Closing Statements and Directed Verdicts

When the attorneys for both sides have presented all the evidence and finished the cross-examination of witnesses, each one makes a closing statement. These closing remarks summarize the facts of the case for the jury and restate whatever remedy was requested by the plaintiff. If the evidence presented substantially proves one side of the case or the other, either party may request a directed verdict. If the judge agrees, the jury is directed by the judge to decide in favor of one of the parties without deliberation.

Jury Instructions

If the case does not merit a directed verdict for either party, the judge instructs the jury on how it should reach a decision about the case. This is called the judge's *charge* to the jury and includes the judge's interpretation of the relevant points of law. After the charge, the jury retires to another room to conduct its deliberations in secret. When a decision has been reached, the jury returns to the courtroom and announces its verdict.

At this time, the judge has the option of accepting the verdict and ordering appropriate remedies or rejecting the verdict. This latter decision is made only when the jury's verdict does not appear reasonable. In such a case, the judge has the option of issuing a judgement notwithstanding the verdict. Such a decision can reject all or part of the verdict or modify it. Either party to the case may request such a decision; however, the likelihood of a judge granting such a verdict is not very great.

THE END STAGE OF A LEGAL ACTION

Appeals

Once a case has been decided and a verdict entered by the court, the losing parties must elect either to accept or reject the verdict. Losing parties that reject the verdict request a "stay of execution," which is then applied to the case while an appeal to a higher court is in progress. Higher courts either accept cases for appeal, i.e., *grant certiorari*, or refuse to consider them, *deny certiorari*. To succeed in an appeal on a case, losing parties must show that a material error was committed during the trial that might have altered the outcome of the case.

A few of the more common examples of material errors include incorrect instructions to the jury (an incorrect charge), allegations that the court failed to follow proper court procedures, incorrect omissions or admittance of specific items of evidence, or the discovery of new evidence that might affect the outcome of the case. In some criminal cases, e.g., murder cases with death sentences, the defendant is automatically entitled to an appeal.

Appellate Procedures

The court procedures for an appeal are quite different from the course of events at a trial. Appellate courts only hear or examine points of law, not questions of fact. It is assumed that only the trial judges or the juries can decide questions of fact, since they heard and saw all the factual evidence in the case. If an appellate court finds that no substantial evidence exists to support a finding of fact by the jury, however, they may overrule the jury's finding.

Another major difference at the appellate court level is that only the attorneys for each side are allowed to present any arguments or material during the hearing. In addition, instead of only one judge being present for the hearing, there are often three judges or, in the case of supreme courts, nine judges.

The appellate court decision may affirm that of the trial court, in which case the verdict remains the same. It also may reverse the decision, or *remand* the case to the trial court for additional evidence or work. As mentioned earlier, it is the opinions written by these appellate court judges analyzing the law and other precedents that become the guidelines for judges' decisions in future cases.

ENFORCEMENT

After a case is decided and the verdict accepted, or after all appellate remedies are completed, a verdict becomes final and it is time for enforcement. It is at this point where veterinarians who have brought a legal action in small claims court for fees not paid are most likely to meet the reality of defeat. Just because parties win lawsuits does not mean they will be able to collect the monies due them.

Some remedies for a failure to pay court-ordered damages, though, do exist. First of all, upon the prevailing party's request, the court can issue *an order of execution* directing the seizure of some or all of the defendant's property to pay the judgment. If the value of that property is insufficient, the prevailing party may try a second tact, i.e., requesting that the court order a *garnishment*. If this request is granted, the court will order someone who owes the defendant money, like an employer, to pay some or all of that money to the plaintiff instead of to the defendant as a means of paying off part or all of the judgment. Keep in mind that if a counterclaim has been filed, in which case the plaintiff in the primary action becomes a defendant in the countersuit, the original plaintiff can end up owing the defendant a sum of money instead of vice versa.

Yet another option is available to people who attempt to collect a judgment. This involves placing a lien on the defendant's property. If the defendant owns property, especially a house or business, this can be an effective method for collecting a debt. *Attaching a lien* to the defendant's property means that, in the event that the defendant ever sells that property, the proceeds must go to pay off the judgment before any money can be kept by or returned to the defendant.

ALTERNATIVE METHODS FOR SOLVING DISPUTES

Very often the complexity of the legal system, the sluggish progression of cases, and the high costs of attorneys' fees for both parties in a dispute discourage people from using the judicial arm of government. Consequently, a brief review of some alternatives is in order.

NEGOTIATED SETTLEMENTS

It is not uncommon for business people to elect to resolve business disputes in a practical manner by themselves instead of through the legal system. The method for resolving disputes may be written into the business's contract, or it may be agreed upon after a dispute occurs.

An example involves a method for arriving at the value of a veterinary practice. It is very difficult to establish a monetary value for the goodwill, equipment, inventory, medical records, and other components of a veterinary practice. Although no one person has any magic formula, there are experienced professionals in the veterinary business services arena who can help in valuing practices.

One way to resolve disputes involving the valuation of veterinary practice partnerships, corporations, or sole proprietorships (in the event of a death, disability, expulsion, retirement, loss of license, bankruptcy, etc.) is to allow a court to determine value. The costs and difficulties of deciding an issue like this via a jury trial can be overwhelming, though.

An alternative to a judicial resolution to this problem is to develop a negotiated method for resolving disputes about value and make it a part of the partnership agreement or corporation bylaws when these documents are created. The following contract clause has been used in numerous business agreements with good success. Its workability has been tested three times, each time resulting in the sale or purchase of an interest in the business at the agreed-upon value:

Annually, at a time not later than four months subsequent to the end of the partnership (or corporation)'s fiscal year, the assets of the partnership shall be valued and an interest rate to be used in a buyout determined.

If the partners (or shareholders) fail to agree on such valuation and/or interest rate, the assets and liabilities of the business shall be appraised by a disinterested third party with expertise in the appraisal of veterinary medical practices, who shall be selected by agree-
ment of the partners (shareholders). All costs of such appraisal shall be borne by the partnership (or corporation).

If the parties to this agreement fail to agree on an appraiser, then each partner may select one appraiser. If an even number of owners exists, then the appraisers chosen by the owners can select one more person to reestablish an odd number of people. These appraisers shall then decide upon a valuation and an interest rate based upon a majority vote. All costs of such appraisal shall be borne proportionately by the partnership (or corporation).

Although in this case the negotiated settlement to a dispute of this type is binding on the parties because the agreement says it is, such negotiation need not be binding. It could be nothing more than a voluntary settlement conference between the parties with or without their legal counsel.

Mediation

Sometimes, because of personal animosities or a stalemate based upon "principles," negotiations between individuals are impossible. To overcome such a situation, the parties may elect to use an intermediary. This person must be a neutral party in whom both sides have confidence. The parties will not be required to accept the mediator's findings or decision, but involving such a person may well be worth the effort. The economic savings in legal fees and court costs plus the potential for an expeditious resolution may mean that a less-than-perfect solution is much better than the alternative of a lawsuit.

The following example is taken from Thomas J. Herron's excellent book on business law:

A recent landlord-tenant dispute illustrates the use of mediation to solve a legal problem. A group of tenants refused to pay their rents because their landlord had failed to make repairs he had agreed to make. When the landlord threatened to evict them, the tenants threatened to file complaints with the city housing authority. Neither side wanted a prolonged struggle. The tenants only wanted the repairs made and the landlord only wanted the rents paid. Instead of pursuing the dispute through legal channels, the parties agreed to turn it over to a local minister for mediation. The parties followed the recommendation of the minister and reached an agreement about the types of repairs that were to be done and the amount of rent that was to be paid.[30]

The potential benefits of time saved and aggravation avoided alone are worth considering mediation of disputes as a viable alternative to a legal action.

ARBITRATION

Arbitration is similar to mediation except that the findings of the neutral arbitrator are generally binding on the parties. Under this system, for example, each party could choose one arbitrator and those arbitrators could select a third. Another method often used is to have disputes concerning contracts decided by a member of the American Arbitration Association. Still another way of gathering an unbiased group to arbitrate a contract dispute is as follows:

Should any dispute arise concerning the scope, validity, effect, or construction of this agreement, then each party shall submit to a presiding judge in and for the county (where the business resides) a list of three attorneys, three business people, and three veterinarians. The presiding judge shall select one person from each party's list of nine proposed arbitrators, and those people selected shall comprise a panel of arbitrators to resolve such dispute. The arbitration shall be conducted pursuant to the rules of the Illinois (or whatever state in which parties reside) Code of Civil Procedure.

Although settling a dispute in this fashion may not be ideal, it is certainly faster and, in all likelihood, less costly than the legal option.

These alternative methods for resolving disputes may look attractive, but before any of them are used, the experience and advice of local counsel should be considered. After all, the legal system has evolved in a fashion intended to protect the rights of all the parties. Its function should not be bypassed without good reason.

CONCLUSION

This chapter provides basic background information about ethics and the law. The information contained herein related to employment contracts and employee benefits will be expanded upon in future chapters as one topic at a time is discussed in more depth. Because laws and precedents vary so much from state to state and year to year, the necessity for the counsel of local attorneys cannot be overemphasized as readers attempt to implement ideas and suggestion that are found throughout this book.

REFERENCES

1. Wilson JF: *Law and Ethics of the Veterinary Profession.* Yardley, PA, Priority Press, Ltd, 1988 (phone 215-321-9488; jwilson@pvmc.net).

2. *Knowles Animal Hospital, Inc* v *Wills,* 360 So2d 37 (Fla 1978).

3. *Campbell* v *Animal Quarantine Station,* 632 P2d 1066 (Hawaii 1981).

4. *Peloquin* v *Calasieu Parish Police Jury,* 367 So2d 1246 (LA 1979).

5. *City of Farland* v *White,* 368 SW2d 12 (Texas 1963).

6. Landers A: *Phila Inquirer* (Box 11562, Chicago, IL 60611-0562).

7. Rollin BE: *An Introduction to Veterinary Medical Ethics: Theory and Cases.* Ames, IA, ISU Press, 1999, pp 5, 8-10.

8. Ibid, pp 8-10.

9. Principles of Veterinary Medical Ethics. *Membership Directory and Resource Manual - 1999 AVMA 48th ed.* Schaumburg, IL, American Veterinary Medical Association, 1998, pp 44-46.

10. Blood DC: *Veterinary Law, Ethics, Etiquette, and Convention.* Melbourne, Victoria, Australia, The Law Book Company Ltd, pp 7-8 (389-393 Lonsdale St., Melbourne, Victoria, Australia).

11. Tannenbaum J: *Veterinary Ethics, Baltimore, MD, Williams & Wilkins,* 1989, p 6.

12. Tannenbaum J: *Veterinary Ethics Animal Welfare, Client Relations, Competition and Collegiality, second ed.* St. Louis, MO, Mosby-Year Book, Inc, 1995, pp 15-16.

13. Estrin R: Harvard offers course on animal law. The Associated Press, June 26, 1999.

14. Wilson JF: Personal experience in teaching at 10 veterinary schools in 1998 and consultant to a 1998 CSU graduate who insisted that this subject be covered in her employment contract.

15. Nolan J: Proctor and Gamble agrees to stop most testing on animals. *Phila Inquirer* Sect C:1, July 1, 1999.

16. *Goldfarb* v *Virginia Bar,* 421 U.S. 773 (1975).

17. *Bates* v *State Bar of Arizona,* 433 U.S. 350 (1977).

18. California Business and Professions Code § 4830.5.

19. *Rules and By-Laws,* Alabama State Board of Veterinary Medicine, Chap 930-X-11(21).

20. Pennsylvania Veterinary Medicine Practice Act, 63 P.S. 166, § 485.1 et seq. § 26.1.

21. Pennsylvania, Massachusetts, Minnesota, Iowa, Wisconsin, Delaware veterinary practice acts or regulations are examples as well as many others.

22. Hannah H: *Legal Briefs.* Schaumburg, IL, AVMA, 1986; Francione GL: *Animals, Property, and the Law.* Philadelphia, Temple University Press, 1995.

23. California Code of Civil Procedure § 340.5.

24. Glendon MA: *Comparative Legal Traditions.* St. Paul, MN, West Publishing Co, 1985, pp 167,168.

25. Leibler E: Personal communication, AVMLA, Lansing, MI. (phone 517-333-7000, fax 517-337-5609, email Eliebler@aol.com.

26. Meyers D: The long paw of the law. *Phila Inquirer,* Suburban Section, Oct 27, 1993, p 1.

27. Levine B: Defending the underdog. *Los Angeles Times,* Section E, Sept 23, 1996, p 1.

28. How to keep a lawyer from running up your bill. *Vet Econ* (Nov):1985.

29. California Business and Professions Code § 4883(1).

30. Harron TJ: *Business Law.* Boston, Allyn & Bacon, Inc, 1981, p 48.

Chapter 2

THE BASICS OF CONTRACT LAW

By James F. Wilson, DVM, JD

The types of contracts that veterinarians most often encounter involve the sales and purchases of goods, the performance of professional services, employment, and real estate. These different types of contracts are controlled by various statutory laws as well as different common law precedents.

Veterinarians often are unaware of the legal requirements and interpretations surrounding contract law until disagreements or misunderstandings occur. It is then that the importance of the legal doctrines associated with contract law becomes evident. This chapter presents basic contract law terminology and principles to help practitioners determine their rights and responsibilities under oral and written agreements. Contract law, however, is often complex and vague, and legal counsel is recommended whenever veterinarians are about to enter into major agreements.

FORMATION OF THE CONTRACT

THE CONTRACT

The term *contract* generally refers to an agreement between two or more parties. This agreement consists of a promise or mutual promises that the law will enforce or the performance of which the law recognizes as a duty.[1] Simply stated, a contract is an agreement that creates an obligation.[2]

TRADITIONAL CONTRACT LAW

Traditionally, agreements were evaluated for five elements essential to the formation of a contract. These include three objective elements: (1) an offer, (2) an acceptance, and (3) consideration; and two subjective elements (4) an intent to contract and (5) a meeting of the minds. Current contract law emphasizes only the three objective elements of an agreement.

THE UNIFORM COMMERCIAL CODE

Modern consumer law is a mixture of old and new law. Unfair or fraudulent business practices that were more prevalent in the first half of this century forced state legislatures and the courts to put consumers on a more equal basis with sellers. That led to the creation of a code of law called the *Uniform Commercial Code (UCC)*, which applies to the sale of goods. This code protects buyers from unfair business practices by requiring that sellers disclose certain relevant information that was not offered during the "buyer beware" era.

The UCC was created during the 1960s to make consumer transactions involving the sale of goods consistent across state borders. The UCC has been adopted as statutory law in all states. It defines goods as

All things (including specially manufactured goods) which are movable at the time of identification to the contract of sale....[3]

The UCC along with court interpretations thereof provide the primary sources of legal information and precedents covering the sales of goods. When the UCC does not specifically address an issue, traditional common law (court-made law) precedents apply.

DETERMINING WHICH LAW COVERS A TRANSACTION

Common law principles apply to contracts for labor, services, or the sale of land. Contracts for veterinary services, however, often include sales of both goods and services combined. In order to determine which body of law applies, it must be determined whether goods or services comprised the predominant thrust and purpose of the sale. When the predominant effort was the sale of goods, the UCC applies. In cases where the principal purpose was the rendering of services, traditional contract law applies.[1]

Throughout this chapter, references are made to the *Restatement of Contracts, Second* as a source of information about contract law. This reference is published by the American Law Institute to inform lawyers and scholars of the law in a general area, how it is changing, and what direction the authors think that change should take. Although the *Restatement of Contracts, Second* is a valuable reference, it is a private legal publication and is not always followed by the courts; thus, contract law precedents vary from one jurisdiction to another.

THE ELEMENTS OF A CONTRACT

At one time, proof of five elements was required to establish an enforceable contract. These consisted of the offer, an acceptance, a meeting of the minds, consideration, and an intent to form a contract. Today, however, only three of these elements must be proved; the concepts of a meeting of the minds and intent to contract are integrated with proof that the offer was an understandable offer and the acceptance a knowledgeable acceptance.

THE OFFER

OFFER UNDER COMMON LAW

The first element required for the creation of a contract is an offer. An offer is a promise or a commitment made in reasonably certain terms to do or refrain from doing some specified thing in the future.[4] When one person demonstrates a willingness to enter into an agreement involving certain definite terms and invites the other party in the bargaining transaction to agree to the same terms, a legally sufficient offer has been made.

The mere statement of an offer price, standing alone, may be held to be a legally unenforceable offer because it omits many terms necessary to the making of a contract.[4] In order for the offer to be considered legally sufficient, it must contain enough information so that reasonable people would understand to what it was they were agreeing. It is in this context that proof of the subjective *a meeting of the minds* element overlaps with the offer element of a contract.

Most offers leading to the purchase of hospital drugs, supplies, and lower-priced equipment, as well as the performance of veterinary services for clients' animals, are presented orally. The same is true for offers of employment between practice owners and support staff. Though personal experience shows that the existence of written offers between practice owners and associate veterinarians has grown in the last decade, there is no hard data regarding the frequency with which such offers are presented.

Offers also are written formally or informally, with great forethought or with none, and placed in the classified sections of newspapers, professional journals or web sites, letters to job applicants or job fairs, or telephone *Yellow Pages*. If words of commitment are used or there is an invitation to take action without further communication, this form of advertising to individuals or the general public also can constitute a valid offer. In some cases, employment contract offers are established merely from sets of notes taken during the course of telephone or in-person interviews.

A legal challenge by a recent veterinary graduate concerned promises supposedly made by an employer participating in a job interview forum conducted at the University of Pennsylvania's winter conference. As unbelievable as it may seem, a key element of evidence regarding the content of the employer's job offer supposedly came from the brief description provided to and printed by the school's director of continuing education prior to the time students signed up for interviews. It seems incomprehensible that the employer and employee in this case had no further discussions or clarifications regarding the terms of their agreement, other than that presented in the job offer. However, such is the case sometimes in the informal world of veterinary practice management (perhaps better known as practice mismanagement?). Because of the limited discussion of the terms of employment, and the lack of clarity in the offer, the parties to this agreement spent a great deal of time, energy, and money hiring legal counsel to pursue interrogatories and depositions, prepare for trial and, ultimately, settle this case out of court, rather than doing what they do best, generating income and practicing veterinary medicine.

It is in the advertising of merchandise or services via newspapers, direct-mail flyers, radio messages, web sites, television commercials, or other means that problems can occur regarding the presence or absence of an operative offer. For example, does a newspaper announcement from a particular veterinary hospital advertising low-cost spays allow any owner of a female dog or cat to walk into that office and say, "I accept your offer to spay my obese bulldog, my in-estrus rottweiler, my pregnant cat or my 12-year-old dog with a draining pyometra for the price advertised on this flyer. Here is the cash you requested. When shall I pick her up?"

In such situations, what looks like an offer may not be a legally operative offer. Instead, it may be only a preliminary invitation for prospective clients or buyers to consider when negotiating the purchase of the advertised service. The *Restatement of Contracts, Second* § 26 addresses this issue:

> A manifestation of willingness to enter into a bargain is not an offer if the person to whom it is addressed knows or has reason to know that the person making it does not intend to conclude a bargain until he has made a further manifestation of assent.

One could argue that most reasonable animal owners should know that such offers for low cost spays could depend on many medical factors. This is especially true with respect to owners of obese animals, females in heat or experienced bulldog owners who are aware of the anesthetic risks associated with the breed. One might expect them to recognize that a further manifestation of assent on the part of their veterinarians might be essential before the low-cost service offers were extended to them and their pets. Nonetheless, one also could argue that naive, first-time owners of obese dogs, bitches in heat, or bulldog owners cannot be assumed to have such knowledge. Thus, unless veterinarians are willing to offer this service to animals of all ages and in all states of physical health as well as to owners of all breeds, an all-inclusive advertisement like this should not be made without a disclaimer denying the offer to aging patients or those with specified medical or genetic maladies.

One does not know what the courts would hold if our hypothetical "reasonable bulldog owner" accepted an offer like this, only to find that the veterinarian wanted to charge more than quoted. As is always the case with the law, decisions are based on an analysis of all the facts as well as the legal precedents.

Some states have consumer laws and regulations that address the issue of operative offers in the advertising of professional services. Massachusetts[5] and California are two such states. Section 17500 of the California Business and Professions Code says the following about offers for services:

It is unlawful for any person...with intent directly or indirectly...to perform services, professional or otherwise...to induce the public to enter into any obligation relating thereto, to make or disseminate...in any newspaper or other publication...any statement concerning such...services...which is untrue or misleading, and which is known, or which by the exercise of reasonable care should be known, to be untrue or misleading...with the intent not to sell such...services...so advertised at the price stated therein, or as so advertised. Any violation of the provisions of this section is a misdemeanor punishable by imprisonment in the county jail not exceeding six months, or by a fine not exceeding...$2500, or both.

Offers that do not state a time within which another party must accept or reject the offer pose another legal hurdle associated with the offer component of a contract. In general, an offer may be accepted or rejected within a reasonable time. Just what would be deemed reasonable is open to legal review, so it is extremely unwise for any business to make an offer without an expiration date. With certain exceptions, offers without expiration dates can be revoked or withdrawn at any time before they are accepted. Offers that have expiration dates may not be withdrawn before that date.

Offers may originate from sellers or consumers. Clients, for example, may drop off pets at clinics for examinations in the morning without ever seeing the attending veterinarians. In doing so, they are saying, "Good morning, Doc. Old 'Crusty' here has been scratching up a storm lately and needs some treatment so all of us can sleep at night. Could you please make a diagnosis and prescribe a treatment? I'll be in late this afternoon to pay you for your services and pick him up."

Consumers who place such orders for specific goods or services, request ambulatory visits for livestock, leave pets at hospitals for care, or mail or leave deposits for product purchases will be held to have made valid offers. Without instructions to call and consult with the offeror about diagnostics, treatments, and fees before proceeding with the agreed-upon services, clients could be held to have provided an implied acceptance to whatever reasonable care the offeree (veterinary practice) provides. Obviously, this is not a smart way to seek care, make diagnoses, nor conduct business. Still, the law often is called upon to resolve dumb things done by parties seeking its intervention.

Under the law, these same consumers may be able to withdraw their offers if they do so before the veterinary practices or sellers communicate their acceptances. If no acceptances are ever communicated by the sellers, no contracts will have been formed, and the consumers would be entitled to refunds of their deposits.[5]

ACCEPTANCE

COMMON LAW ACCEPTANCE

Once a valid offer has been made, the next essential element in the establishment of an enforceable contract is proof of an acceptance. An acceptance has occurred when the party to whom the offer was made makes the return requested in the offer.[6] In most cases, this return occurs via the payment of money. Under common law, an acceptance must conform precisely to the terms of the offer. If it varies from those terms, it fails as an acceptance and instead becomes a counteroffer.[7,8]

It is through this traditional common law process that practitioners can find themselves faced with offers and counteroffers to the point that they no longer know whether they are the offeror or the offeree. They may offer to perform specified veterinary services for stated fees and then find that they are being asked to accept a client's offer to pay for those veterinary services under entirely different payment terms than they had originally intended. At this point veterinarians may elect to counter the offer with a different payment plan or a less-expensive treatment protocol.

It is through this offer and counteroffer bargaining process that misunderstandings occur which lead to disputes. When veterinarians realize that this is happening, it is time to produce a written estimate. Only then can it be shown that sufficient common ground existed to constitute a meeting of the minds and a valid acceptance.

ACCEPTANCE IN IMPLIED VERSUS EXPRESS CONTRACTS

It would seem that proof of an acceptance would be a fairly straightforward component of a contract, free of much legal wrangling. If the words "I accept" are uttered, it is a simple matter. Words to this effect indicate a willingness to provide the consideration requested (usually to pay the bill). This form of acceptance is called an *express acceptance* and establishes an *express contract*.

In many cases, however, no words or signatures on a document are provided, and then the process is more complicated. Yet courts still may find that an acceptance can be inferred from the actions of the parties even if no express acceptance is proved. In such situations, the acceptance may be an *implied acceptance* and the agreement is then called an *implied contract*. If a contract is implied, the terms agreed upon and whether the entire agreement or only parts of it were accepted may still be called into question.

As with offers for practices to provide veterinary care, acceptances by clients are implied if, for example, animals with medical problems are dropped off at veterinary hospitals with information about their symptoms, but with no direct communications between the doctors and the animals' owners. Equivalent examples in large animal practice would be where cows are left in stanchions with notes attached to adjacent posts by farmers describing their symptoms. If these clients are off working and are unavailable for consultation, acceptance of the care rendered can be implied. The extent of the medical care that a court might allow in cases like this, and for which it might require payment, may be in question. Nonetheless, an implied contract for some medical care certainly exists.

In both of these examples the presence of an implied acceptance is enhanced if similar transactions had occurred previously between the clients and their doctors and full payment for the veterinary services had been made. The theory is that ratification of prior treatments by payment without any challenge is grounds for implying an acceptance for similar requests in the future. Clients who do not wish to make such implied acceptances need to inform their veterinarians that no diagnostic procedures or treatments are to be performed until further discussions are held and express authorizations for those services is given.

WHEN IS AN OFFER ACCEPTED?

A key question that arises with the formation of contracts entails *when* an offer was accepted. Generally, this is dependent on the facts of the situation. To illustrate the difficulties associated with this key question, two examples will be used, the first related to the delivery of veterinary care, the second related to employment contracts.

A well-to-do horse owner with a Grand Prix quality jumper calls her veterinarian, Dr. Meanswell, because her horse, "Skylark," appears to be suffering from colic. Dr. M's receptionist, Ms. Doesgood, informs the owner that Dr. M is attending another emergency halfway across the county at the moment but should be about ready to wind things up at that site. Ms. D tells the owner that Dr. M should be able to make it to her location within an hour. The owner, relying on this information, tells Ms. D that she's counting on that and will wait until Dr. M arrives rather than call another doctor.

The hour goes by, during which time Ms. D is unable to contact Dr. M. She also fails to call the stable manager back to inform her of the impending delay. Two more hours pass, at which time the owner calls Dr. M's office fuming, "Where the heck is Dr. M? Skylark is in agony and looks like he's 'going down.' How much longer will it be?" To that Ms. D replies, "I'm not sure because I can't seem to reach Dr. M. However, I'm sure she can make it within another hour."

By the time Dr. M arrives an additional two hours later, poor Skylark is agonal. Appropriate treatment is rendered but he dies that evening. The irate owner elects not to pay Dr. M, so eventually Dr. M turns this client over to a collection agency. In protest for what the client believed was inappropriate conduct by Dr. M and her staff, she files suit against the practice for a breach of contract and malpractice.

The breach of contract charge is based on Dr. M's failure to arrive at the time initially promised by Ms. D. The allegations contain two components. The first is that, because of the delay in treatment, Dr. M was unable to initiate treatment in time to save Skylark's life. The second is that, because

she relied on Dr. M's estimated time of arrival, the owner chose not to search for a second veterinarian who, in her judgment, most likely could have initiated treatment in time to save Skylark's life.

Was there a breach of contract in this case? Depending on the owner's ability to prove the facts exactly as they have been presented, the answer most likely is yes. This is precisely why most tradesmen, moving companies, telephone repair people, and other providers of on-site household repairs or delivery people are so reluctant to set precise times of arrival. Their fear is that if they miss the target by several hours or more, they will have breached their contracts and could be held liable for the value of the lost work time of those customers who have missed work to accommodate them and then were forced to twiddle their thumbs for lengthy periods.

With these contract principles in mind, it is advisable for ambulatory clinicians, as well as those with fixed facilities, who agree to appointed times for their visits to

- use caution giving clients specific times at which they will arrive to provide the care for which they have been contracted,

- have staff members contact, or at least attempt to contact, clients and provide updated expected times of arrival for doctors when delays are anticipated,

- inform clients whose animals need emergency care of the nature and expected time of the delay and encourage them to seek emergency services elsewhere if that is the most medically prudent choice, and

- apologize profusely for their tardiness if and when they finally arrive.

The second example focuses on situations encountered repeatedly in the authors' consulting business. It involves offers of employment by practice owners, apparent acceptances by associates and, then, decisions by either party to withdraw the offer.

The most common situations occur similarly to the following. Dr. Ownsmore offers full-time employment to Dr. Greenhorn, spelling out the elements of the agreement quite clearly. Dr. G consults with his legal or practice management advisor and identifies several items in the offer that need clarification. He calls Dr. O and requests an increase in compensation, a reduction in the restrictive covenant terms, and clarification of the CE allowance and work schedule (a counteroffer). To those requests Dr. O responds, "Gee, those sound reasonable, but I'll have to think them over, talk with my office manager, and get back to you."

Because Dr. Greenhorn never heard Dr. Ownsmore say, "No, we won't be able to meet those requests," he assumes Dr. O will accept the changes without a lot more negotiating. However, because Dr. G still has not heard a definitive, "okay," he puts off decisions with other employers who are pressuring him for an answer to their offers, trying to keep those doors open, even though his top choice is to work for Dr. O.

Three days later, Dr. O calls and says, "We've talked it over and we can't meet all of your requests. How about meeting us halfway?" To that, Dr. G says, "I'm going to need to talk further with my advisors, but that probably will be acceptable."

It takes Dr. G three days to contact his advisors, who advise against taking the job because, in their minds, the restrictive covenant is still unreasonable. Dr. G decides to take the job in spite of their advice and calls Dr. O to tell him the good news. Much to Dr. G's surprise, Dr. O says, "Gosh, Dr. O, we have been able to find a veterinarian with three years experience that meets our needs much better than a new graduate, so we signed a contract with her yesterday. I'm sorry we just couldn't work things out with you. Thank you for the interest in the position; we'll keep you in mind in case something comes up next year."

In many cases the process described in this situation goes on for several weeks, and the parties who thought they had found the nearly perfect match are terribly discouraged and angry about what happened. As discussed later in the chapter, if no one relied excessively on the broken promises inherent in these offers, neither party would have a legal cause of action. Instead, this is just part of a "welcome to the wonderful world of contract negotiations" situation. All parties must understand that each of these offers and counteroffers were merely operative offers unless they had "drop dead" points at which the offers were withdrawn or until one of the parties accepted the conditions orally or via a written document. It is a good example, however, of the pitfalls inherent in the formation of contracts and why written offers with endpoints linked to their acceptance are as critical as written acceptances.

OFFER AND ACCEPTANCE UNDER THE UCC

Most contracts between veterinarians and clients are for combinations of services and goods. Practitioners provide services in the form of professional time for examinations, surgery, dentistry, and diagnostic procedures. Sometimes, though, they also dispense large-dollar volumes of goods in the form of vaccine, medications, pet food, and supplies. The cost of these goods in many cases exceeds the cost of veterinary services.

As previously discussed, the type of contract law governing such transactions varies. If sales of services predominate, the contract is regulated by common law principles. If the major portion of the agreement consists of the sale of goods, it is regulated by the UCC.

Unlike common law, the UCC makes no attempt to define an offer and, under its principles, a valid contract may be present even in the absence of certain traditional contract terms or elements. If it can be found that the parties intended to make a contract and that an agreement existed based upon language used by the parties or by implication from other circumstances, such as a "course of dealing," a "usage of trade," or "a course of performance," a contract for the sale of goods will be enforced.[9] However, the more terms that are left open, the less likely it is that the parties intended to have a contract and the less likely it is that a court will find in favor of the existence of a contract.[10]

Meeting of the Minds

Proof of the subjective *meeting of the minds* component of the offer and acceptance process is derived from the discussions and actions of the parties. It can be seen from the new legal concepts embodied in the UCC that the precise language of the contractual agreement is less important than the intent of the parties as illustrated by their actions. Thus, in contemporary thinking, it is less critical to subjectively establish what each party was actually thinking than it is to show objectively what reasonable people in the position of the other parties would have concluded from the course of events.

It is under the element entitled *meeting of the minds* that written fee estimates for sales of products to clients and the provision of veterinary services to patients become critically important. Likewise, written job descriptions and outlines of salaries, benefits, and work schedules are essential to convince job applicants, judges, and juries that the parties understood the employment relationships into which they were entering.

Without written evidence helping to support a meeting of the minds, it is difficult for attending veterinarians to establish medical priorities and set forth the various diagnostic and treatment options for clients to consider. It is equally difficult for practice owners to solidify good working relationships with new employees. The result is that clients become angry because they did not comprehend the outcome or total costs for veterinary services, or new employees lose faith in their employers.

Because of the deficiencies inherent in oral discussions, establishing a legally acceptable meeting of the minds without a written document is difficult. And, without clear proof of this element, it is much more difficult arguing the merits of an oral contract than a written one. It is also why experienced clinicians routinely use formal written estimates as valuable medical decision-making and legal defense tools. Similarly, simple letters on practice stationery, or even hen scratches on restaurant napkins outlining salaries, benefits, and work schedules for prospective employees can increase trust and reduce differing recollections of what the contracting parties agreed upon.

In summary, when written memoranda of peoples' thoughts are created, the likelihood of a meeting of the minds increases and opportunities for disputes decrease. Moreover, the probability of courts finding understandable offers and knowledgeable acceptances is greatly enhanced.

Intent

The more traditional, subjective view of contract law required the presence of an intent to contract, the fifth element for the formation of a contract. The rationale for this element was that valid contracts could not be formed if the parties did not intend to form one. However, proving to a court what the parties to the agreement intended or did not intend is difficult, especially when the parties themselves may not have known precisely what they intended at each point in time.

Although practitioners may still find this subjective element to be up for legal discussion, the newer trend, as seen in the UCC, is to approach the law of contracts objectively. Under this theory of contracts, less importance is placed upon a party's intent and more emphasis is placed on what a reasonable person in the position of one party would conclude from the conduct of the other.

CONSIDERATION

The fourth and final element required to form a contract is consideration (sometimes called *legal detriment*). This is the factor that justifies the enforcement of a promise or the thing bargained for or given in exchange for the promise. Consideration means that people do or promise to do something that they were not already legally obligated to do, or refrain or promise to refrain from doing something that they had a legal right to do.[4]

In simple terms, consideration is a benefit conferred to the promisor and a detriment incurred by the promisee. In a marriage contract, the consideration consists of the exchange of promises under the direction and supervision of a person legally authorized to conduct marriages. In most other transactions the promise to pay money to obtain goods or services constitutes consideration. In a minority of cases, the exchange of consideration involves trading services for services, e.g., legal or carpentry services for veterinary services, or goods for services, e.g., art work, wood carvings, draperies, or pottery for veterinary care. This is the world of barter, an exchange the Internal Revenue Service dislikes unless the value of such exchanges is reported as income to the parties but, nonetheless, the application of legitimate contract law.

An issue occasionally encountered under this contract law element involves how much benefit or detriment must exist in order to establish or modify a contract. Historically, the courts have held that if contracts were freely made by competent parties, the fact that they were not supported by sufficient consideration was not a satisfactory reason to refuse to enforce them.[11] More recently, though, courts have refused to enforce contracts, or particular clauses within them, if they have found the terms to be unconscionable under the circumstances. Agreements that exceed the limits of any reasonable claim or expectation can be classified by courts as unconscionable. Whereas under common law this doctrine can vary from one jurisdiction to another, the UCC gives it explicit recognition.[12]

There are several other issues regarding the subject of consideration. Two of them that have particular application in the veterinary business arena are discussed below.

The Preexisting Duty Rule

There is a well-established rule of contract law that a promise to do what one is already legally bound to do is not binding for lack of consideration. The rationale given is that no legal detriment exists.

This rule comes into play, for example, if veterinarians elect to accept less than full payment as payment in full for debts owed by clients. The general rule is that partial payment of an amount that is admitted to be due is insufficient consideration to support a promise by a creditor to discharge the rest of the debt. For example, a client has owed Dr. Jones $200 for the past two months and does not dispute the amount owed. Dr. Jones is tired of waiting for the money so she calls the client and is in the process of getting put off for another month when she decides to offer a compromise. Dr. Jones says, "If you will pay me $100 within the next two days, I will accept that as payment in full for the entire debt."

If the client pays the $100 within the two-day time limit, does it mean that Dr. Jones cannot collect the remaining $100? In most jurisdictions, the parties to a contract can agree to an arrangement like this, and the creditor who made such an offer can promise to accept the lesser amount as payment in full. However, because the debtor is already under a legal duty to pay the full amount, there is a lack of consideration to be able to enforce this new agreement. As a result, legally, Dr. Jones could accept the lesser amount and still sue for the balance.[13] It is certainly not recommended that this course of action be pursued, but under the preexisting duty rule, the law would support it.

In other cases, because of inadequate or incomplete estimates or varying recollections of the negotiation process, the amount of a debt legitimately owed is disputed. In such cases, debtors often try to renege on full payment by sending amounts less than those which are claimed to be due, clearly indicating on their checks that the payments being sent represent full payment. In such cases, this offer to pay in full and the creditor's acceptance of the lesser amount constitute a full discharge of the remainder of the unpaid account. This is because by accepting payment and, thus, precluding the need for further squabbles, billings, and the ongoing risk of late or nonpayment, the creditors can be held to have received consideration for accepting this offer, even if it is for less than full payment.

Promissory Estoppel, or Action in Reliance

Another doctrine of contract law that can have an impact on veterinarians involves *promissory estoppel* or *action in reliance*. This legal doctrine could have been invoked as a result of the offer/counter-offer/counter-counteroffer hypothetical example presented earlier in the chapter.

The *Restatement of Contracts, Second* defines this doctrine as follows:

> A promise which the promisor shall reasonably expect to induce action or forbearance on the part of the promisee or a third person and which does induce such action or forbearance is binding if injustice can be avoided only by enforcement of the promise....[14]

In nonlegal language, this means that, although there may have been no agreement ironed out by the parties, justice requires the enforcement of one's promise when another party has justifiably relied upon that promise and changed its position, incurring substantial detriment.

An example of the application of this doctrine to veterinary medicine is a one-year offer of employment to a graduating veterinary student starting a month after graduation. The student relies on the offer, which includes a salary of $3,500/month, and tells the employer, "I will be there on July 1st." A number of details concerning the term of the contract and benefits are vague, and no contract is ever signed.

The student rejects several other job opportunities and stops looking for employment. After graduating, she notifies her future employer that she will be driving 400 miles to the town where the job is located in search of an apartment. The prospective employer is out of town at a seminar the weekend she arrives but knows the applicant is in town. Three days before the new veterinarian is to start work, the intended employer contacts the new graduate and informs her that he cannot hire anyone due to a slowdown in the business.

Did a contract exist? Is the new graduate entitled to damages because of a breach of contract? In analyzing the facts of this hypothetical situation, the new graduate incurred considerable debt and personal expense looking for a place to live and turned down another offer because she thought she had a job. The employer knew of the prospective employee's efforts to find a place to live and said nothing to discourage that effort. Based on these facts, a court would very likely find that a contract had been formed. This is precisely the type of setting in which the doctrine of promissory estoppel could come into play to support the existence of consideration.

STANDARD FORM CONTRACTS, OR CONTRACTS OF ADHESION

The world of commerce could not function without the use of standardized printed contract forms. Anyone who has purchased a car, appliance, or house is familiar with them. It is commonplace for such forms to be accepted and signed whether or not they are read or understood.

These printed forms are frequently referred to as *adhesion contracts* or *contracts of adhesion*. An adhesion contract may be defined as a contract written exclusively by one party (the *dominant party*) and presented to the other party (the *adhering party*) under circumstances in which there is no realistic opportunity to negotiate.[4] The consequences of signing an agreement vary under the UCC as compared with common law precedents. In practice, even if people are able to read and understand these contracts, they are still helpless to vary them in any way. The only recourse usually offered is to sign the form just as it is.

The common law rule was that "one who signs a contract which he had an opportunity to read and understand is bound by its provisions."[15] That rule is formulated on the rationale that signed contracts would not be very reliable if parties were allowed to claim at a later time that since they did not read or understand the contracts, they should not be bound by them.

The unfairness of this rule was dealt with in 1960 with the famous case of *Henningsen* v. *Bloomfield Motors, Inc.*[16] In that case the court refused to enforce a warranty disclaimer found in fine print on the reverse side of a purchase order for a car. The theory invoked was that a disclaimer that forced buyers to accept an unalterable contract on an unconditional basis was against public policy.

The UCC takes the same approach by including in the code what it calls the *doctrine of unconscionability*. This legal precept affords consumers who have little or no bargaining power and who accept form contracts that are procedurally or substantively unconscionable the right to resist their enforcement.

There are several types of situations where provisions within adhesion contracts are not enforced by the courts. These include situations in which

- Provisions protecting the dominant party, like disclaimers of warranties, are buried in fine print on the back side of the form or in the middle of a long paragraph.

- Written provisions are legible but are presented in such a way as to make it unlikely that they would come to the attention of the other party.

- The dominant party misrepresents to another party what is embodied in the document. The other party signs the document without reading it and then later discovers that the representations were false. In this type of situation, one party is negligent and the other is fraudulent.

There is a trend away from strict enforcement of the duty-to-read rule with adhesion contracts.[17] The theories differ, but the result is that provisions that operate unfairly or oppressively will not be enforced against an uninformed party or someone who could not reasonably have been expected to know of it.[17]

CAPACITY TO CONTRACT

There are three basic situations wherein questions regarding the capacity to make a valid contract would be questioned. These are minority, mental disability, and intoxication.

MINORITY

Under common law rules, people lacked the legal capacity to enter into contracts until the age of 21. Most states now have statutes setting the age of majority at 18, although for some purposes a few may still require people to be 19.

The law does not say that minors cannot enter into contracts and uphold them. The law does, however, grant people the right to avoid or disaffirm any contracts made while they were minors. Specific state statutes allow minors to enter into some types of valid contracts and have them enforced against them. Two of the more common types are contracts for motor vehicle liability insurance and contracts with institutions of higher learning for the purpose of financing an education.

If minors enter into contracts, only they—not the adults with whom they contracted—may disaffirm or void the contracts. This is true in the majority of jurisdictions even if the minors misrepresent their ages at the time they entered into the contract. Surprisingly, minors who disaffirm contracts are not required to return property they obtained and no longer have in their possession. If they do have the property contracted for, they are required to return it, but they are entitled to recover any consideration paid. Contracts entered into during the age of minority may be disaffirmed at any time during that minority or within a reasonable time after reaching the age of majority.

The law carves out a separate niche for items classified as "necessaries" of life. Minors may be held liable for the fair market value of necessaries, but the party claiming against them has the burden of proving that the items furnished were necessaries that a legally responsible parent was unwilling or unable to supply.[18] It is very doubtful that veterinary services would ever be classified in this narrow group.

It is not uncommon for veterinarians to be approached by minors seeking medical care for their animals. The best way to effect an enforceable contract with these individuals is to contact a parent or guardian and have them provide the required acceptance. If parents have ratified contracts initiated by their minor children in the past by paying for services on a timely basis, the argument can be made that the parents have appointed them as their agents. It may be a satisfactory policy for practitioners to depend on this course of dealing with the children of parents who have reliably paid in the past if the costs for services to be rendered are reasonably low. The safest

course always will be, however, to ask youthful-looking people how old they are and for proof of age if they appear to be less than 18. If it turns out they are minors, clinicians should proceed with veterinary care only after contacting a parent or guardian for authorization to render the requested services.

MENTAL DISABILITY

People who lack the required mental capacity to make a contract can avoid or disaffirm contracts just as minors can. Mental illness, retardation, and senility are the most common reasons for releasing these people from their contractual obligations or decisions. The test is whether the party seeking to avoid the contract was capable of comprehending the nature and quality of the transaction entered into and its probable consequences. Also at issue is how heavy a duty is placed on the other party to foresee and comprehend the extent of the mentally disabled person's mental capacity. Contracting parties cannot be held to a rigid standard to foresee at what point a person slips from a mentally competent state to incompetence. Obvious mental disorders, however, must be recognized.

Because of the large population of elderly people, senility is the incapacity that veterinarians are most likely to face. Watching clients' memories and health fail is difficult. The concurrent failure of their animals' health because of their inability to properly care for them is disheartening. Sometimes, the only morally and contractually acceptable way to deal with these situations is for veterinarians to seek out other family members who can make decisions for them.

In a contract setting, senility becomes important in at least two primary matters: (1) contracts for expensive care in which, because of a mental disability, clients cannot remember what they agreed to (and they refuse to pay for those services), and (2) when agreements are being made to euthanize patients belonging to senile or mentally ill owners. The former of these is the less serious one because it may simply mean that veterinarians will have trouble collecting debts owed. The latter constitutes a worse hazard, because euthanasia cannot be reversed. Extra precautions are needed when the mental competence of owners to make decisions about euthanasia is in question.

In order to prevent either the unnecessary death of an animal or a major family feud, animals should not be euthanized until practitioners are certain that a concurring family member agrees with the action requested. In some cases practitioners may be wise to wait until the next day before performing euthanasia in order to provide sufficient time to contact someone else in the family or the client's legal guardian.

INTOXICATION OR SUBSTANCE ABUSE

In most cases the courts do not look favorably upon intoxication or being "stoned" as an incapacity. If the state of inebriation or mental incoherence is extreme, however, the affected person is not unlike the mentally disabled person who cannot understand the nature and consequences of the contract and, thus, cannot assent to the agreement.

The modern view of voluntary intoxication or substance abuse as a grounds for avoiding contracts focuses considerable attention on whether the sober party or a reasonably sober party in a similar position should have been aware of the distorted mental capacity. A side issue that is also considered by the courts is whether the sober party took unfair advantage of the other party's intoxicated or mentally incoherent state.

If a contract is voidable because of intoxication or substance abuse, when affected people become sober, they can either ratify or disaffirm the agreement in much the same manner as mentally disabled people can. If they disaffirm the contract, they must return the consideration received. If the consideration has been used or wasted before the intoxicated or stoned people become sober, they do not need to make restitution.[18]

Inebriated or "doped out" clients are not uncommon in veterinary medicine. When alcohol is the culprit, the outward evidence of intoxication is reasonably obvious. When drug abuse is the cause of the mental incoherence, the mentally disabled state may not be as noticeable. Any time that there is serious doubt about drug or alcohol intoxication, the same concerns regarding euthanasia or incurring major expenses for medical services discussed under mental disability should be considered.

STATUTE OF FRAUDS

Many people are surprised to learn that the majority of oral contracts are valid and enforceable. History has shown that the larger the value or the longer the term of a contract, the more likelihood there is for fraud to be associated with it. Because of this concern, in the 1600s the English enacted a statute known as the *Statute of Frauds*. This law required the production of a written memorandum before the courts would enforce certain kinds of contracts. The basic tenets set forth in that law are still applicable today.

TYPES OF CONTRACTS COVERED

Most American jurisdictions have retained the original wording of the English statute. The most common types of contracts that must be in writing are (1) contracts for the sale of real estate, (2) leases for longer than one year, (3) contracts not to be performed within one year, (4) contracts to answer for the debts of another, and (5) contracts for the sale of goods over a specified price. The law says that these types of contracts are "within the Statute of Frauds" and are therefore unenforceable without a written document.

Although each of these types of contracts has a body of law interpreting the Statute of Frauds' application to it, one which needs some further explanation is that pertaining to the sale of goods. Where written contracts are required, the UCC separates sales of goods into different categories. Those categories with special significance to consumers are sales of goods costing more than $500,[19] contracts involving securities,[20] security agreements,[21] and sales of other types of personal property. In the context of a veterinary practice, this would not include sales of goods incorporated within and linked to services, such as radiographs, surgical implants, injections, and IV catheters and fluids.

Under the UCC section covering the sale of goods valued at more than $500, two of the rules are that the written agreement must be signed by the party to be charged, and it must specify the quantity of goods sold.[22] As for the sale of personal property, the Code requires that contracts involving the sale of personal property valued at more than $5,000 must be written to be enforceable.

Remedies for a Failure to Comply

Most courts hold that an oral contract that falls within the Statute of Frauds is unenforceable if no sufficient written memorandum exists, but it is not void or ineffective. This is an important consideration, because it means that the courts will uphold oral contracts that have been fully performed. For example, an oral contract that required more than one year for performance is enforceable if one party has fulfilled the term and has fully performed the other requirements of the agreement.

The doctrine of promissory estoppel reappears under the Statute of Frauds. If one party has detrimentally relied on a promise or acted in reliance and in doing so has substantially performed the requirements of an oral contract, those actions will take the case out of the Statute of Frauds. In other words, under the Statute of Frauds, an oral contract that should have been written in order to be enforceable becomes enforceable in order to avoid injustice to the injured party.[23]

Parol Evidence

The parol (oral) evidence rule is another complex legal doctrine worthy of discussion because it is often referred to in contract law and in the context of a claim for breach of contract. When two parties have made and signed a written contract, and included a clause within the agreement stating that the writing represents the entirety of the contract, oral testimony aimed at altering or contradicting the terms of the writing will not be permitted. Such clauses are part of what is known as *boiler plate* in contracts. This means that it is consistent from one contract to another without any room for the person who receives the offer to negotiate alternative language. An example follows:

> *Contract Terms To Be Exclusive: This agreement supercedes any and all other agreements, whether written or oral, between the parties hereto with respect to this employment agreement and contains all of the promises and agreements between the parties. Each party acknowledges that no representation, inducements, promises or agreements have been made, orally or otherwise, by any party or anyone acting on behalf of any party, that are not embodied herein. All other agreements, statements or promises not contained in this agreement shall be invalid.*

Strict enforcement of the parol evidence rule would create numerous hardships because it is impossible for most written agreements to clearly include everything to which the parties are agreeing. As usual, the law provides some exceptions to strict application of the parol evidence rule. Parol (oral) evidence is admissible to explain ambiguous language in a written contract and to prove fraud, duress, and mistakes. Fraud in this context can be misrepresentations in the written contract that do not reflect an accurate prior oral understanding of the parties. This can include contracts where the writing omits terms upon which the parties have agreed or terms upon which the evidence shows they have not agreed.

In sum, parties to contracts should not be allowed to lie and thereby win their lawsuits; but neither should they be allowed to win because the rules of evidence keep the court from hearing additional information about the agreement they thought they were entering into. Although written documents are often the most credible evidence regarding the terms of a contract, additional evidence that would help a court decide the merits of the case should be allowed. The parol evidence rule and its exceptions blend the merits of the written word with the need for some oral explanation to provide a better form of justice for all concerned parties.

REMEDIES FOR BREACHES OF CONTRACT

When a party to a contract fails to perform a contractual duty and has no legal excuse for that failure, a breach of contract has occurred. In most cases, it is impossible for the courts to require specific performance of the contract as it was written or agreed upon. Consequently, an attempt is usually made to assess the damages and award monetary compensation to the party who suffered a loss because of the breach.

DAMAGES

Whenever a breach of contract has been proved, the nonbreaching party is entitled to a verdict for at least some damages. It is easy for a jury to say, "Yes, there was a broken promise, a breach of contract, an injustice, but we cannot see where any significant damage was incurred because of that." It is because of situations like this

that attorneys are often forced to inform clients that the legal costs incurred to pursue a case probably will be greater than the damages likely to be awarded. Unless the legal principle is extremely important, what is otherwise a legitimate case will not be worth pursuing. If the court decides a breach occurred but damages were minimal, an award of *nominal damages* is made. A sum of $1 is common for cases awarding nominal damages.

Compensatory damages are awarded when the plaintiff is found to have sustained considerable financial detriment. This can be one of the most serious and difficult elements of a legal action to prove.

When considering compensatory damages, courts have many possible approaches for arriving at an amount. The following situations are but a few examples of the many approaches:

- Where there is a failure to perform labor or services required under a contract, as in building or construction cases, plaintiffs may recover the reasonable costs for locating a replacement contractor and completing the contract. When applied to veterinary employment contracts, damages for employers could potentially include the added costs of hiring more expensive relief veterinarians to fill shifts left uncovered by the premature departure of associates. It could also include costs to advertise, interview, select, and train replacement veterinarians as well as lost profits associated with understaffing. With respect to losses incurred by employees from terminations that are held to be breaches of contract, they could potentially recover lost wages; lost earnings resulting from the loss of experience, as in an internship; and costs incurred searching for and locating a replacement job.

- Where a defendant's performance under the contract is completed but defective, the measure of damages is the reasonable cost of repairing the defect. The most likely application of this measure of damages would occur in equine reproduction and food animal herd health or production medicine services where veterinarians failed to provide all services for which they had contracted.

- When it is too impracticable to repair or remedy the defect, the measure of damages is the difference between the value of the work as completed and the value it would have had if the contract had been properly fulfilled.

- Where specific damages for a failure to fully perform under the contact have been established in advance and stated in the contract, those damages are called *liquidated damages*. The purpose for this type of damage determination is to compensate and not to punish. If a breach occurs and the amount of damage is reasonable in light of the anticipated or actual loss incurred, the measure of damages allowed will be the preset amount established by the contract.

There are many other methods to determine the value or extent of damages or to fit the injustices created by various types of contract breaches. Only competent legal counsel can evaluate and advise practitioners or staff members who need additional help in such matters.

SPECIFIC PERFORMANCE

The emphasis of law generally is not to compel people to perform precisely what was promised in a valid contract. Instead, courts try to establish a monetary value for the damages incurred. This is because it is virtually impossible to force people to get along or perform an agreement that will meet the exact expectations and requirements of each party.

There are, however, some circumstances wherein damages are simply inadequate to compensate the nonbreaching party. It is in these situations where the remedy entitled *specific performance* can be utilized.

When the court elects to grant a request for specific performance, the breaching party is ordered to comply with the precise terms of the contract. This remedy is granted most frequently in breaches of contract involving real estate sales. The rationale is that real estate is unique, and money alone cannot adequately compensate the plaintiff. Furthermore, after the sale goes through, sellers and buyers no longer have to work together as they would in employment contracts.

Specific performance is never allowed with breaches of employment contracts because of the impossibility of forcing people to work together without discord. With contracts pertaining to personal property, specific performance can be invoked by the court if it can be shown that the property is unique or of limited supply. Heirlooms are a common example, but champion or unique animals also can be the subject of a plea for specific performance. For example, if someone purchases a champion ram at the National Columbia Show and Sale and the seller refuses to transfer title to that ram to the buyer, offering a substitute animal of equal or higher quality instead, a plea for specific performance may be the most equitable solution. It is well known that national champions are unique and that they provide owners with special breeding and marketing capabilities. It is likely that in such a case, a court would order the breaching seller to transfer title of this specific champion rather than try to arrive at monetary damages.

RESTITUTION

Restitution is a contract remedy that can be requested as an alternative to monetary damages or specific performance. Restitution is appropriate if the breaching party has been unfairly enriched by the acts of the nonbreaching party. The purpose of this remedy is to require breaching parties to give up their unfair gains. Damages in these cases are measured by valuing the defendant's unfair gains—not simply by compensating plaintiffs for their provable losses.[24] This remedy is similar to the unjust enrichment doctrine (discussed later in this chapter).

An example wherein restitution could be employed as a remedy follows:

Dr. Able agrees with the seller of some real estate to buy one acre of land upon which a veterinary hospital will be built. The seller assures Dr. Able that the city will allow the construction of a veterinary facility at that location. Relying upon this assurance, Dr. Able accepts the seller's offer and leaves a $10,000 deposit with the seller, who agrees to hold that amount in an interest-bearing escrow account until the sale is completed.

After six months of research and haggling with city planners, Dr. Able is informed that obtaining a use permit for a full-service veterinary hospital is virtually impossible. Dr. Able contacts the seller, informs him of the situation, and demands that the $10,000 be returned along with six month's worth of interest and $1,000 for time and expenses. The seller informs Dr. Able that he cannot do this because he used the money to buy stock in a bioengineering company about to start an FDA phase II clinical trial with genetically engineered stem cells that are expected to repair nerve damage. Unfortunately, the seller's stock carries with it a two-year restriction on its transfer or sale.

Dr. Able sues for breach of contract, and the suit drags on for a year and a half. At the time of trial, Dr. Able lists his damages as (1) the $10,000 down payment, (2) $1,000 for his time and effort, and (3) $2,200 for 2 year's interest on the $10,000 at 10%. Meanwhile, the bioengineering company has hit the jackpot with an FDA approval, and the stock is now worth $40,000.

Dr. Able has a cause of action for damages for breach of contract that amounts to $13,200 (the sum of the above figures). Dr. Able also has an alternative claim in restitution for $40,000 (the current value of the down payment that the seller invested in the stock). Under the restitutionary remedy for determining damages from this breach of contract, Dr. Able most likely can recover the full value of the investment made by the seller with the $10,000, because he breached the contract and misused Dr. Able's money.

An entire body of law exists on the subject of restitution as a means of measuring damages. Veterinarians should be aware of this alternative type of remedy for breaches of contracts that focus on the defendant's gains and not the plaintiff's losses.

THE DUTY TO MITIGATE DAMAGES

When a contract is breached, severe hardship can be created if a nonbreaching party relies only on lawsuits to recoup damages and does nothing to limit the damages caused by the breach. To prevent injustices, courts have established requirements that parties suffering breaches must attempt to mitigate or minimize any damages incurred.[25]

The earlier illustration in the section on promissory estoppel wherein the new graduate acted in reliance on the contract offer from the veterinarian 400 miles away is a good example where the duty to mitigate damages might come into play. (For the purposes of this example, it is assumed that the court would find in favor of the existence of a contract in that case.)

To mitigate damages, the new graduate could try to find another job in the area where she had made arrangements to live (if, for example, she signed a lease for a one-year term), so as not to incur damages for breaking that lease. Alternatively, she could break the lease, taking the loss, and attempt to find a job elsewhere so that she did not lose the $3,500-per-month salary for an indefinite period of time. She would not have to take the first job that came along but could hold out for a reasonable time to find a job similar to the one offered by the veterinarian who breached the agreement. Costs of job searching might also be recoverable if she could show that those expenses were incurred in a diligent attempt to mitigate the damages. Whatever the case, she may not, however, sit back and just let damages cumulate without risking a court's denial of her claim for failing to attempt to mitigate damages.

THE LAW OF AGENCY

An area of the law to which veterinarians and their staff repeatedly are subjected is the law of agency. This involves situations wherein owners have given other people the authority to act on their behalf in the request for and purchase of veterinary goods and services. In some cases, the principal:agent relationship will have been created via formal written contract, as with some equine stabling and training agreements. In other cases, it could be via settlements of pet custody battles in divorce cases or through coownership agreements for breeding animals. All too often, however, there is no clear, written principal:agent contract and, instead, veterinarians are forced to rely merely on statements of clients presenting animals for treatment rather than formal documents. In these cases, an agency relationship must be implied by the information provided by or actions of the parties.

AGENCY AND CONSENTS FOR ROUTINE CARE

The key point involving agency relationships is that when they exist, the agents have the power to consent to treatment and bind the principals (the owners) to payment for services rendered even when the ani-

mals' owners did not know of the request for treatment or costs incurred.

Obviously, the best way to verify the existence of an agency relationship between clients requesting treatments for animals and the owners who are expected to pay for their care is to ask for and see a copy of the contract establishing it. This is rarely possible because such contracts often are not stored near the site where the animals are housed, nor are they brought with clients to a hospital setting. The result, then, typically is that

- agents simply claim they have the power to request veterinary services,

- practitioners assume such statements are true and provide the care requested,

- practices send bills for services to the parties identified by the agents, and

- owners of the animals in question pay the bills, verifying and ratifying the existence of the agency relationship.

Despite efforts to avoid these predicaments, unpaid bills can be a consequence of agents who have made false claims or practitioners who make erroneous assumptions about agency relationships. Thus, when clinicians or office managers are skeptical of requests for veterinary services by people unwilling to claim ownership of patients or financial responsibility for the services they request, and no agency-verifying documents are available, it is best to call and talk with the purported owners prior to the provision of care. Such calls serve three purposes. First, they provide owners with tentative diagnoses, recommended courses of treatment, likely prognoses, follow-up care anticipated, and estimated costs. Second, they help verify that the clients requesting services are entitled to serve as the owners' agents. And third, it allows staff members to make arrangements for payment of current and future services requested by the agents.

Because of the ambulatory nature of their practices and work patterns of their clients, large animal practitioners and house call small animal clinicians frequently face requests for care by agents. Not to be left out, small animal practitioners whose clients are leaving on vacations, business trips or medical leaves of absence often wish to preauthorize needed medical care or named agents who could make decisions for them in their absence, too. For small animal practitioners who like to plan ahead, hand written notes can be drafted into medical records identifying agents and owners can initial such entries. For small and large ambulatory clinicians who do not have their patient's medical records in the vehicle with them, consent forms like that in Figure 2.1 work well and can be presented at the time new clients are acquired or sent out with their billing statements.

AGENCY AND EMERGENCY CARE

When patients require emergency care, it is always best to provide stabilizing care first and call for verification of the agency relationship immediately thereafter. As explained in the next section covering the law of unjust enrichment, in case owners deny the existence of agency relationships, records of treatment and efforts to contact owners should be documented carefully. To avoid problems with authenticity and documentation of agency relationships in emer-

gency care situations, practices are advised to use forms like the that in Figure 2.2 or draft notes into patients' medical records authorizing such agency relationships with specified parties.

Many of the same problems with medical decisions and fee authorizations by agents arise when ambulatory clinicians arrive on the scene of an emergency and are faced with medical crises that would benefit by or require referrals to specialists. Once again, these practitioners face the dilemma, "Just what would Mr. or Mrs Jones want me to do under these circumstances?" Since referrals to specialists often entail expenses far greater than that to which clients are accustomed, it is important to know what clients would desire under these circumstances. The best way for handling this is to use a consent form like that in Figure 2.3:

AGENCY AND CONSENTS FOR EUTHANASIA

Major crises related to the law of agency occur most often regarding decisions involving euthanasia. In general, the person in whose name an animal is registered on the patient's medical record is considered the owner. Thus arises a quandary when Mr. Ferrell delivers what admittedly is his wife's cat to your veterinary practice and during

---

Ambulatory Practice Consents For Routine Veterinary Care

I, the owner of the following animals (horse, cow, flock of sheep, dogs, cats, etc.), or any other animals I may own in the future, hereby consent to the provision of **routine** veterinary services by (practice name) when such services are needed for my animal(s). In the event I am unavailable, I hereby authorize (name of relative, friend, neighbor, or trainer/manager) to act as my **agent(s)**, and request care as needed in his or her judgment. I agree to pay the reasonable fees for these veterinary services within 30 days after receiving a billing statement.

_____

Signature of Owner or Agent   Date

Figure 2.1. An ambulatory practice consent form for routine veterinary care

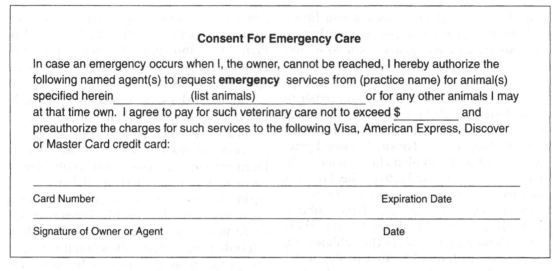

Figure 2.2. A consent form for emergency care

the next three days, you consult on the phone about "Blackie's" medical care only with Mrs. Ferrell. Suddenly, near the end of the third day, as Blackie is failing, Mr. Ferrell calls and indicates that he and Mrs. Ferrell have decided it is time to put Blackie to sleep.

What are you and your staff to do? If you heed his request without talking to his wife, you have no assurance that this is a communal decision. If you call Mrs. Ferrell, she may object to this request and you are placed in the middle of a conflict. The need for forced communications between parties with equal authority who are providing conflicting requests is enhanced in this hypothetical situation because of the finality of the request for euthanasia. It is one thing not to be paid for one's services because of conflicts involving the law of agency. However, a much larger problem looms when the requested treatment is euthanasia.

Although there is a presumption that the party who registered the animal at the time of the first visit and signed the initial treatment consent form is the owner and ultimate decision maker, this presumption can be overcome via oral or written comments from other family members alleging to be the responsible owner. Thus, practitioners and staff are advised to proceed

slowly with requests for euthanasia until all ambiguities regarding ownership and agency have been addressed.

When situations like this arise, it is advisable to have the ultimate decision maker come to the practice in person and sign the euthanasia consent form. This helps substantiate the practice's effort to prevent disputes. It also diminishes the validity of any claims for professional liability caused by a staff person's alleged substandard judgment regarding a life and death decision.

THE LAW OF UNJUST ENRICHMENT

The law of unjust enrichment is a valuable doctrine of contract law with which practitioners should be familiar. Its use comes into play most frequently when emergency care for animals is required but none of the previously discussed agency relationships exist. It is a portion of the law of restitution created to fill a void between contract law and tort law (the law of negligence). Under this legal theory, defendants are required to repay money or restore property because it would be wrong and against

---

Consent To Refer Case To Specialist

If an illness or injury suffered by one or several of the previously named animals, or any other animals I may own in the future, is so serious that it requires referral to a specialist, I authorize the attending veterinarian to refer such animal(s) for such specialty care to one of the following (indicate your choice by filling in or circling one of the following):

a.) the_____ (practice name) referral hospital,

b.) the referral hospital of Dr._____'s choice.

c.) the referral hospital selected by one of my above-named agents,

d.) under no circumstances will I approve of a referral seeking specialty care.

I hereby impose a $_____limit on such specialty care before I or my agent must be contacted to proceed with further veterinary care.

Signature of Owner or Agent   Date

Figure 2.3. A consent form to refer cases to specialists

public policy for them to retain any benefit or value.

During their practice of veterinary medicine, practitioners are called upon repeatedly to render veterinary services without the authorization or consent of an animal's owner. The petition for care can come in an emergency or nonemergency situation and often occurs without any assurance of payment for services. The request might be made by a friend, relative, or neighbor caring for someone's horse, dog, cat, or livestock; by a boarding kennel or stable acting as a bailee; or by a helpful person who picks up an injured animal for someone who does not have a regular veterinarian. Although the law imposes no legal duty to be a good Samaritan, there is a logical expectation that doctors and nurses will assist injured people and veterinarians will assist injured animals, and the law does not discourage that expectation. The law of unjust enrichment further recognizes that average people seek to have such care administered if they are around to request it, and that veterinarians

and other health professionals are in the business of providing medical services for pay, but not gratuitously.[24]

The law of unjust enrichment was established by the courts to deal with situations in which any of the above situations occur. The basic philosophy is that the law should not allow one person to be unjustly enriched at the expense of another.

So that justice is exercised only in those cases where it legitimately applies, there are certain limitations placed on this doctrine. The following critical factors are considered by the legal system before it applies the law of unjust enrichment or quasi contract.

- **Value:** The more valuable the animal is, either from its visual appearance or from statements made about the animal by a minor, a friend, a neighbor, an office coworker, the manager of a boarding facility, or anyone else who knows about the animal, the better is the chance that a court will allow a recovery. Value need not be based entirely on economic value. It also can be based on emotional value to the owners through the apparent depth of the human-animal bond. With respect to companion animals, this can be shown by rabies, licensing, or pet health insurance tags; collars; tatoos; microchip identification; or just good grooming and the appearance of good behavior.

- **Severity of the Emergency:** The more emergent the animal's needs are, the more leeway exists to provide the required emergency medical care. In such cases radiographs showing major skeletal or chest injuries, blood and/or urine values, detailed medical records, photographs, the presence of witnesses, and anything else that helps document the life-threatening situation becomes important. Most owners do not balk at minor fees for services rendered without their knowledge; however, convincing evidence that the patient's life was in danger must be presented in order to justify major expenditures for emergency care.

- **Attempts to Reach the Owner:** The veterinarian's attempt to reach the owner prior to rendering medical care is evaluated. Documentation of efforts made to reach an accountable person must be shown and must be believable. Notations on medical records as to who attempted to call the owner, what number(s) were called, what time of day it was, and how many attempts were made to reach the owner are all important facts to list.

Because practices rendering emergency services often are asked to provide care for stray animals brought in by good Samaritans, it is advisable to have poster board, magic markers, and nails or carpet tacks available at all times. This allows staff members to create signs describing the appearance of lost pets and announcing phone numbers and locations where the animals are being kept. Then the parties who transported the injured strays can be asked to place the posters at sites near locations where the animals were found. This helps return pets to their owners and increases the chances that the veterinary practice will recover fees for the emergency care rendered.

- **Stabilizing Care:** Lastly, the extent of emergency care required to stabilize the patient is considered. If at all possible, once patients are stable, it is best not to proceed with extensive care until owners have been contacted. For example, if a dog had a fractured tibia and fibula that was serious but not comminuted, the court might well allow recovery for the costs incurred applying a Robert Jones bandage and treating the concomitant shock. The court most likely would balk, however, at a claim for reimbursement for emergency compression plating or pinning unless extenuating circumstances were present. A caveat here is that the more identification a pet has, such as a collar, rabies or license tag, tatoo or computer chip, and the better it appears to be cared for, the more leeway practices have in providing advanced, rather than merely stabilizing, emergency care, and recovering for such efforts.

In short, the legal system encourages good Samaritans to render life-saving medical care without authorization from the owner when certain circumstances exist. The law frowns on the unjust enrichment of one party at the expense of another person who has shown that he or she is reasonable, practical, and well meaning.

PERSONAL SERVICE CONTRACTS

Contracts to purchase veterinary supplies from vendors and provide veterinary services to clients are the contracts most frequently encountered by practitioners. The next most common group is contracts with employees. Disputes over the terms of employment agreements are not uncommon and frequently require considerable management time to reconcile. The disagreements may be merely disagreements without animosity; they may result in major misunderstandings, bitterness, and hard feelings; or they may develop into lawsuits.

REASONS WHY PRACTITIONERS AVOID EMPLOYMENT CONTRACTS

Unfortunately, many practices do not utilize employment contracts. The most frequent reasons that practitioners cite for having no contracts are that

- they believe that such business formalities are time consuming, and they simply do not want to afford the time.

- they do not wish to spend money hiring attorneys to draft contracts.

- they have never delineated the terms they want included in their employment contracts. They prefer, instead, to have the flexibility to decide employment issues as the need arises.

- they have functioned effectively for years without them and don't feel they need them for the future.

- they feel that an atmosphere of distrust is generated when they suggest the need for a formal written agreement, especially for employees who have been with the practice for several years.

PROBLEMS WITH RECOLLECTION

Most new employees come from a pool of applicants. Thus, employers often have discussions regarding salary and benefits with many different people before one is ultimately hired. Practitioners should be concerned about the information provided during the employee-selection process, because things said initially can be inter-preted and remembered quite differently by the prospective employee than they are by the employer.

Once new employees are working and have been paid for their services, it is apparent that some type of contract has been formed. This is so even if the terms of an oral agreement are unclear. If the agreement exceeds one year in length, it is unenforceable under the statute of frauds unless a written memorandum exists. Since most employment contracts are for less than one year, the oral agreements are perfectly valid. Unless some written agreement exists, though, the terms of the contract are still open for interpretation.

EMPLOYMENT CONTRACT TERMS

Employment contracts can be oral or written, lengthy or short. Determining which components are the most critical is futile, because different people will find different elements more important. The major ingredients to include in a written contract or that should at least be discussed in an oral agreement as well as clauses to explain each of these items are found in subsequent chapters.

EMPLOYMENT CONTRACTS AND COVENANTS NOT TO COMPETE

Each year many veterinarians seek employment with established practices. It is not uncommon for these professionals to encounter clauses in agreements presented for them to sign containing promises not to compete with their employers after they leave the practice. These contract clauses go by several interchangeable titles, including *covenants not to compete*, *restrictive covenants*, and *noncompetition clauses*.

Professionals have entered into agreements containing restrictive covenants for many years. Because of the increase in competition between practices during the past 20 years, it cannot be assumed that all existing practices will continue to grow and prosper even when former employed veterinarians open practices nearby. For this reason, practice owners are more likely to insist on noncompetition, nonsolicitation, and confidential information clauses in employment contracts in the future than they were in the past. These contract clauses are enforceable in most states and are discussed in depth in Chapter 9.

Summary

Contract law is a vital part of the veterinarian's daily business existence. Thus, the more practitioners know about contracts, the less likely it is that they will be subject to time-consuming controversies which detract from their primary professional goal—the delivery of veterinary services.

References

1. *Restatement, Second, Contracts* § 1; p 1.
2. *Black's Law Dictionary*, ed 5. St. Paul, West Publishing Co, 1979, pp 291-292.
3. UCC § 2-105(1).
4. Schaber, Rohwer:*Contracts in a Nutshell*, ed 2. St. Paul, West Publishing Co, 1984, § 7; § 131, p 232; § 48, 49.
5. Alperin HJ, Chase RF: *Consumer Law*. St. Paul, West Publishing Co, 1986, § 3, pp 4-5.
6. *Restatement, Second, Contracts*, § 50(1).
7. *Restatement, Second, Contracts*, § 58.
8. *Restatement, Second, Contracts*, § 59.
9. UCC § 1-205(1),(2) and 1-201(3).
10. Alperin HJ, Chase RF: *Consumer Law*, St. Paul, West Publishing Co, 1986, § 4, p 7.
11. *Restatement, Second, Contracts*, § 79.
12. UCC § 2-302(1).
13. *Voight & McMakin Air Conditioning, Inc* v *Property Redevelopment Corp*, 276A.2d 239 (D.C.App 1971).
14. *Restatement, Second Contracts*, § 90(1).
15. *Paterson v Reeves*, 304 F.2d 950, 951 (D.C.Cir.1962).
16. 32 N.J. 358, 161 A. 2d 69 (1960).
17. Alperin HJ, Chase RF: *Consumer Law*. St. Paul, West Publishing Co, 1986, pp 10-11.
18. Alperin HJ, Chase RF: *Consumer Law*. St. Paul, West Publishing Co, 1986, § 23, p 40; § 26, p 43.
19. UCC § 2-201.
20. UCC § 8-319.
21. UCC § 9-203.
22. UCC § 2-201 [1].
23. Alperin HJ, Chase RF: *Consumer Law*. St. Paul, West Publishing Co, 1986, § 12, p 25.
24. Hunter HO: *Modern Law of Contracts, Breaches and Remedies*. Boston, Warren, Gorham, and Lamont; § 7.02 (4), pp 7-8; § 9.01(4) p 9-6.
25. *Restatement, Second, Contracts*, § 347, 350.

Chapter 3

COMPENSATION

By James F. Wilson, DVM, JD

It is important to recognize from the out-set that this chapter and many of the others in this book are geared to issues and ideas encountered in private practice rather than in public and corporate forms of veterinary employment. The reasons for this are that (1) there tends to be remarkably more diversity and negotiation with respect to compensation and fringe benefits in private practice than in public and corporate employment; (2) approximately 75% of the jobs for new graduates are in private practice; and (3) most veterinarians who accept employment opportunities in public or corporate practice, such as in universities, government, the military, or industry, find themselves in preestablished, tiered salary and benefit programs with less opportunity for negotiation than in private practice. The types of private practices where these issues surface include small, large, equine, ambulatory, and exotic animal practices; emergency clinics and critical care centers; specialty practices; and situations where veterinarians serve as relief doctors.

Although fringe benefits, work schedules, and restrictive covenants are essential bargaining points in employment contracts, and are often more important than money, most offers and negotiations start with discussions about salary. Thus, compensation is addressed first in this book, followed by a host of other benefits and supplementary issues in subsequent chapters.

Experience has shown that because the veterinary profession is such a fragmented, one to four doctor-sized business environment, practice owners often lack information about industry standards for salaries paid to veterinary associates, board-eligible and board-certified specialists, practice managers, part-time doctors, and relief veterinarians. This chapter provides information based on consultations with over 600 veterinary employees and employers and cites references that practice owners and managers can use to locate additional information. Traditions and trends affecting the veterinary profession also are discussed.

TRADITIONS AND TRENDS

Unlike much of the American work force that is paid on an hourly basis, veterinarians traditionally have been paid salaries based on yearly, monthly, or daily calculations. This custom has, in part, been forced on the profession because of the difficulties encountered in trying to schedule the delivery of veterinary services into the standard 8:00 a.m. to 12:00 noon and 1:00 p.m. to 6:00 p.m. time blocks.

Animals become ill during all hours of the day and night, and worried or harried owners seek veterinary services when they perceive medical problems exist or when their personal schedules permit. This imprecise demand for services is exacerbated by the fact that animals cannot talk and, thus, cannot tell their owners where their injuries or discomforts are located or how serious those ailments are. Additionally, since veterinarians are licensed professionals and since most practice managers have jobs that meet the executive or administrative tests established by the Fair Labor Standards Act, neither of these groups is eligible for overtime, unless it is a condition of their contract. All of these factors have driven the profession toward salaried rather than hourly compensation for veterinary associates and practice managers.

The problem with the salaried method of compensation is that it tends to attract workers with a "warm body" mentality, i.e., those who want the security of finite working hours and a steady stream of income, irrespective of the professional or financial success of their employers. Such compensation systems have customarily rewarded employees based on seniority rather than productivity. Although this seems acceptable to employed professionals, it is unacceptable and has become financially unrealistic for many employers. Hence, the major trend in compensation today is toward base salaries, or salaries based on percentages of income production, whichever is higher. The subject of percentage-based compensation will be discussed in great detail later in this chapter.

Two 1995 *Philadelphia Inquirer* articles addressed the strong trend in the American work force away from "warm body" compensation.[1,2] The first article stated that the average American employer's habit of paying workers a little more each year is fading and being replaced by one-time bonuses and project incentives. A survey of nearly 1,400 companies in 1995 revealed that 41% of them offered some form of variable pay to nonexecutive employees, up from 35% in 1994. The article went on to say that, although bonuses and one-time incentive payments may give employees more money than they earned the previous year, such

plans leave base pay at the same level. This keeps the employer's payroll obligations consistent but makes it difficult for employees to plan ahead financially.

The second article reported that from 1981 through 1989, 52% of personal income gains were paid in the form of salaries or wages. By 1993, though, only 38% of such gains came in the form of salaries or wages. The rest of the gains were paid as incentives and bonuses. The good news in all of this was that companies were beginning to offer the opportunities for employees to share in their company's success along with the shareholders and top executives. Of course, if these companies did not experience the financial success they had hoped to see, the risk of no gain also was being shared with the employees.

The end result of this shift in compensation format is that workers who receive some of their compensation in the form of productivity incentives are now being forced to think like business owners rather than employees. This has been good for the economy, business managers, employees, and company partners or shareholders. The trend toward incentive-based compensation reported in these articles also has been occurring in the veterinary profession.

BASE SALARIES FOR VETERINARIANS

The most complete data on veterinary compensation traditionally has been published by the AVMA's Center for Information Management. The basic new graduate information on this subject usually can be found in one of the December or January issues of the *Journal of the AVMA*. These annual reports cite starting salaries and educational indebtedness for new graduates.[3] Information about salaries for private practitioners generally is published in *JAVMA* every two years.[4] More detailed data are available in the excellent AVMA book published every two years entitled *Report on Veterinary*

Compensation[5] and the American Animal Hospital Association's *Compensation and Benefits—An In-Depth Look.*[6] Practice managers would be wise to regularly purchase these references. Additional data are published intermittently by the Veterinary Hospital Management Association in its *Compensation and Benefits Survey,*[7] by Tom Lynch, M.A.,[8] and by *Veterinary Economics.*[9]

EDUCATIONAL DEBT

A growing concern has been the rapid increase in educational debts for new graduates relative to starting salaries. Between 1983 and 2008, starting salaries for all new United States graduates increased 310%, from $19,872 to $61,518. During the same time period, mean educational debt for those who had debt increased from $18,897 to $119,803, a whopping 634%.[13] A closer analysis of this trend shows that debts from 1984 to 1990 climbed from approximately $20,000 to $30,000, followed by an additional $10,000 increase from 1990 to 1994, and a third $10,000 increase to nearly $50,000 between 1994 and 1996.[3,10] Since debt increased for 1998 graduates at nearly the same pace as it did for '97 graduates, another $10,000 was added to this total in the years 1997 and 1998.[11] That has been followed by the addition of another $60,000 between 1998 and 2008[13] Needless to say this is a frightening scenario, especially since debt has been exceeding increases in starting salaries by more than a 2:1 ratio for over a decade.

So why has this debt skyrocketed? Student loan volume exploded after 1992 when Congress tried to take some of the sting out of college tuition inflation by opening up federal loan programs to more middle-class families.[12] Between 1992 and 1994, borrowing under federal student loan programs rose 57%. Of the $183 billion lent between 1966 and 1994, 22% was in the last two of those years.[12]

The volume of federal funding for student loans has continued at this brisk pace since 1994 with a resultant rapid rise in the cost of an education. As one author puts it, there has been a fundamental shift in the way higher education is financed in this country. [12] "In the past," said Patrick Callan, executive director of the California Higher Education Policy Center in San Jose, "every generation took on most of the responsibility for educating the next. Now the young are paying for it themselves, out of future earnings. Besides, the days when students could cover tuition with summer jobs are over."[12]

Other causes of student debt include:

- Costs for a college education are rising twice as fast as the Consumer Price Index. State and federal governments are allocating more money for healthcare for an aging population than to educate the next generation. Colleges also complain that compliance with government regulations is costly, eating up more than $0.12 of every tuition dollar at private universities.[14]

- Because of the expanded curricular demands, students appear to have less time to work while in veterinary school today than in the past.

- The affluence of today's parents has spoiled students. Many do not want to give up the good life they have had growing up. Some borrow to support this lifestyle rather than survive on a shoestring. However, as the recession of 2008-10 closes in, most are living an austere existence, fearful of the inordinate debt they are cumulating.

- There are very few, if any, G-I Bill students with military experience and governmental subsidies for education among today's veterinary classes. This is a significant change from the 1950s, 60s, and 70s when many draftees pursued college and graduate educations with federal assistance.

- There are more financial aid programs available today than there were 15 to 25 years ago, and those in existence have much higher borrowing limitations. Financial aid increased to $143 billion in the 2008-09 school year, nearly double that of a decade ago.[15] Additionally, the financial aid system seems to discourage saving and encourage borrowing, with the effect that "students are mortgaging themselves for a future they may not be able to afford."[15]

- On-campus transportation and security costs as well as demands by students and their parents for healthcare services, writing and tutorial centers, computer labs, restaurant-quality food, and quality recreational areas also contribute to the rising costs of tuition.

An important feature of the United States veterinary graduate educational debt dilemma is that debt loads are remarkably uneven, depending heavily upon the school from which a person graduated. Veterinary graduates paying the lowest tuition in 2008-09, $9,212 per year at North Carolina State can leave school with as little as $78,000 average debt. Others graduating from private schools or state schools, paying non-resident tuitions of over $35,000 (and total yearly costs of as much as $62,000), have educational debts of $250,000 and more.

Interestingly, as reported at the Elephant in the Room Symposium at NAVC in 2008, American Association of Veterinary Medical Colleges data shows that between 2004 and 2008, the cost of tuition, fees and expenses for a veterinary education rose at an annual rate of 12.75% for residents and 10.66% for nonresidents. Additionally, during this time, interest rates for graduate student loans rose from less than 2.5% in 2004 to 6.8% for students entering school after July 1, 2006. Whereas the average veterinary graduate's debt in 1983 was $18,897 and 95.1% of starting salary, by 2008, that debt number has risen to $119,803 or 194.5% of starting salary.

A synopsis of tuitions and annual total costs of education by veterinary school for the entering class of 2012 is presented in Table 3.1.[16]

An analysis of Table 3.1 shows that tuitions for resident students in the Canadian veterinary schools are remarkably lower than those of United States' schools. Because of this situation, educational debt loads have not been nearly the problem for Canadian graduates as they have for United States grads.

1997 Tax Relief Act and Beyond

Because of the budget deficits of the 1980s, Congress passed the Tax Reform Act of 1986, eliminating the interest deduction on educational debts. As the federal budget deficit soared during the 1989 to 1992 recession, Congress had no opportunity to restore educational debt as a tax-deductible expense. Finally, after several years of strong national economic growth and concomitant reduced federal budget deficits, the Tax Reform Act of 1997 provided some tax relief for those with educational debts.

Since 1998, the good news was that graduates who were not claimed as dependents on someone else's tax return were able to deduct student-loan interest for qualified higher education expenses after they graduated. Loans for tuition, fees, room and board, books, and supplies constitute qualified expenses. As much as $2,500 of interest can be deducted in 2008. Additionally, indebted graduates need not itemize deductions to claim this tax break. The bad news, however, is that this deduction starts phasing out for single people with adjusted gross incomes (AGI) above $55,000 and joint filers reporting AGIs of more than $110,000. The deduction disappears completely for single people with AGIs of $70,000 and married couples with $130,000,[17] meaning that single veterinarians with AGIs of

Table 3.1. First-Year DVM Student Expenses
Resident and Nonresident Students (Class of 2012)

Schools	Tuition and Fees		Other Expenses*		TOTAL COSTS	
	R	NR	R	NR	R	NR
Auburn University	$12,250	$36,890	$16,095	$16,095	$28,345	$52,985
University of California-Davis	22,409	34,654	23,530	23,530	45,939	58,184
Colorado State University	16,546	43,748	13,706	13,706	30,254	58,154
Cornell University	25,100	37,100	16,500	16,500	41,600	53,600
University of Florida	21,041	42,066	13,228	13,228	34,269	55,244
University of Georgia**	13,222	35,622	11,028	11,028	24,250	46,650
University of Illinois-Urbana	21,392	39,856	15,474	15,474	36,866	55,330
Iowa State University	15,886	37,082	17,364	17,364	33,250	54,446
Kansas State University	17,773	39,973	16,035	16,035	33,808	56,008
Louisiana State University	12,669	35,069	23,992	23,992	36,661	59,061
Michigan State University	20,510	42,578	16,460	16,460	36,970	59,038
University of Minnesota	23,041	41,700	16,890	16,890	39,931	58,590
Mississippi State University	13,156	31,898	21,454	21,454	34,610	53,352
University of Missouri	17,320	33,035	17,240	17,240	34,560	50,275
North Carolina State University	10,637	33,400	17,718	17,718	28,355	51,118
The Ohio State University	23,598	55,440	17,336	17,336	40,934	72,776
Oklahoma State University	14,490	31,770	13,000	13,000	27,490	44,770
Oregon State University***	17,605	33,952	N/A	N/A	17,605	33,952
University of Pennsylvania	33,712	40,868	22,125	22,125	55,837	62,993
Purdue University	15,546	37,260	13,080	13,420	28,626	50,500
University of Tennessee	15,348	40,724	18,884	18,884	34,232	59,608
Texas A&M University	13,742	24,542	14,910	15,146	28,652	39,688
Tufts University	32,620	38,306	18,601	18,601	51,221	56,907
Tuskegee University	18,080	22,380	27,647	27,647	45,727	50,027
VA-MD Regional VMC	17,336	38,270	16,430	16,430	33,766	54,700
Washington State University	17,951	43,195	16,257	16,257	34,208	59,452
Western University	36,310	36,310	24,324	24,324	60,634	60,634
University of WI-Madison	17,220	25,292	14,220	14,220	31,440	39,512
Average U.S. Schools	**$19,161**	**$36,892**	**$16,911**	**$16,926**	**$36,073**	**$53,841**
University of Calgary	7,419	N/A	11,130	N/A	18,549	N/A
Universite de Montreal-Quebec	6,528	52,000	122	878	6,650	52,878
University of Ontario	6,851	52,879	1,639	N/A	8,490	52,879
University of PEI	3,200	N/A	1,100	N/A	4,300	N/A
University of Saskatchewan	9,614	49,006	15,321	16,728	24,935	65,734

R = Resident, NR = Nonresident

Note: Information in this table appears courtesy of the Association of American Veterinary Medical Colleges.

*Other expenses include room & board, books & equipment, personal, transportation, health, and other expenses.

**The University of Georgia lists tuition and fee for both residents and non-residents at $13,222 but then lists other fees for non-residents at $22,500. We have added this to the $13,222 for non residents to more accurately reflect the cost of their tuition and fees.

***Oregon State University did not report numbers for anything included in "Other Expenses", which resulted in this being marked "Not Available". This gives the appearance that it is markedly less expensive to attend school here, which may not be the case. Not available has also been marked for the Canadian schools that did not report any numbers in certain categories.

$65,000 lose two-thirds of this deduction and those with greater than $70,000 lose it entirely.

Therefore, even though this "tax relief" provides some assistance for today's debt-laden veterinary graduates during their first few years after graduation, before their adjusted gross incomes exceed $70,000, it is little more than a Band-Aid for most young veterinarians, whose annual interest payments normally will exceed $7,500 on their national average $119,803 loans.

An additional tax benefit came into existence in 2002. As of 2009, up to $2,000 of tax relief is available through the Lifetime Learning Tax Credit. This allows a dollar for dollar tax credit for qualified tuition and fees paid in a given tax year to be credited against other federal income taxes. To qualify for this credit, taxpayers must have an AGI below $48,000 for single filers and $96,000 for joint filers. Since new graduates only work half years after graduation, most qualify for this tax credit if they paid their tuition for the winter and spring terms after January 1.

The Impact of High Student Debt

Why is educational debt load important? Initially, it is because it impacts new graduates' ability to balance their budgets on a traditionally low associate veterinarian salary. Additionally, high debt discourages or makes it impossible for veterinarians to purchase practices within the first 5 to 15 years after graduation. For many young graduates, the responsibilities of supporting a family, paying off $80,000 to $250,000 of student loans, saving for retirement or a down payment on a home, and saving money to purchase a veterinary practice make it increasingly difficult for them to become practice owners.[18] Moreover, since many of today's students marry classmates, the debt load for them often is doubled.

Many of these students and couples have trouble paying their educational debt, and thus they do not qualify for loans enabling them to purchase homes or veterinary practices. Additionally, tough current federal government policies will not allow them to discharge these debts through bankrupty. On the other hand, the most entrepreneurially driven and best budgeters and savers will see that the only way they can repay their huge loans will be to buy practices and take control of their financial destinies. Whether large numbers of graduates of the early 2000s and beyond can do that, though, is yet to be determined.

Addressing the Debt Issue

The challenges of excess debt present an obstacle for the future of veterinary practice ownership which leaders of the profession must address. Among the options to reduce the risks of this debt are the following:

1. Veterinary schools should make applicants fully aware of the costs of a veterinary school education and the financial rewards and concomitant economic picture they can expect after graduation — before they sign their acceptances.

2. Students must learn, with a school's help, to manage their costs of living while in veterinary school and minimize their accumulation of debt.

3. Schools must provide curricular time and enthusiastic faculty to teach personal finance and business management so that graduates have a better understanding of the financial ramifications of membership in the veterinary profession.

4. Veterinary practices must raise fees sufficiently to allow them to pay salaries that are high enough that young doctors can pay off their heavy debt loads and have a life, or they will leave this profession en masse for greener financial pastures.

5. Practice owners must provide better training and mentoring of young associates so that they can become more financially successful veterinarians. They also must leverage staff and deliver services more expeditiously so as to compensate these young, highly indebted graduates in a manner that allows them to pay their debts and save for the future.

6. Veterinary school administrators and faculties must focus on ways of minimizing the high costs associated with today's traditional, antiquated, lecture-based delivery of veterinary education. Students, on the other hand, must develop study habits that allow them to learn materials independently, instead of via conventional spoon-feeding methods.

7. The profession must help promote a risk-sharing, third-party payment system of pet health insurance that will enable it to deliver veterinary care at fees that allow graduates and practice owners to charge more realistically for the knowledge, skill, and technology they possess.

THE COMPENSATION NEGOTIATION PROCESS

At some point during the interview process, one party or the other must initiate a discussion of compensation. Since nervous job applicants need to know how much money is being offered, but often are reluctant to ask, it is advisable for employers to broach the subject first. Even if employers do, though, applicants need to have planned their responses. For example, a practice owner might say,

"We probably ought to talk a bit about money at some point. Our plans have been to offer a new graduate like you the same salary we see as the average salary published in *JAVMA*. That means we're offering $70,000. How does that sound to you?"

Other veterinary employers who are less inclined to give away their hands might initiate salary discussions as follows:

"I'm sure you're wondering about salary. We're basing it on experience, personality, references, and other factors. I guess the most important thing, though, is determining what you're going to need. What's it going to take to bring you on board?"

Pow! There it is, applicants! Your future employers are hoping you will show your cards before they have to show theirs. What are you going to say? How much will you need to earn to make ends meet? What do you know about your own personal expenses? Unfortunately, no matter how much young associates want or need jobs, they often are unprepared to answer this question.

Because this scenario plays out so frequently, it behooves job applicants to spend some time determining how much money and benefits they need before they begin the job hunt and, most certainly, before they accept a job. That means establishing a personal financial budget, a topic discussed in considerable depth later in this chapter. The following sections focus on questions, other than those related to money, that employers and employees should be discussing prior to or during the interview and negotiation process.

QUESTIONS EMPLOYERS SHOULD BE ASKING

To select the person who is best fit for the job being offered, employers should ask themselves the following questions before they begin the search process:

1. Why am I (we) hiring a new person? Is it to have more time off or because the practice needs an infusion of new energy and ideas? Do we need another body to alleviate the stress of our emergency call schedule? Is a departing associate being replaced, or is another person being added because the practice has become so busy our clients are not receiving the quality of time and care they are demanding? Is it because of a need to find

someone willing to purchase all or part of the practice within a few years, thus providing me with an exit strategy?[19]

2. What volume of personal and professional development time am I (or other owners of our practice) willing to provide for our new hire? This question entails determining how much supervisory time and effort employers are willing to invest mentoring recent graduates. Because work experience in veterinary practices has not been a primary veterinary school admission criterion in recent years, and animal rights issues have decreased the numbers of animals available for teaching surgical skills, the bad news is that many of today's graduates have considerably less hands-on surgical and anesthetic experience than did graduates from the 70s and 80s. The result is that many of them also have less confidence than those earlier graduates and, thus, a greater need for mentorship and an intensive three-month initial training period. The good news, though, is that the diagnostic and medical skills of today's students tend to be excellent and, except for developing the time-management skills they will need to succeed in the private sector, they do quite well with clients.

3. By what date must we find someone? Is the practice willing to subsidize and train an associate through the slow months so we can have the extra help needed for the busy season? Unfortunately, many practitioners start looking for associates and veterinary technicians too late to make sound choices. The booming economy and shortage of veterinarians and technicians that has surfaced on both coasts of the United States in the late 1990s has exaggerated this problem.[20,21] Proper planning is the only way to prevent the burnout brought on by staff shortages and exacerbated by the inability of finding qualified people in a timely manner.

4. Who shall we hire? Will we accept a well-educated but inexperienced new graduate? Is the practice so busy we don't have time to train a new grad and must hire someone with experience? Do we need a woman, or a man, for better balance in the practice, providing options for gender-sensitive clients?

5. Where shall we look for the next associate? Is it better to hire someone who was trained at a different veterinary school than the current staff, knowing that that may provoke conflicts in diagnostic and treatment protocols, or should the practice choose someone who has the same alma mater as the rest of the doctors? If the sale of my practice to this new associate is a desired option, shall I recruit a new graduate primarily from the schools with the lowest tuition and, thus, lowest debt? Shall I inquire as to the extent of the applicants' debts and take their answers to that question into consideration when selecting the best new associate who could be a potential buyer for my practice?

6. How will my staff feel about a "wet-behind-the-ears" new graduate and how many additional, if any, support staff must be hired to make this new doctor productive? Will the personality and work ethic of our new hire blend with the personalities of existing loyal and competent staff members?[22]

7. Who are the character, work habit, and technical skill references for the top candidates? How well do they know the applicants, and what are they saying about them? In this day and age of self-centered people, embezzlers, and employees of all ages with chemical dependencies, no employer should hire any employee without speaking first with that person's references.

8. When dealing with new graduates, what do their classmates say about them? Are they enthusiastic, caring, concerned, outgoing, likeable people or nitpicking, whining, untrustworthy, alcohol and drug dependent, emotionally unstable, antisocial hermits?

QUESTIONS EMPLOYEES SHOULD BE ASKING

As associate veterinarians, office managers, and support staff enter the negotiation stage of their selection of employers, they should think beyond merely locating jobs and consider the myriad other issues associated with employment.[23,24] Issues to consider are the following:

1. What am I looking for in a job?

- Money - the most money possible?
- Experience - a high-volume practice where I am exposed to high numbers of cases, or a lower-volume practice where there is time to learn more from what I do?
- Mentorship - somebody willing to listen to my ideas and teach me the technical skills I lack?
- Work schedule - no more than 40 hours per week?, 40 to 45 hours per week?, 45 to 50? Am I willing to work more than 50 hours per week?
- Fringe benefits (covered in Chapters 4 to 7)?
- A training program for new associates? The better the training program offered by the practice, the more rapidly new doctors can become happy, productive members of the team.[25] New graduates must understand, nonetheless, that training programs for young doctors do not exist in most privately owned practices.
- A practice, business, and personal philosophy in harmony with my own?[26]
- An opportunity to develop my surgical skills, or interest in exotic animals, reproduction, animal behavior, complimentary or alternative medicine?
- Nights and weekends with no emergency duty requirements, or opportunities for emergencies where I can bond with clients, develop my emergency medicine skills, and earn some additional money?
- Two days off together each week and at least every other or every third weekend off so I can have a life?

2. Where am I looking?

- Close to family — or far, far away? (the Virgin Islands, Alaska, Guam?) During the formative years of their marriage, newlyweds are encouraged to move at least 300 miles from the locale in which either party grew up or from either set of parents. This forces them to develop new friendships as married couples, without the baggage of pre-existing friendships of either party or their families.
- A region or area of the country with affordable housing for young veterinarians?
- In the mountains, near the ocean, in the country, in a city, in the suburbs?
- Where there is good job and personal security?
- Where I don't have to commute through heavy traffic more than 15 or 30 minutes?

3. Why am I looking for a job?

- Because that is why I went to school for the past 7 to 10 years and I can't wait to start putting all this education and knowledge to work.
- Because I have this horrendous debt staring me in the face and no one else has offered to pay it.
- Because my parents (spouse? children?) expect me to start using my education and pay my own way.
- So that I can complete the American dream of owning my own business by buying a practice or starting one from scratch.

4. With what kind of employer will I seek work?

- Private practice - small, large, mixed, equine, emergency, specialty, exotic animal?

- The public or corporate industry sector?

- An employer offering advanced training in the form of an internship, residency, or postdoctoral training?

- Does the practice have a niche that needs filling? Would my interest and experience in dentistry, behavior, emergency care, sports medicine, avian and exotic animal medicine, equine or bovine reproduction, computers, production medicine, or ophthalmology be of special value?[27]

5. Can the employer provide references from former employees for me to call? Since employers routinely ask for references from applicants, it is appropriate for applicants to ask for references from them.

  - Is the employer willing to provide references? If the employer seems unwilling to provide references or has trouble producing any former employees who could serve as references, proceed with caution.

  - When did the reference with whom you are speaking last work for the employer, and how freely does the person provide frank and open commentary?

  - What are those people saying about the job, hours, quality of veterinary care and support staff, and harmony of the work environment at the practice in question?

6. How well does the practice appear to be organized, and what is the perceived quality of veterinary care being delivered?

  - Review some medical records. Are they legible, have cases been SOAPed, could you provide follow-up care based on what you can read on the record of ongoing cases?

- Look at some radiographs and other images. Are films properly labeled? Are the exposure, positioning and labeling appropriate? Does the practice routinely take two or more views of all limbs and body cavities?

- How often does the practice perform biopsies and pursue histopathologic diagnoses? Does the practice perform aspiration biopsies and cytology and, if so, are specimens read in house or sent to credible veterinary laboratories?

- Examine the quality and age of the practice's instruments and equipment. If it is an ambulatory large animal practice, are hoof testers and trimmers functional? What type of in-house or portable radiographic equipment, cassettes, and film processing system does the practice use? Are the vehicles in good shape? How well are the ambulatory Bowie or Leboit boxes maintained? If it is a small animal practice, how many surgery packs are present? What types of surgeries are done in house and what types are referred? What types of lab work are done in house? What is the practice's policy on referrals to emergency and specialty clinics?

7. Size up the staff. Knowing that highly successful small animal veterinary practices employ from 3.2 to as many as 5 support staff members per full-time veterinarian, as opposed to the average of 2.7 for average practices, how many support staff are there per doctor in this practice?[28]

  - How many staff members are certified veterinary technicians (or registered veterinary nurses)? Does the practice encourage and provide financial assistance for the continuing education of its support staff? At what financial level?

- How long have staff members worked at the practice, and do they like working there? What is the level of tension or harmony among workers? Is the staff encouraging you to or discouraging you from working at the practice? Questions of support staff often provide better answers than those of overly enthusiastic, sometimes unrealistic, employers.

IS THERE ROOM FOR NEGOTIATION?

Regardless of the circumstances, the art of negotiating a salary by either party should start with the same question: "Is there room for negotiation?" In some cases, because of finances, the answer may be "no." This is especially true when solo veterinarians are hiring their first associates or multi-doctor practices are hiring their first office managers. Budgetary constraints under these circumstances may be heavy, leaving little room for upward salary negotiations. The "no" answer also may apply, however, when young associates with large educational debts cannot accept the low salaries offered and still make ends meet.

Whatever the case, much time and considerable hard feelings can be saved if both parties are aware that there either is or is not room for negotiation. To be cognizant of the financial considerations required for negotiations, both parties should have pursued some form of budgetary review before the hiring or job selection process began. Employers should be asking the subsequent economic and ego-related questions to assure themselves that they can hire and retain associates. Associates, as discussed later in this chapter, should be answering the questions asked previously, especially, "how much money will I need to survive?"

WHAT DOES IT TAKE TO SUPPORT A DOCTOR?

Among the budgetary rules of thumb to be considered when practice owners seek to hire additional associates are the following:

- According to one source, small animal practices typically need the addition of 1,200 to 1,300 clients to support an additional doctor.[29] In the author's experience, small animal practices generally need between 800 to 1,200 animal owners per veterinarian to support each full-time equivalent (FTE) general small animal practitioner, depending on the demographics of the trade area, average client transaction fee for the practice, and the type and quality of medicine provided. The numbers of clients needed for large animal or mixed animal practices vary remarkably by region of the country, species of animals serviced, species mix, and style of practice, e.g., "fire engine," nutrition, reproduction, herd health, or management consulting. Because of this, only vague rules of thumb exist for large and mixed animal practices.

- Additional issues involve the affluence of the small animal clients in a mixed practice, and the breakdown of the practice, i.e., predominantly large versus predominantly small; mostly equine versus large volumes of backyard small ruminants. Increased numbers of exotic livestock such as ostriches, emus, llamas, white tail deer, bison, and alpacas in the trade area also can affect the practice's income and need for additional manpower. Some basic criteria to be used when hiring additional large or mixed animal practitioners follow:

  › If the business is a predominantly large animal practice, it is likely to require 1,200 to 1,500 transactions per FTE veterinarian per year (1,000 of which are related to large animal calls).

> If the practice consists of predominantly small animals, it probably will require 2,500 to 3,500 transactions per FTE veterinarian (approximately 2,000 of which are created by the small animal side of the business).

> If it is a dairy practice, as few as 6 to 10 herds or as many as 150 herds may be needed per doctor, depending on the size of the herds in the area.

> If it is an equine ambulatory practice, it most likely will require 500 to 800 clients per doctor, depending on the numbers of stables in the trade area.

- Small animal practices in stable populations should generate 20 new clients per month per doctor.[29,30] In trade areas with considerable turnover (near military bases and college communities), this number may need to be in the range of 30 per month per doctor to sustain adequate growth.

- In general, practices should have 2,750 to 4,200 client transactions (invoices) annually per general small animal practitioner to sustain each FTE veterinarian. The actual number needed depends upon the style and philosophy of the practice. It could be as high as 6,000 in a high-volume, low-fee general practice; as low as 2,200 in a low-volume, high-fee general practice; or between 700 and 1,200 in a specialty practice. For an excellent resource that reports data on this subject by region of the United States and Canada, see AAHA's publication entitled *Financial and Productivity Pulsepoints*.[31]

- Small animal practices generally require between $325,000 and $450,000 of potential gross income production collected per full time veterinarian (exclusive of sales of over-the-counter products) to be able to employ each additional full-time associate.[31] Large

animal practices should generate a total of $220,000 to $280,000 of revenue per doctor.

- Unfortunately, as practices grow, many owners find themselves near burnout and want to hire additional veterinarians to relieve the workload before it is economically viable to do so. What they often find after expanding is that their practices do not produce nearly enough total income to accommodate the additional full-time veterinarian(s) they hired. The question these practitioners must ask themselves when their practices do not fulfill the previous criteria is, "Am I ready and able to incur a significant cut in personal income in order to reduce my workload?" If the answer is "no," it probably is time to hire a part-time doctor or share an associate with another practice rather than hire a full-time person who will be asked to leave within six months to a year.

- A different approach to evaluating the economic viability of hiring additional associates is to assume that 50% of households have pets, that there are 1.6 pets per household, and that 75% of pet owners use companion animal veterinary services.[32] If, as AVMA marketing research shows, a city has 14,000 households, 5,200 will have pets that will see a veterinarian annually ([14,000 x .5] x .75). Since households typically average 1.6 pets per household, this results in 8,400 pets visiting a veterinarian annually.

> Knowing that the 2006 average annual household expenditure was $356 per dog and $190 per cat, and using an average mix for a practice of 60% dogs to 40% cats, one can estimate that each household spends an average of $290/pet for veterinary care. Multiplying that by 8,400 pets in the trade area generates $2.44 million in veterinary revenues. When that $2.44 million is divided by, for example,

five practitioners working in two to four practices in the area, it results in the potential for $487,200 of revenue per full-time doctor.[33] Since that exceeds the $325,000 to $450,000/doctor figure cited above, it would appear this community could expand from a four-practice, five-doctor community with relative ease.

› Expanding to six doctors in the trade area ($406,000 of revenue/ doctor), however, might result in economic difficulties, unless the local population were growing. Expanding to seven ($348,000/ doctor) most likely would create economic difficulties for all of the practitioners in the area.

• In many cases, employers must review their fee schedules and consider their willingness to increase fees to enable them to add another veterinary associate. One of the benchmarks to look at when considering expansion is the average client transaction (ACT) for the practice and each doctor in it. Examples of low, median, and high ACTs by region of the United States and Canada can be found in AAHA's *Financial and Productivity Pulsepoints*.[34]

• Employers also must evaluate their paraprofessional staffing needs in light of hiring an additional veterinarian.[22]

• Practice owners, spouses working in the business, and managers must be willing to look at the existing case distribution and determine the owner's, spouse's, receptionist's, or manager's willingness to allow new doctors to have carte blanche access to existing and new clientele. This is a "where is my ego" question. If owners are unwilling to pass along clients to their new associates, the move to add another doctor probably will not work. Additionally, if the egos or insecurities of the owners, established associates, or owner's spouses will not tolerate the successful

bonding of their favorite clients with new associates, an expansion with new doctors will be unsuccessful. In general, associates should be cautious of signing on with practices where spouses are deeply involved in the financial and personnel management of the business. Although some produce highly satisfactory results, the authors' experience is that the majority do not.

• Lastly, practice owners must be financially astute enough to estimate and project their practices' gross and net incomes for the next year or be willing to seek some advice before expanding. This is essential to assure themselves that sufficient monies will be generated by the additional associates to enable their practices to pay realistic salaries and still produce enough income to meet their needs as owners. In many cases, this cannot be determined without input from a CPA or practice management consultant, i.e., someone more familiar with budgets and projections than are many practice owners. In the end, the volume of cash flowing to the bottom line will have a major effect on whether employees who are hired will be low, middle, or highly paid associates and whether they are likely to survive as employees into a second year.

CAVEATS REGARDING NEW ASSOCIATES

Years of experience advising new graduates and practice owners about contract and employment relationships have taught the authors three things: (1) nothing is ever quite as it seems to be, (2) the majority of new graduates will not last longer than one year at their first place of employment, and (3) many veterinarians who become the first full-time associate added to a solo veterinarian practice also will be gone in a year or less.

The first reason for these caveats is that no matter how diligent employers and applicants are with their selection process, it is impossible to know the moral and ethical fiber of each other or fully evaluate differences in practice philosophies, technical skills, or work ethics prior to initiating an employer-employee relationship. Living by the rule that one will never accept a job or hire an associate without spending at least two full days working together in the practice goes a long way toward reducing wrong decisions.

The second reason is that employers hiring their first associates have nothing with which to compare the personality, competency, and ability of their initial veterinary employees. This frequently leads to misguided expectations, difficulties with communications, and failed working relationships.

The third reason is based on the fact that new graduates have no practices with which to compare the management style, numbers and abilities support staff, work load, medical quality of the business, or practice philosophies of the owners. It is because of these inherent difficulties that turnover always has been and most likely always will remain higher than desired by both sides.

The Next Step

Having established some criteria for the hiring of additional veterinarians, it is now time to look at the types of expenses veterinary practices normally experience in their operations. Only by understanding the basic economics of veterinary practices will readers have a reasonable grasp of the levels of compensation that are achievable for associate veterinarians, support staff, office and veterinary managers, and practice owners.

The Five Tiers of Owner Compensation - "Practice Management 101," or "Where Does the Money Go?"

To better understand the economic impact of adding or decreasing the numbers of owners, associate veterinarians, and/or support staff members in a veterinary practice, it helps to have a basic understanding of veterinary economics, or "where does the money go?" Table 3.2 presents the expenses and cash flow for an average two-doctor small animal veterinary practice.

Expenses vary among practices, of course, depending on the age and size of the facility; rent; volume of lease-hold improvements required; level of compensation and benefits provided for professional, management, and support staff; volume of new equipment leased or purchased; and marketing, accounting, and legal expenses. The ranges presented here are intended simply to help owners, new graduates, practice managers, and experienced veterinary employees understand the basics of practice economics.

Practice expenses fall into two major categories:

- the cost of professional services (also called *direct* or *inventory costs* by many management consultants), and

- general and administrative expenses, commonly called *indirect costs* or *G&A expenses.*

To be more useful, G&A expenses are subdivided into five subcategories, consisting of (1) compensation for professional staff, (2) compensation for support staff, (3) expenditures for management, (4) occupancy expenses (rent or mortgage), and (5) other miscellaneous G&A expenses. What is left over after all expenses are paid is the "net" or "book profits" of the business. Table 3.2 illustrates the interaction and effect of these expenses on practice profits.

Table 3.2. Breakdown of Expenses in a Small Animal Practice Showing Owner's Net Income

A $1,000,000/Year Practice			
	Range	Our Percentage	Our Example
Income from operations (including 7.5% non-Dr. revenue)	100%	100%	$1,000,000
Expenses			
(-) Direct Costs (costs of goods sold - COGS)	18-21%	20%	$200,000
Expenses directly related to the generation of income. Includes drug and laboratory costs, pet food expenses, and anesthesia, surgical, medical, and radiological supplies			
(-) Indirect Costs (general and administrative expenses - G&A)			
Compensation of professional staff (18-23% of professional revenues) (In this example, owner/associate are pd. 20% of $925,000 Dr. produced revenue - 7.5% of $1,00,000, $75,000 is non-Dr. production)	18-23%	18.5%	$185,000
Compensation of support staff (17-23% of gross income)	17-22%	21%	$210,000
Compensation for owner's management duties (2-4% of gross income)	2-4%	3.5%	$35,000
Occupancy expenses (rent or mortgage - 4-8% of gross income)	4-8%	6.5%	$65,000
Other general and administrative costs - health, liability, & business insurance; office and medical records; accounting & legal; payroll taxes; CE; advertising; dues; auto; phone; computer and other equipment maintenance; property taxes; building maintenance; bank charges & interest; depreciation; and misc.	12-21%	16.5%	$165,000
Total Indirect Costs (General and Administrative expenses)	53-79%	66%	$660,000
-Total Direct and Indirect Costs from Above	71-100%	86%	$860,000
= NET INCOME (return-on-investment and/or profits)	0-29%	14%	$140,000

Nearly 30 years ago, the American Animal Hospital Association generated a standard chart of accounts to establish which expenses should be entered in each of the categories and subcategories listed in Table 3.2. That chart of accounts is the gold standard by which all practices are encouraged to track income and expenses. To assist in the cumulation of meaningful financial data regarding their businesses, all veterinary practice owners and certified public accountants involved in veterinary financial management are encouraged to use that chart of accounts.

In the economic analysis of practice income, most practice owners traditionally have stopped at the net income or net profit figure. To be more accurate and to allow for more equitable compensation of owners, though, the practice's net income must be broken down into its components. Table 3.3 and the explanations that follow elucidate the complexities of determining the true profitability of small businesses in general and veterinary practices in particular.

THE LOGIC OF FAIR COMPENSATION FOR SOLO AND MULTIPLE OWNERS

Note: It is important for readers to recognize that this section of the book represents solely Dr. Wilson's personal views and those of his management consulting partner, Dr. Larry McCormick, based on Dr. Wilson's 10-year ownership of a veterinary practice with three different partners and his management consulting relationships with many multi-owner veterinary practices. In each of these consulting situations the owners sought assistance mediating disputes about compensation that were antagonistic enough to precipitate the dissolution of the business. What follows represents hundreds of hours of thought and consulting effort identifying the inequities and proposing solutions to the problems of owner compensation in multi-owner partnerships and corporations.

To understand "where the money goes" more fully, the categories identified in Table 3.3 must be further analyzed and explained. Since veterinary practices are small, closely held businesses, the objective of this net income analysis is to fairly compensate owners based on the particular functions each performs and the value they bring the practice. Table 3.4 defines the five tiers of compensation which should be considered in establishing owner compensation policies. These five tiers of compensation are viable for owners of veterinary corporations, partnerships, limited liability partnerships, and limited liability companies; however, one of the reasons for adopting a partnership or limited liability form of ownership is because it is somewhat easier to draft agreements and distribute the five tiers of income via those business structures than it is with corporations.

Briefly, the types, or *tiers*, of compensation pertaining to particular functions that practice owners provide are as follows:

1. Veterinary Salaries - First and foremost, practices must allocate fair compensation for each owner's efforts as a practicing veterinarian in the business. In many cases, this is done by determining the volume of income produced and collected by each owner and allocating a premium veterinary salary equal to 22% of that amount as realistic compensation for that person's effort and success as a veterinarian.

2. Management Salaries - Next, compensation must be allocated for the time, effort, and accomplishments of each owner's management of the business. After subtracting these two tiers of owner compensation and all other business expenses,

Table 3.3. Breakdown of Expenses to Establish Net Income and Profits

Income from operations
Expenses
(-)   **Costs of professional services (direct costs)**
(-)   **General and administrative expenses (indirect costs)**
1. Fair compensation for veterinary staff
2. Compensation of support staff
3. Compensation for owner's management duties
4. Occupancy expense (if not allocated as an expense, rent must be paid to owner)
5. Other general and administrative expenses including cost of perks
Net Income
(+)   Perk income (legitimate IRS business expenses which also fulfill personal needs of owners)
Revised Net Income
(-)   Profits expected as a return on investment in the practice
(-)   Equitable distribution of profits among owners

Table 3.4 . Identifying the Five Tiers of Owner Compensation

Income from operations	
Expenses	
(-)	**Costs of professional services (direct costs)**
(-)	**General and administrative expenses (indirect costs)**
	Tier 1 Fair compensation for efforts as a veterinarian
	Owners receive 22% of their veterinary production as tier one compensation
	Tier 2 Compensation for owners' management efforts and duties
	Note: If practice owners own the real estate but do not pay themselves rent, they must deduct the fair market value of the rent before arriving at the net income.
Net Income	
(+)	Tier 3 Value of perk income to owners (Legitimate IRS business expenses that are personal in nature for owners).
Revised Net Income	
(-)	Tier 4 Profits reflected as a return on investment in the practice
(-)	Tier 5 Equitable distribution of remaining profits among owners based on contributions

the remaining practice income is called its *net income*.

3. Perquisite Income - Perquisite or "perk" income for owners also must be measured and equalized among the owners. Perks are those expenses that were personally incurred but were paid for by the business. As such, they are tax deductible to the business. Under the strictest of IRS interpretations, these could be considered net profits of the business or taxable income for the recipients. However, as with many IRS interpretations, some business deductions are neither black nor white, but grey. In such cases, the IRS allows the deductions because they had important business value even though the payment of such expenses reduced the recipient's personal expenditures and tax liability in the process. Occasionally, the perks of the practice eat up most or all of profits, leaving nothing left over. In most cases, though, additional monies are available for distribution as Tier 4 or 5 compensation.

4. Profits Reflected as a Return on Owners' Investments in the Practice - This component of a practice's net income has

little to do with owners' veterinary or management skills and, instead, has everything to do with the money these parties have tied up in their investments in the practice. To determine what percentage of the profits is linked to the owners' investment in the business, valuations of practices must be determined annually. Owners can expect a 10% to 11% annualized return on investment (ROI) from this tier of income, comparable to what they would make via dividends, dividend reinvestments, and stock appreciation from a long-term blue chip portfolio in the stock market.

5. Equitable Distribution of Remaining Profits Among Owners - Two methods are suggested for sharing profits in excess of the expected ROI on investment and perks. These are based either on each doctor's percentage of business ownership, or are determined by agreements among the parties regarding the value of contributions such as

- personal, professional, or financial skills;

- amount of time devoted to the promotion of the business (through such methods as community service, leadership, or public speaking);

- important speaking engagements, personal and business contacts, and networks that lead to referrals to the business (the "rainmaker" factor); and

- personal liability or collateral pledged for debts of the practice.

To maintain a harmonious co-ownership, the parties must recognize that extensive efforts by one person in one of these categories are unlikely to offset that person's need to shoulder an appropriate share of the practice's workload. Hence, too much rainmaking may produce tremendous business growth but generate acrimony among the other owners who are holding down the fort. This is especially true if the people performing most of the work are minority owners who do not share equitably in Tiers 4 and 5 of the business's profits.

AN IN-DEPTH LOOK AT THE FIVE TIERS OF OWNER INCOME

TIER 1 - COMPENSATION FOR VETERINARY EFFORTS

To establish fair compensation for owners' efforts as veterinarians, practice managers should consider what it would cost to replace the owners should they cease to perform their jobs as practicing veterinarians.

As discussed earlier, wages for veterinary owners are established by determining what competitive salary would be required to hire an equivalent veterinary associate. Although many practices at the end of the first decade of the 2000s pay veterinary salaries as fixed amounts ranging from $70,000 to $95,000 annually, an appropriate salary for most small animal veterinarians falls in the range of 18% to 22% of professional revenue generated. According

to 2007 AVMA statistics, the mean professional income for all veterinarians in private practice (average of the entire database) varied from a low of $107,330 for predominately large animal practitioners to a high of $139,612 for large animal exclusive practitioners. During that year, the mean professional income for all veterinarians in private practice was $115,447,[4] while the median (equal numbers of salaries above and below a mid point) was $91,000[4]. It has been theorized that the large variance between the median and the mean occurred because the income of a few highly compensated professionals more than offset the high number of low-paid veterinarians.

A more recent study of equine practitioners showed that associates under the age of 30 had a mean salary of $48,280 while those over 60 earned $160,240. The overall average for equine practitioners was $111,340.[35]

The most recent survey for small animal veterinarians showed 378 owners receiving an average salary of $126,299 and a median of $105,000, with associates earning an average of $71,316 and a median of $70,000, based on 340 responses.[36]

Variations in compensation for owners depend on

- their levels of experience and self-esteem;

- the fee schedule for the business;

- the affluence of the practice's trade area and clientele;

- the quality, quantity, and longevity of support staff at the facility (the higher the volume, better training, and longer term employment for support staff, the lower the compensation percentage for the doctors);

- the energy levels and physical, mental, and family health of the parties;

- individual variations in time-management efficiencies;

- the quality, size, and aesthetics of the physical plant in which such people work, and

- the personality, popularity, and drawing power of each owner.

Historically, most small animal practices pay their associate veterinarians salaries equal to approximately 20% of revenue generated and collected. Of the 44% of United States practices that pay based on personal production, the vast majority of them pay between 18% and 22% of production.[37] This number is stated as a percentage of the doctor-produced revenues, not the gross income of the practice.

Considerable differences in doctor-generated revenues exist among practices because of variations in fees and the volume of invoices from sales of over-the-counter merchandise, pet food, prescription refills, lab work, and vaccinations performed without veterinary examinations of patients, as well as boarding, grooming, and obedience training. In the average small animal practice, 80% to 95% of practice gross income is derived from the direct efforts of its doctors and, thus, veterinary salaries are based on or are at least related to this number. Furthermore, because 5% to 20% of most practices' income results from the efforts of its support staff, total professional salaries are reported as a percentage of doctor-generated revenues and not as a percentage of the practice's gross income.

Because of their experience, technical acumen, time-management skills, and long-term association with the clientele, practice owners often are paid premium wages for their veterinary efforts and expertise. This is reflected in their salaries of 22% (and occasionally even 23%) of their professional revenues generated, rather than the more standard 20% received by most veterinary associates. This veterinary salary is paid in addition to fringe benefits such as health coverage, vacation, CE allowance, sick leave, professional liability coverage, professional licenses, and dues. If practice owners do pay themselves premium salaries of 23% of the revenues they generate, which when averaged with salaries for nonowner associates comes to approximately 21% of the practice's gross income, other expenses must be reduced by an equivalent amount for the practice to maintain the same level of profitability (Table 3.2).

It is important to recognize that according to the 2007 VHMA Compensation and Benefits survey, full-time associates who were paid on a percentage of gross income earned the highest salaries, $86,383. This was $17,630, 25%, more than salaried associates.[38]

TIER 2 - COMPENSATION FOR MANAGEMENT

Determining fair compensation for owners' efforts as managers is more difficult. A starting reference is to compare the salaries to be paid to the parties in question with those earned by people in similar management positions in the profession or salaries earned by office managers in other types of businesses. Yearly salaries in the first decade of the 2000s of $42,000 to $60,000, or hourly rates of $22 to $35 plus benefits, would be exceptional. Although these may seem low when compared with the value of the owners' time attending cases, premiums can be added to these basic management wages, when appropriate, to account for an owner's or manager's experience, leadership, knowledge of the profession, marketing or computer skills, ability to fill in as a practitioner when the practice is short-handed, and the volume of the practice's net income. The above salaries gleaned from the authors' consultations correspond closely with the median salaries of $36,000 and $49,400 for full-time office managers and hospital administrators paid by the 92 practices surveyed for AAHA's *Compensation and Benefits* booklet.[36]

For simplicity, management salaries for owners often are based on the practice's gross revenues. Unfortunately, this method of determining salary is somewhat inappropriate because tying a manager's compensation to gross revenues implies a direct cause-and-effect relationship between the practice's total revenue; the manager's effort, contribution, and success in each revenue center of the business; and the net earnings of the enterprise. In most cases, this does not reflect reality.

In an ideal world, the majority of management pay would be linked to net income. This method of determining compensation poses its own set of dilemmas, though, because expenses for purchases of equipment, drugs, and biologicals; facility and equipment repairs; lease-hold improvements; owner bonuses; and other expenditures vary remarkably from year to year. Tax benefits gained from using year-end profits to pay some of the next year's expenses also can skew the numbers. This negatively affects the current year's net income even as it positively affects the practice's future. Such yearly fluctuations make accurate calculations of net income difficult and inconsistent.

Additionally, it may be appropriate to pay a higher percentage for full-time doctor-owner-managers of multi-million dollar practices. In these cases, management compensation might consist of 3.5% of the first $1 million of practice revenue followed by a gradually decreasing percentage, i.e., 3% for the next $1 million, and 2.5% for successive millions. This is because the veterinary owner or manager's total workload does not necessarily parallel the growth in practice income and may not increase proportionately with each successive million dollars of gross revenue.

It is unquestioned that a manager's salary should be linked at least in part to the business's net earnings rather than its gross revenues. The problem is this leads to disagreements regarding the justification for various practice expenditures. It also predisposes owners and managers to conflict each time they attempt to determine the business's net income.

To avoid such conflicts and reduce the time needed and difficulties encountered in analyzing the business's net income and profits each year, most veterinary practice management consultants use the simple formula wherein practice owners receive between 2% and 4% of the practice's collected gross revenues. The exact percentage to be paid these owner-managers is decided on a case-by-case basis depending on the gross income of the practice, the amount of time required to complete the job, the bargaining power of the owner-manager, and the numbers of experienced and capable nonveterinary managers assisting with management.

The usual range for total management expenses, including support staff engaged in management duties, is 4% to 5.5% of the practice's gross revenues. This number includes an allocation of 0.5% to 1.5% for the managerial efforts of the veterinary chief of staff, head technician, head receptionist, inventory manager, and staff members other than full-time office managers. Practices with full-time office managers pay owners closer to the 2% figure for their efforts, while practices without office managers may pay owners as much as 4% for management.

After specifying the percentage of income allocated for a practice's management, multi-owner practices can divide the 2% to 4% among themselves based on the difficulty and volume of managerial duties assigned to and completed by each owner. Management responsibilities are listed below.

Financial Management

- Establish an annual departmentalized budget.
- Set up internal controls to prevent embezzlement.
- Review all accounts payable.
- Balance and reconcile the checkbook.
- Review and evaluate income by department; determine if each is profitable.

- Consider various pension and profit-sharing options and oversee administration of the one selected.

- Produce monthly and annual financial reports with assistance of the practice's CPA.

- Establish an inventory control system for all OTC products, dispensable products, and hospital supplies.

- Work with doctors to review, update, and evaluate the effectiveness of and compliance with the practice's established fee schedule. Adjust fee schedule twice yearly.

- Maintain a hospital credit policy, establish credit application forms, and monitor accounts receivable.

- Select and monitor a collection agency to pursue past-due accounts receivable.

- Work with a CPA to produce and review all federal, state, and local income, sales, and use taxes.

- Review existing insurance coverage, meet with insurance agents, and determine which company provides the best medical, hospital business package, life, disability, workers' compensation, and professional liability coverage.

- Determine whether it is more economical to hire an automated payroll company to do payroll or complete this task in house. Select payroll company with assistance of a CPA, should that be the decision.

- Attend continuing education programs focusing on business tax planning and financial affairs.

- Track perk income taken by each owner.

Personnel Management

- Develop and enforce consistent personnel policies.

- Listen to and resolve staff complaints.

- Develop and implement a cohesive staff training program.

- Develop and maintain a hospital procedure manual.

- Be responsible for hiring and firing of support staff; assist with hiring and firing of employed veterinarians.

- Create and review job descriptions for all support staff members.

- Implement a routine performance appraisal system for all employees.

- Handle personnel regulatory matters dealing with I-9s, OSHA, Toxic Hazard Communication Act, payment of overtime, sick leave, pregnancies, etc.

- Establish contracts for employed veterinarians and any support staff who should have them.

- Oversee the scheduling of support staff.

- Review and tabulate the employee payroll and report hours to in-house payroll personnel or the automated payroll service.

- Help employees develop personalized continuing education plans.

- Develop support staff compensation incentive programs.

- Attend continuing education seminars devoted to personnel management and motivation.

Marketing Management

- Revise and/or develop practice brochures, newsletters, and handouts.

- Review and develop client reminders and written communications.

- Select and oversee appropriate size and content of Yellow Page ads or entries.

- Develop client education messages printed on client receipts.

- Create and/or implement training programs to improve the marketing skills of support staff members.

- Review effectiveness of current point-of-purchase sales area for over-the-counter products and determine whether this should be further developed.

- Review various types of external marketing techniques such as elementary school visitations and presentations by staff members, open houses, membership of veterinarians in local service clubs, etc.

- Attend continuing education programs dealing with marketing of veterinary services.

Maintenance Management

- Develop and oversee a maintenance plan for the physical plant and all hospital equipment.

- Locate and keep a list of qualified plumbers, electricians, flooring contractors, and other handymen as needed.

- Fix equipment or furnishings in need of repair or determine who is best qualified to make such repairs and arrange for repairs to be completed.

- Evaluate cost benefit and cost effectiveness of new equipment purchases.

- Obtain prices on competitive equipment before any purchases are made.

- Maintain a warranty and repair file for all purchased or leased equipment.

- Maintain all documents pertaining to the lease of the physical plant and equipment.

- Fix or hire someone to repair any problems that occur with the phone system and/or intercom.

Computer Management

- Oversee computer-generated reminder systems and target mailings.

- Review new versions of computer programs offered by vendors; determine what types of software or hardware upgrades should be made.

- Resolve problems with computer glitches, disk drives, printers, cables, batteries, back-up systems, memory cards, etc.

- Develop an effective computer training program to educate new personnel as expeditiously as possible.

TIER 3 - EQUALIZING OWNERS' PERKS

Once expenses have been paid by the practice and net income is determined, the next category of owner income to be addressed is perquisite income. In reality, this income is not available for year-end owner distribution because it is comprised of general and administrative expenses already paid by the practice on behalf of the owners throughout the fiscal year. Rather, this is the time to take stock of who has received what perks over the year, and ensure that those perks are equally or, depending on ownership percentages of the parties, at least fairly divided among the owners.

Determining the volume of perquisite money entails identifying the disbursements paid under one or more of the initial six categories of tax-deductible business expenses shown in Table 3.2 that are personal to each owner. Examples include payment for personal tax preparation in conjunction with the business tax return, some of the business auto expenses, a health club membership, home landscaping, the purchase of a new computer that eventually finds its way to an owner's residence, or at least a portion of expenses for attendance at a continuing education seminar on a Carribean island or cruise with great lodging, food, drink, and free time.

As long as the payment of such expenses meets the IRS demands for documentation and business purposes, compensation for owners in this manner is a viable means by which they receive tax-free income. Since owners may wish to take some of their income or profits via these nontaxable perks, tracking of such expenses by owners is essential to keep distributions equitable.

Solo owners often extract net income from businesses via nontaxable perks without measuring the volume of the personal benefit (but be warned, this can incite an IRS audit). When these owners wish to sell their practices, though, they must identify all perk income they have received in order to maximize the revised net income of the business upon which the practice's goodwill value is predicated. Only by completing this procedure can sellers prove to buyers that the practice is more profitable than it appears on paper in the profit and loss statements and the tax returns. (Revised profits, known in the appraisal industry as *excess earnings* or *excess income*, are those monies available for distribution to owners after paying the legitimate business expenses of the business.)

For solo owners, decisions regarding the payment of personal expenses through the business can be made with relative ease because they must answer only to themselves and their spouses. In this case they alone run the risk of an IRS audit. However, when multiple owners are involved, decisions must be made as to

- the willingness of each owner to subject the business to an IRS audit triggered by excessive business expenditures for personal use;

- the volume of time and money expended tracking and equalizing each owner's perks (in other words, are the tax benefits worth the costs incurred);

- the allocation made for perk income to minority owners compared to that for majority owners; and

- the allocation of perk income based on hours worked as veterinarians, income produced for the practice, or the total contribution and effort of each owner on behalf of the business.

Although no hard data on this subject exist, the authors' experience is that most multi-owner practices share perk income based on hours worked and contributions to the practice. Some, however, base it on ownership. Sharing perk income according to hours worked and contributions to the practice benefits minority owners because this income is paid as a routine expense of the business without regard to ownership interests of majority versus minority parties, before the revised net income is distributed via Tier 4 ROI and Tier 5 profits.

One must keep in mind that if no personal expenses (perk income) had been paid on behalf of the owners, this money would have percolated through to the business's bottom line for distribution under Tiers 4 and 5. Therefore, if perk income is too high, practices may not produce any of the revised net income illustrated in Table 3.4. If, on the other hand, perk income is exceedingly low and the practice is a profitable one, the cash available for disbursement as Tier 4 ROI and Tier 5 profits can be significant.

TIER 4 - PROFITS REFLECTED AS A RETURN ON INVESTMENT IN THE PRACTICE

The presence or absence of owner income in Tiers 4 and 5 serves as a basic assessment of the value of continuing the business. If owners' feelings about practice ownership focus primarily on the enjoyment of secure jobs, the freedom of being one's own boss, or serving animals and animal owners as they see fit, it may not be important for them to produce any profits in this category. However, if owners do not enjoy the management headaches and stresses of ownership, and they are astute enough to realize that the business is producing no "risk reward" ROI profits for their effort, worry, and capital investment, they may as well sell their practices, take jobs elsewhere, and invest the proceeds in another medium. In essence, unless a practice produces a net income sufficient to provide an acceptable return on investment, the risks are not worth the effort required to own and manage that practice.

Payment of this fourth tier of owner compensation is based on establishing an annual valuation for the practice and, hopefully, providing owners with a 10% to 11% ROI each on their portion of the current year's value. This ROI is similar to the 10.5% annual return on investments, with reinvested dividends, reported from 1930 to 2001 in the S&P 500 Composite Stock Index.[39]

To be functioning like publicly traded companies, practice owners should be reinvesting continually in the practice's equipment, knowledge base, and lease-hold improvements. Through good planning, practitioners can establish budgets that allow for the production of at least 10% in annual revised net income, which is then available for distribution to the sole proprietors, partners, or members of limited liability companies as Tier 4 ROI. To avoid the IRS interpreting this as taxable income in a corporate setting, upon which corporate taxes would be owed, tax advisors for corporations simply label and pay it as employment compensation bonuses.

For practices that are expanding, net income could be allocated entirely to investments in the business, with nothing going to Tiers 4 and 5 owner compensation. For mature, stable businesses, where the owners need income for personal needs, Tiers 4 and 5 money could be distributed entirely as ROI bonus compensation. For those in between, it could be partly for Tier 4 ROI compensation and partly for investments in the business such as new equipment and lease-hold improvements. If their practices are unable to provide them with this type of minimum 10% to 11% ROI, owners may be better off selling and investing the money in the stock and bond markets, where economic risks exist but far less work is required to produce a consistent ROI.

As mentioned previously, for this system to work, owners must value their businesses annually. This may sound like a difficult, expensive, and atypical way of compensating owners. Furthermore, it requires carefully drafted partnership, LLC, shareholder, and employment agreements between shareholder veterinarians and the corporations they own to prevent confusion and establish the legal requirement to compensate owners in this fashion. Nonetheless, only when this has been done can distributing Tier 4 revised net income be a reality-based allocation. Additionally, annual valuations serve as good management tools, because if the business's value is not increasing, corrections to inadequate practice income growth or excessive expenses can be made immediately, thus averting financial troubles or embarrassments later.

For tax purposes, Tier 4 revised net income distributions must be paid as distributions of profits in partnerships and as "bonus income" to the shareholders of corporations. As such they are taxed as ordinary income to recipients and are not classified as dividends to shareholders. This prevents the double taxation problem inherent in corporate dividends and keeps this income eligible for personal contributions to retirement plans. Differences in tax consequences and tax planning occur between S-Corporations and C-Corporations, so owners are advised to seek the advice of their CPAs before proceeding too far down this path.

To understand the logic of this calculation, owners, associate veterinarians, practice managers, and support staff must realize that Tier 4 profits in the form of ROI are based solely on ownership and have no relevance to each owner's role or function in the practice. In fact, even if owners do not work at the practice, they still are entitled to a share of the business's profits as a return on their investment.

Tier 5 - Equitable Distribution of Remaining Profits Among Owners

After perk income has been equalized and ROI profits distributed, the remaining monies are the "true profits," "bonuses," "risk reward profits," or "gravy." The volume of income in Tiers 4 and 5 determines the value of continuing in business. Because of the significant risks and headaches endured in owning and managing a business, many practice owners believe they should be entitled to additional personal income above and beyond a 10% to 11% Tier 4 return on the value of their investment.

Sometimes, though, there are no profits produced for distribution as Tier 5 compensation. This could be because there is nothing left after paying for owner perks or Tier 4 ROI, or it could be that the owners are plowing the extra profits back into the business, thus directly increasing the value of its tangible assets (inventory, instruments, or equipment) and, ultimately, the potential value of its intangible assets, i.e., its goodwill. This would be akin to the tactics publicly traded companies like Disney, Microsoft, Cisco Systems, and Intel use wherein they pay low dividends but invest heavily in research and development and buy back stock to drive the value of the company's shares upward. With this technique, small dividends are paid that produce little tax consequence to shareholders until the stock is sold, at which time the gain is taxed as capital gain, at considerably lower rates than the ordinary income rate for dividends or bonuses. (In 2009 the differential rates were 15% for capital gains, depending on the length of asset ownership, and 15% to 36% for ordinary income, depending on the taxpayer's tax bracket.)

Tier 5 profits or bonuses present owners with decisions as to their distribution. Much more than the equitable distribution of perk income, the manner by which this business income is divided in multi-owner practices impacts the motivation each owner has to work for and stimulate growth in the practice's gross and net revenues. Traditionally, profits or bonus calculations and distributions have been linked to ownership. From a rational and motivational perspective, though, it is recommended that the distribution of Tier 5 profits be based partly or entirely on each owner's contributions to and commitment and efforts in support of the business. The following examples illustrate various avenues for handling the distribution of this fifth tier of owner income.

- If ownership is equal among the parties and each contributes reasonably equal time, effort, and income production to the practice, Tier 5 profits could be split evenly.

- As with perk income, when allocating profits in situations where ownership or contributions to the success of the business are unequal, owners should consider measurable factors such as (1) the salaries they were paid for their Tier 1 efforts as veterinarians versus the salaries they should have earned in that capacity if they had been paid at the standard owner rate of 22% to 23% of professional revenues generated and (2) the volume of personal assets placed at risk as collateral for debts of the practice.

- Not as easily quantified but also of importance are the business contacts, name recognition in the trade area, and business-enhancing volunteer efforts in the community (the "rainmaker factor").

With the Tier 5 equitable distribution of profits approach advocated here, the division of profits or bonus money is based on assessments of contribution rather than being linked strictly to ownership. Although this process provides room for discord because of its subjective nature, its precepts require that owners evaluate their business contributions annually. In doing so, the less productive, less active, and less financially or emotionally committed owners must assess their conduct and, if adjustments are needed to bring them back into parity with co-owners, they must make those adjustments before they are entitled to more of this fifth tier of owner income. To better explain these concepts, a series of hypothetical examples follows.

Example 1: If one owner was on a leave of absence for several months during a stipulated time period—depressed because of family strife; off work because of a personal or family illness, a pregnancy, or other disability; or partially retired—the owners would consider such decrease in value and productivity or absence from the practice when allocating Tier 5 income. Alternatively, they might decide not to add insult to injury and allocate this tier equally.

Example 2: If two junior owners each own 15% of the business but produce more income and devote more time and energy to the practice than the senior, 70% owner, the parties could decide that each owner should receive one third of the equitable distribution of profits among owners rather than splitting this tier 15:15:70. In doing so, they would be demonstrating that the junior owners' commitment and productivity were more important than their financial ownership. Reallocating practice income through an equitable distribution of a fifth tier of compensation helps motivate minority owners to continue their efforts.

Example 3: A practice has three owners, two of whom own 45% of the practice and one of whom owns 10%. Dr. A (45% owner) handles most of the personnel, marketing, financial, and operational management duties and generates a mere $160,000 of income for which he receives a veterinary salary of $35,200, or 22% of income generated. Dr. B (45% owner) handles most of the computer management and generates only $250,000 of professional revenues for his $55,000 veterinary salary. Dr. C, the newest kid on the block, and only a 10% owner, is an extremely efficient young mother with a charismatic personality, superb veterinary skills, and great delegational abilities. Furthermore, staff members love working with her, which helps enable her to generate $500,000 of professional revenues for the practice. For this she receives a veterinary salary of $110,000.

A simple question that comes up repeatedly is, "Which doctor produces the most revised net income (Tiers 4 and 5 profits) for the practice?" Although it is nearly impossible to answer this question short of doing a time:motion study, in all likelihood, Dr. C generated the most profit. However, if the practice pays her Tier 4 ROI profits and her Tier 5 equitable distribution of profits based on her 10% ownership, she most likely will be an unhappy camper.

Dr. A will argue that it was his management that made the practice profitable; Dr. B will argue that it was his marketing skills; and Dr. C will argue that since she completed the work load that produced 18.75% more income than the other two owners combined, she must have produced far more profits for the business than they did. However, when she receives only 10% of both Tiers 4 and 5 income, she most likely will not be excited about continuing her incredible production efforts, even if she earned a much higher veterinary salary than either of them.

With this new "equitable" system for allocating Tier 5 profits, she might well be eligible for one third or even one half, rather than 10% of them and, thus, could feel good about the financial recognition provided for her efforts. Meanwhile, Drs. A and B should be happy to share more of the Tier 5 profits with Dr. C because her terrific productivity helped enlarge their Tier 4 ROI profits, which were based entirely on ownership.

Example 4: Assume for this example that the two veterinarians in Table 3.2 were partners in the business rather than employer and employee. Partner # 1 covers the expenses of her horses with approximately $4,000 of food, housing, and veterinary care paid by the practice. Partner # 2 has three children and needs every dime of income from the practice he can muster. At year's end the two prepare to divvy up the $26,400 of Tier 5 profits and the $6,000 of perk income. If the partners each had received $1,000 of the $6,000 in routine perk income, Partner # 2 would lag behind Partner # 1 by $4,000 in total compensation and benefits received from his ownership of the practice.

To correct this inequity, this $4,000 would be deducted from the $26,400 cash portion of Tier 5 profits, resulting in $22,400 to be divided equally among them. Each partner would thus receive an $11,200 distribution of this tier of income in the form of a bonus. However, because Partner # 2 got only $1,000 of perk income, he would receive an additional $4,000 of cash (for a total of $15,200 of the Tier 5 profits) in order to equalize the distribution of profits in this category. It should be noted that in this process, Partner # 1 received much of her profits as nontaxable perk income, while Partner # 2 gets more cash but must pay more in taxes. The following mathematical calculations illustrate this distribution.

Profits available for equitable distribution among owners = $32,400

Less Perks	($6,000)
Profits	$26,400 ÷ 2 = $13,200 each

Dr. A had an extra $4,000 in perk income, so one-half of this must be added to Dr. B's share of the profits while the other half is subtracted from Dr. A's profits

$13,200 for Dr. A	$13,200 for Dr. B
- $2,000	+ $2,000
$11,200 profits for Dr. A	$15,200 profits for Dr. B

To check one's figures, simply add each owner's perks to these numbers and see if the total equals the total risk reward profits.

$11,200 for Dr. A	$15,200 for Dr. B
+ $ 5,000 perk Income	+ $1,000 perk income
$16,200 for Dr. A	$16,200 for Dr. B

$16,200 x 2 = $32,400 = total Tier 5 profits

Because contributions by multiple owners change over time, the calculations by which this distribution of risk reward profits is made should be updated every one to three years to reflect activities and events that have transpired since the previous assessment. The detriments of this process are that time, effort and, in some cases, interpersonal conflict, are required to address these issues every year or two, and that changes occurring during previous time periods do not affect the financial outcomes of the parties until later. The benefit is that it is a systematic way for distributing Tier 5 profits as bonuses based on the value each owner brings to the business.

At this point, it should be apparent that practices that fail to produce adequate gross income to provide Tier 4 returns on owners' investments and, therefore, produce no Tier 5 profits, may not be providing a fair return on each owner's investment in the business nor any compensation for the risks associated with owning a small business. In essence, unless all profits are being poured back into the practices, such businesses may be functioning as nonprofit veterinary practices. When this untenable result occurs, owners and managers have several options:

- Accept the result and assume that their ownership interests in the practice serve primarily to provide a desirable way of life and a secure job rather than a valuable investment in a business;

- Evaluate the volume of net income being reinvested in the business and its effect on enhancing the sales value of this asset,

- Raise fees sufficiently so the practice produces an acceptable ROI and a higher level of profits for the owners in the following years;

- Increase productivity sufficiently to produce profits in subsequent years;

- Cut expenses adequately to produce ROI and profits; or

- Pursue a combination of these higher-fee, increased-productivity, and decreased-expense actions.

Compensation for Young Associates: How Much Money Will I Need?

One of the most daunting tasks for new graduates, and even for experienced job applicants, is determining how much personal income will be required to cover living expenses, pay off debts, save for the future, and "have a life." Although an entire text book could be written on personal finances alone, the fundamentals included herein should be of help to veterinary job applicants in determining their economic needs and comparing various job offers.

The Importance of a Budget

Veterinarians entering the job market cannot begin to consider jobs or job offers until they have calculated their personal budgets. The primary reason for understanding one's financial picture becomes apparent during contract negotiations. During the interview process, conversations almost always get around to the inevitable question, "Well, just how much money are you going to need, Dr. Newgrad?"

If the answer to that question is based upon desires, guesses, or science fiction, no one wins. This is because the question "How much will you need?" did not address the inherent subquestions, such as how much will you as a new graduate need to

- survive financially;

- move to this location, rent an apartment, pay security deposits, and become financially secure;

- feel good about the compensation the employer has proposed for your skills, talent, knowledge, personal efforts, and educational and experiential preparation;

- pay off your educational debts in 10 years, buy a house, support a family, and plan for retirement; and/or

- be happy with your day-to-day employment rewards and living arrangements.

Fourth-year students, new graduates, interns, or young associates who have not determined how much they will need to balance their budgets prior to a job interview are at a serious disadvantage and suddenly are placed in a position where they have limited bargaining power. After years of living on a student's budget, salaries of $65,000 per year may sound terrific—until applicants discover that it will be impossible to find a place to live; buy food; cover the costs of an auto; pay state and federal income taxes, FICA (social security taxes), and Medicare; and make payments on their educational debts for less than, for example, $78,000 per year.

Not only is this not a good scenario for applicants, it does not bode well for employers. More than likely, they will lose their newly hired doctors soon after they start, when the associates inform them they have located other jobs where the salaries being offered provide them with livable wages, or the same wage, but with a more lenient work schedule. When that occurs, all the training employers have put in is lost, and considerable time is required to search for, select, and hire another associate.

Third-year students enrolled in the professional foundations classes at the University of Pennsylvania (a course focusing on resumes; budgets; financial planning; stress management; and interviewing for, selecting, and negotiating for one's first job) have been required to complete personal budgets for the first year postgraduation since 1988.

For many, this is the first time they have faced the results of the massive debt loads they have been accumulating since their preveterinary days. It forces them to sit down with spouses or significant others to match expected monthly expenses with potential income. At that point they must accept the financial responsibilities and realities commensurate with graduation.

For the majority of students with educational debt, creating a budget is a disheartening experience. Fortunately, several teachers of practice management and personal development at other United States veterinary schools also require budgets. Students and employers all would be better served if this were a required element of every school's curriculum. After all, if young veterinarians are unable to understand the economic consequences of their own budgets, they cannot be expected to understand the financial limitations under which their employers operate.

SOURCES OF SAMPLE BUDGETS

New associates need to recognize that they cannot begin evaluating job offers and negotiating compensation without developing a personal budget. Without a knowledge of the expenses they will incur for housing, utilities, phone, food, transportation, healthcare, insurance, gifts, vacations, repayment of educational and credit card debt, and taxes, they may find that they have accepted a job that will not allow them to survive financially.

The easiest way for United States students to create a personal budget is to use the budget program available at www.finsim.umn.edu. This has been developed by David Lee, DVM, MBA, Hospital Director at the University of Minnesota, with assistance of the author. It is sponsored by Veterinary Pet Insurance. Thousands of veterinary students have been using this program since 2004.

After completing this budget, users need to go to one of several websites that allow

them to compare cost of living issues. The calculator that is currently the most valuable can be found at www.bestplaces.net/col. First, enter a city and state in the current city and comparison city fields. Then, enter the number developed from the www.finsim.umn.edu budget in the annual income field and click compare. A second cost of living calculator can be found at www.bankrate.com/brm/movecalc.asp. The best option is to use both and average the two.

An alternative to utilizing the computer program is to initiate the budget process with the sample found in Figure 3.1. Data from existing expenses can be tabulated and entered into the columns on a monthly or annual basis. Most people completing this assignment are amazed at two things, these being how fast the little things add up, and what an enormous chunk of their income goes to taxes.

LOCATING AND APPLYING THE TAX MULTIPLIER

After expenses have been entered on the budget document in Figure 3.1 and a person's total fixed and variable expenses are calculated, the next step is to study Table 3.5 for single people and Table 3.6 for married couples to locate the appropriate tax multiplier. These numbers have been established by performing the longhand tax calculations discussed later in the chapter. The numbers found in these charts reflect the impact that federal income taxes, social security, Medicare, and an average state income tax of 3.5% have on a person's total fixed and variable living expenses. It should be noted that state taxes vary considerably, from those states with no income taxes, like Texas and Nevada, to those with a graduated income tax up to 9%, like California.

Table 3.5 is for use by single people with no children, i.e., only one dependent; Table 3.6 is for married couples with no children who file joint tax returns. Because of the

My Budget For First Year After Graduation

Household Expenses	Budget ($)	
	Monthly	Yearly
Fixed or Committed Expenses		
1. Mortgage or rent		
2. Real estate or property taxes		
3. Homeowners or renters insurance		
4. Savings		
5. Debt reduction - personal (credit cards, etc.)		
6. Debt reduction - educational debt total: $_____,000		
- monthly payment: $ _____.00 over ___ years		
7. Debt reduction - other		
8. Automobile (monthly payment)		
Total Fixed Expenses		
Variable Expenses		
9. Food		
10. Telephone		
11. Electricity, gas, or oil		
12. Water		
13. Cleaning - laundry		
14. Auto - gas, commuter expenses		
a. Car washes, maintenance, and repairs		
b. Insurance, license, registration, etc		
15. Physicians		
16. Dentists (include dental prophy)		
17. Optometrists		
18. Prescriptions, vitamins, aspirin, etc.		
19. Clothing -		
a. Self,		
b. Spouse/significant other		
c. Children		
20. Personal (haircuts, hairdressers, cosmetics, etc.)		
21. Repairs and home improvements (appliances, painting, lawn care)		
22. Home furnishings		
23. Education (books, newspapers, periodicals, etc.)		
24. Recreation (sitters, meals out, movies, concerts, sports, clubs, etc.)		
25. Charitable contributions (church, schools, veterinary school)		
26. Gifts and flowers		
27. Animal food, care, and veterinary bills		

Figure 3.1. Establishing a budget

Variable Expenses (cont.) Household Expenses	Budget ($)	
	Monthly	Yearly
28. Miscellaneous (bank service charges)		
29. Vacation		
30. Moving expenses and security deposit		
31. Other		
Total Variable Expenses		
Total Fixed & Variable Expenses:		
Multiplied by multiplier from one of the charts that follow: Multiplier		
Income Needed Before Taxes (see chart):		
Variable (Nontaxable) Benefits Hopefully Provided By Employer		
32. Dues & licenses (veterinary associations, etc.)		
33. Continuing education		
34. Health insurance		
35. Pension		
36. Relocation reimbursement		
37. Other misc. benefits (health club membership, dental/vision coverage, etc.)		

Figure 3.1. Establishing a budget (cont.)

variable levels of tax-deductible interest expenses on residences, property taxes, and state income taxes paid by homeowners, neither of these tables are accurate for taxpayers who own homes and itemize deductions on their tax returns. They also do not consider the impact of newly passed tax deductions for educational interest nor the tax credits of the Lifetime Learning Credit.

Only after job applicants have completed their personal budget calculations can they begin interviewing for jobs with enough knowledge and bargaining power to begin contract negotiation. An important byproduct of creating this budget early on is that they will have initiated planning for their financial future at the beginning of their careers, rather than halfway through, as so often is the case.

An inherent problem with this approach is that students, interns, and residents who have completed their education with minimal debt are at a serious bargaining disadvantage compared with their companions who have large debts. This is because they can survive on considerably lower salaries than their heavily indebted classmates. One questions whether they should be paid less than their debt-laden counterparts, or whether their colleagues should simply accept their plight, accede to standard salaries for graduates with limited debt, and live like paupers.

In general, then, employers and employees must wrestle with the following questions: Should young associates accept lower salaries only because they have no or minimal debt? Are associates with no debt worth less than those who have debt? In other words, when selecting and compensating associates, which is more important—knowledge, technical skills, and ability, or educational debt?

To be pragmatic, new grads and associates with significant debts simply cannot accept the traditionally low salaries offered by private practices and make ends meet. The trend, then, is that the needs of these

Table 3.5. A Non-Home-Owner Single Person's Before-Tax Income Needs Based onTotal Fixed and Variable Household Expenses (TFVHE)*

TFVHE	x	Multiplier	=	Income Before Taxes
$19,750		1.252		$24,725
$24,425		1.281		$31,200
$26,800		1.310		$35,100
$31,200		1.339		$41,800
$36,160		1.368		$49,500
$41,100		1.397		$56,530
$42,350		1.405		$58,550
$43,600		1.411		$61,520
$44,850		1.417		$63,550
$46,100		1.423		$65,600
$47,350		1.429		$67,650
$48,600		1.434		$69,700
$49,850		1.439		$71,725
$51,100		1.444		$73,800
$52,350		1.447		$75,850
$53,600		1.451		$77,750
$54,850		1.454		$79,745
$56,100		1.457		$81,745
$57,350		1.460		$83,750
$58,600		1.464		$85,775
$62,350		1.474		$91,975

* These calculations do not allow for interest deduction on educational loans nor tuition credits that have been offered by the tax code since 1998. Graduates who can use those tax breaks can deduct between $500 and $2,500 from the "income before taxes" calculation depending on their tax brackets, volume of educational interest paid, and payment of tuition in the tax year.

new grads drive up their salaries as well as those of all new associates. When one thinks about it, this is the only practical solution to the serious financial challenges facing new graduates. Clearly the inverse will not work, because that means that students with low debt who accept low salaries would drive salaries down as a result of their remarkably lower budgetary needs. Furthermore, an erosion of salaries would do noth-ing but reduce the quality of men and women applying for and graduating from the country's veterinary schools.

Lastly, if salaries were to drop to meet the lower economic needs of minimally indebted graduates rather than rise, the result would create an untenable situation for those young associates who have debts above $90,000 or $160,000 and cannot survive on the traditionally low veterinary sala-

Table 3.6. Non-Home-Owner Married People's Before-Tax Income Needs Based on Their Total Fixed and Variable Household Expenses (TFVHE)*

TFVHE	x	Multiplier	=	Income Before Taxes
$36,300		1.253		$45,475
$42,290		1.273		$53,800
$47,350		1.291		$61,100
$51,050		1.303		$66,525
$53,535		1.309		$70,075
$56,000		1.315		$73,625
$58,485		1.323		$77,400
$59,725		1.326		$79,200
$60,965		1.329		$81,000
$62,205		1.332		$82,875
$63,445		1.335		$84,700
$64,685		1.338		$86,550
$65,925		1.341		$88,400
$67,165		1.344		$90,250
$68,405		1.347		$92,100
$69,645		1.349		$94,000
$70,885		1.352		$95,850
$72,125		1.356		$98,050
$73,365		1.360		$99,750
$78,325		1.360		$106,500

*These calculations do not allow for interest deduction on educational loans nor tuition credits that have been offered by the tax code since1998. Graduates who can use those tax breaks can de duct between $500 & $5,000 from the "income before taxes" calculation or more depending on the couple's tax bracket and whether one or both spouses have educational debt interest or tuition.

ries. (Note: Over half of the University of Pennsylvania's graduating class of 2008 had educational debt exceeding $150,000!)[18]

In sum, there appear to be two directions for this situation to go. Either students with low debt can continue to accept lower salaries because of their lesser financial needs, to the detriment of their debt-laden colleagues; or alternatively, to be considered average job applicants, students with low educational debt can draft budgets as if they have debt equal to that of the average new

graduate and bargain for higher salaries accordingly.

This entails the creation of budgets with expenses of $1,379/month allocated to cover the 2008 national average debt of $119,803. Instead of placing this expense entry on line 6 of the budget in Figure 3.1, the same number is placed on line 4, entitled "savings." The justification for such serious savings is to (1) use much of this money to fund an annual $2,000 IRA contribution; (2) save for the purchase of a house; or (3) save to fulfill the dream of starting, buying into, or buying an owner out of a veterinary practice. By budgeting in this manner and requesting higher salaries to cover their savings, debt-free graduates more effectively finance their futures while helping their indebted classmates earn salaries sufficient to cover their higher costs of living.

Using the Budget as a Negotiating Tool

Unfortunately, most private practitioners do not read each year's *JAVMA* reports on starting salaries and educational debt, and those who do often read only about the mean starting salaries, not the mean debt. Furthermore, even if practitioners did read and consider these reports, only rarely would they take the time to calculate the pretax financial consequences of such debt. Thus, most practitioners are unaware of the financial predicament faced by the new generation of veterinarians.

Many new graduates at the 20 veterinary schools where the author teaches each year are now using their financial data to their advantage in interviewing for jobs. Their technique involves preparing a bare bones budget and placing it in a pocket or purse before leaving for a job interview. Then when the question comes up, "Well, Dr. Newgrad, what do you need for a salary?" they pull out their budgets and say, "Gee, I'm so glad you asked. According to my budget, it looks like I'll need $75,000. Would you mind going over this document with me to help me determine whether it is an accurate reflection of the costs of living in this community?"

Reportedly, employers' responses to this approach have ranged from,

- "Wow, I can't believe that," to a disappointing

- "There's no way I can afford to pay that kind of salary around here. I can't afford to hire you," to

- "How on earth did you accumulate that kind of debt?" to,

- "I'm impressed that you have developed your own personal budget. No one suggested that to me when I graduated." This is followed by close scrutiny of the budget, and the comment in many cases that, "There's no way I could live on that budget. Are you sure you can? You know, that number is going to be pretty hard for us to hit, but since it looks conservative at best, and you are our top candidate, we'll have to see what we can do to help you meet it."

This technique, in use and taught at Penn and nineteen other schools, helped one couple named Sheri and Dave fulfill their budgetary requirements that were $8,000 higher than their employer had planned to pay. His rationale? He liked both of them, was impressed with their organization and understanding of money, and felt that offering the two of them what their budget showed they needed before they left his practice would save him considerable time and effort. Needless to say, they accepted.

Another Penn student named Robert was able to land a job for $4,000 more than the employer could have offered two other candidates of relatively equal experience and ability. According to his employer, Tom, "I felt if Robert knew that much about his finances, he was bound to be interested in and understand the financial headaches of my practice, too." Several years and a couple of jobs later, Robert ended up purchasing one of Tom's practices, and Sheri and Dave bought one of their employer's practices. All three of these young associates understood money and what it would take to gain the trust of the sellers who hired them as associates and, eventually, financed the sales.

What is the worst that can happen to savvy applicants who bring their budgets to the interview? Employers could say, "Well, I appreciate that you have a lot of debt and some pretty ugly monthly payments, but that's your problem, not mine. You'll have to find some other employer who is willing to pay you what you need." Or one might hear, "Sorry, but we just can't afford you." In that event, one simply has to keep looking, perhaps in more distant communities where the demand for veterinarians exceeds the supply. As of the early 2000s, the geographic locations with the highest demand and salaries are the mid Atlantic states from New York to Virginia, and Southern California where, according to UC Davis statistics, there is only 1 veterinarian per 10,000 people, less than half the national norm.[40]

To prevent new graduates from using their debt as a crutch justifying their entitlement to a higher salary, young graduates must learn to see it as a financial goal they must attain. With this mindset, they can ask prospective employers to work with them to help them achieve the compensation they need. For example:

- Could they be paid for attending emergency cases to help build their employers' practices, bond clients to those practices, and supplement the salaries being offered?

- Could they enhance the unacceptably low salary being offered by working under a percentage-based compensation formula after they have been at the practice for three or six months?

- Could they earn additional money by working one shift more than other employees being paid the proffered salary?

- Would it be possible to commence employment at the salary being offered but receive a significant raise halfway through the contract year, when their student loans start coming due?

- Would the employer mind if they moonlighted at an another practice or emergency clinic in the area to supplement their income?

All in all, creativity, including refinancing educational loans from 10 years to 15 or 25, will be essential for many of today's young veterinarians to meet their high educational debt loads. Creativity, that is, plus hard work, austerity, good luck, and a good financial game plan.

APPRAISING AN EMPLOYER'S BENEFIT PACKAGE

Work schedules and the mix and volume of employee benefits vary remarkably among practices. Consequently, employees and employers must recognize that salary may not be as important as either of these elements.

It is essential that applicants analyze not only which benefit issues are most important to themselves but also the financial effects of one employer's benefit plan versus that of another. For people with preexisting medical problems, the provision of group health coverage, paid by an employer, may be the most important. Mothers and fathers of young children may find that for them, work schedules, number of hours worked, and childcare allowances are most critical. For people with sufficient income to enable them to limit their work time, paid and unpaid vacation time could be number one.

A key issue for applicants is the effect of receiving these benefits tax free. An earlier discussion using the charts in Tables 3.5 and 3.6 showed that employees must multiply their total fixed and variable expenses by 1.25 to 1.4 to account for income, social security, and medicare taxes. Thus, benefits that qualify as business expenses for employers but produce nontaxable income for employees can save employees 25% to 40% of the value of the benefit in state and federal taxes.

Tables 3.7 to 3.11 identify key benefits offered by veterinary employers and provide reference points establishing the approximate value of each. Four of the initial six benefits covered under this section—(1) health, disability, and life insurance; (2) continuing education: (3) dues, licenses, and fees; and (4) professional liability insurance—are discussed in considerable depth in other chapters in this book. A brief discussion of these four is provided here as well, along with a more extensive discussion of emergency duty pay and an introduction to percentage-based compensation. Employers should use Figure 4.1 in the next chapter to show associates the total value of their compensation and benefits.

HEALTH, DISABILITY, AND LIFE INSURANCE

Health coverage can be provided through group plans offered by employers or via individual plans purchased by employees. Health coverage is available as traditional major medical insurance; limited network health maintenance organizations (HMOs); or hybrids of the two, known as *preferred provider organizations* (PPOs). (See Chapter 5 for much more information on health coverage.) Group plans usually are available to veterinary employers through state and national veterinary associations. Costs for group plans provided by employers generally are less than the individual plans purchased by employees, and they provide broader coverage. Employees usually receive better coverage if their employers provide coverage for them as a member of a group policy rather through individual coverage. Also, employer-sponsored health care plans are tax deductible for employers and tax free for employees.

An example of the costs of a popular group health, disability, and life insurance plan available through the AVMA can be found in Table 3.7.

CONTINUING EDUCATION

Another key benefit that varies among practices is the amount of time off granted for continuing education (CE) and the volume of expenses reimbursed. Stipends for CE vary remarkably based on the profitability of the practice and the importance placed upon this benefit by the employer. Some employers maintain that recent grads do not need CE because they just learned all the latest medicine. Other employers understand that CE

focused on subjects where their young doctors feel inadequate improves morale and produces financial dividends for the practice.

Those who attend scientific symposiums on a regular basis know that the education gained through conversations with colleagues in the hallways, over lunch, during happy hours, or by reading the scientific proceedings of the convention often is as valuable as that acquired in the classroom. Moreover, experience has shown that employers who value CE and are willing to invest in it for their employees almost always are the best employers. A review of Table 3.8 and the additional materials on this subject covered in Chapter 7 will help establish an economic value for this benefit when comparing employment offers.

DUES, LICENSES, AND FEES

Often overlooked but critical to the future of the profession is membership in national, state, and local veterinary associations. A voice in governmental affairs is essential for every profession, and only through the oversight of associations and their political action committees (PACs) can veterinary medicine defend its legal and political interests (see Chapter 7).

Although veterinary medical association dues are considerably lower than dues in other professions, they are proportionate to the relative earnings of veterinarians and expensive if paid with after-tax dollars. Therefore, employees find it highly advantageous to have their employers cover these expenses along with their state licensing fees and Drug Enforcement Agency registration fees using pretax dollars. For examples of the professions norms, see Table 3.9.

PROFESSIONAL LIABILITY INSURANCE

Professional liability insurance is covered in depth in Chapter 7. The value of its payment by employers as a pretax benefit for their employees is shown in Table 3.9.

Table 3.7. Valuing Insurance

Health/Disability/Life Insurance with 2008 rates		
Assume a 30-year-old single DVM making $72,000 per year with $1,000 deductible AVMA GHLIT PPO plan paid by employer. During first year post graduation, all DVMs are provided lowest rate, *Area 1*, at an average cost of $2,886/year. Thereafter, premiums are based on area of residence. In this example, rates would increase to $5,034/year at the highest rated *Area 7* in the second year.		
		Annual Cost
Health Insurance - see www.avmaghlit.org for plans and rates	**1st Year** Area 1	**2nd Year** Area 7
Platinum PPO Plan, $1,000 deductible; 80/20 coinsurance	**$2,886**	**$5,034**
Pays 80% of expenses up to $5,000, 100% thereafter		
Note: A variety of even higher deductible policies have lower premiums		
Long-Term Disability Income Insurance		
Selected from various plans offered by AVMA GHLIT		
Plan 2: $3,600 monthly benefit + cost of living adjustment with 30-day wait period	$1,196	$1,196
Plan 3: same policy but with 90-day wait period	$1,030	$1,030
Average cost:	**$1,113**	**$1,113**
Life Insurance		
$200,000 min., nonsmoker (not needed for educational debts)	**$152**	**$152**
Range for Value of Insurance Benefits/Year	**$4,151**	**$6,299**

EMERGENCY DUTY PAY

Less of a benefit and more an additional obligation of employment, emergency duty pay is an important item for negotiation. In many cases, the only way indebted young associates can balance their budgets is to earn supplemental income from their provision of emergency care. Thus, emergency duty pay can be a critical factor when selecting a job.

Emergency duty pay varies according to the type of veterinary employer. Because there are virtually no emergency clinics in large animal practice, emergency duty is considered to be an essential component of employment. In small animal practices, the need for employees to provide emergency coverage varies as follows:

- never needed because all cases are referred to emergency clinics,

- rotating emergency duty among the doctors owning or working for multiple practices in a given city or area (which can make for infrequent emergency duty but high emergency caseloads whenever one is on call),

- weekend and overnight coverage is shared with other veterinarians in the practice, or

- selective acceptance of cases, with those not requiring extensive care or received before 10:00 p.m. or 11:00 p.m. shared between the practice owners and associates and all others referred to emergency clinics or other practices.

For practices that encourage or require employees to provide emergency coverage, it is important to define what constitutes an emergency. The failure to do so can result in employers being angry that their favorite or

Table 3.8. The Value of Continuing Education Benefits

Continuing Education 2009		
Assume norm during the first year of employment is 3 days with pay. By 3rd year it's likely to be 5 days - but if on production, probably without any additional pay.		
	Ranges Offered	Average First Year Benefit
Value of Benefit Offered	$300 to $2,500	**$750**
Average Costs for Attending a National Meeting:		
Registration	$250 to $400	
Airfare/airport parking	$350 to $600	
Hotel/motel (4 days including hotel taxes)	$420 to $700	
Meals	$150 to $250	
Car rental/shuttle costs at destination	$50 to $200	
Total Costs of Attendance	$1,220 to $2,150	

financially strapped clients were charged an expensive emergency examination fee. Conversely, it can result in frustration for young associates who classify situations as emergencies based on client desires, necessitating additional compensation by their employers, only to discover that the employers feel that the cases need not have been seen as emergencies in the first place and, thus, no emergency fee should have been charged.

As a means of providing strong incentives for employed associates to see emergency cases, work them up appropriately, and provide the level of care and concern that bonds these animal owners to their practices, it makes good sense for employers to pay handsomely for their associates' emergency treatment time. After all, in most cases employers have minimal or no overhead during these off hours, and they should appreciate having someone willing to share emergency call duty and bond clients to their practices. Notwithstanding this positive incentive to see emergencies, however, employers often guard the interests of their clients carefully. Thus, their countervailing fear is that they need to prevent employed veterinarians from taking advantage of their clients because of a desire to receive the higher rate of compensation reserved for emergencies. To help alleviate these conflicting concerns, the following definition of *emergency* can be included in employment contracts or veterinary practice policy manuals:

Emergency Defined: The provision of emergency care includes taking histories, referring patients when justified by the history and time of day, performing physical examinations, and providing or performing those diagnostic procedures and therapeutic measures that are essential to stabilize and/or manage patients until the practice reopens for business. When questions exist regarding the need for emergency care, the desires of the animal owners shall take top priority.

Employers and employees need to address and clarify policies regarding referrals of patients to emergency clinics or specialists. Under professional liability law, veterinarians have a legal duty to offer referrals in situations where their practices lack sufficient equipment, facilities, expertise, or off-hours staff to provide the medical services and observation needed. This is partic-

Table 3.9. Valuing Dues, Licenses, Fees, and the Professional Liability Insurance Benefit

Dues, Licenses, and Liability Inurance Premiums - 2009	
Dues and Licenses	**Annual Cost**
AVMA, state VMA, local VMA, specialty associations (most associations have discounted rates for new graduates)	$675
Veterinary license ($100-$200/state)	$100
DEA registration ($551 for 3 years)	$183
Value of Dues & Licenses Benefits:	**$959**
License Defense Policy - $25,000 for legal counsel and expert witnesses Available with purchse of AVMA professional liability policy	**$69**
Professional Liability Insurance Policy www.avmaplit.com Assume: Individual policy needed in addition to employer's coverage	
Small animal practitioner coverage	
$300,000/900,000 (incident/aggregate)	$212
$1 million/$3 million (example used here)*	**$246**
Mixed, predominantly small animal practice	
$300,000/900,000	$301
$1 million/$3 million	$364
Food animal practice	
$300,000/900,000	$821
$1 million/$3 million	$1,015
Equine exclusive practice	
$300,000/900,000	$2,212
$1 million/$3 million	$2,921
Total Value (dues, licenses, insurance) small animal example*	**$1,274**

*2009 figure for small animal practice associates

ularly important for doctors at practices without weekend or overnight staffing who hospitalize critical patients. Practice owners may have left critical patients alone at night for years, but young associates may find this policy untenable when they know that diagnostic procedures, treatments, and overnight patient observation are available at facilities within a reasonable drive of the practice.

Methods for compensating employees who provide emergency care vary remarkably from large to small animal practices and from general practices to specialty practices. The most common methods in use are as follows:

1. as part of the associate's basic salary: This undesirable policy appears to be more common in large animal than small animal practices. It is discouraged, as it gives associates no financial incen-

tives or rewards for seeing emergencies. When employers who have this policy were asked why they do not to provide additional compensation for emergencies, the answers ranged from (a) "because we don't charge our clients an additional fee" (amazingly enough, this occurs commonly in large animal practices but rarely in small animal practices), to (b) "because I'm already paying a top dollar salary and don't feel I need to pay anything extra," to (c) "because we see so few emergencies it is not worth tracking," and (d) "because no one paid me for emergencies when I first went into practice, so why should I pay anyone else?"

2. a set fee per case, e.g., $50 to$75 per case attended: Such policies tend to be minimally motivating, because they provide only a fixed amount of compensation for

clinicians, regardless of the amount of time and effort required to treat cases and communicate with owners.

3. the full emergency examination fee for each case seen: As in Numbers 4 and 5 below, this assumes practices have emergency examination fees above and beyond their office call and examination fees. For example, many small animal practices charge $44 (or $1 times the cost of a 2009 first class postage stamp to keep pace with inflation) for their routine office visits and examinations and then add emergency fees to that amount equaling $60 to $75 for calls prior to 11:00 p.m. and $100 to $130 after 11:00 p.m. The result is that associates who see emergencies receive $60 to $130 for each emergency case they attend, regardless of the time required to provide the needed care. Under this arrangement, there is a viable financial incentive to see cases but no financial reward for providing the extensive in-house diagnostics or time-consuming observation and treatments required by some.

4. 35% to 50% of the emergency examination portion of the call fee plus all fees paid by clients for in-house diagnostic procedures and treatments rendered prior to the time the hospital reopens for business: Although this formula provides less compensation for merely seeing patients, attending doctors are rewarded financially for sticking around and working them up. The concern for employers, of course, is that by assigning all of the fees for treatments to the doctors, employees might easily be inclined to overdo the volume of diagnostics and treatments offered, padding their pockets in the process. Furthermore, such generous compensation packages transfer much of the income from practice owners to emergency clinicians, wiping out profits and, in some cases, resulting in financial losses for practice owners.

5. 100% of the emergency examination call fee plus the same 18% to 22% of the fees for all items identified under the doctor's routine, daytime, gross billable income

definition discussed later in this chapter: This fairly common method of emergency compensation simplifies the computer entry and tracking of such income so receptionists don't have to remember different formulas for day care versus emergency care. It also minimizes employers' worries about their associates' inclinations to run up the emergency fees to earn extra income.

6. provide a base compensation of $50 to $80 per night or $120 per weekend merely for taking emergency call and, in addition, pay attending doctors as per either Numbers 2, 3, 4, or 5 above. Under this highly motivational arrangement, employees generally receive this base level of emergency on-call pay or their earnings under Numbers 2 through 5 above, whichever is greater.

The rationale for providing attractive emergency compensation is multifold. Traditionally, on-call doctors have been compensated only for cases examined and treated. Since only one in three or four small animal emergency calls received requires an office visit and one in two or three large animal calls requires an ambulatory visit, doctors spend lots of on-call time waiting for or triaging calls for which they receive no compensation. Consequently, it seems only proper that they receive ample compensation for the cases they do attend.

Additionally, since most veterinarians who attend emergency patients are expected to restrain their patients themselves or have clients restrain the animals, with no assistance from support staff, practice owners have essentially no extra overhead associated with these cases. Furthermore, unless doctors are adequately compensated for emergency duty, they lose out all around, spending hours fulfilling their on-call duties in order to service one client's request for legitimate emergency assistance. They must answer and triage all calls and, when necessary, drive to the ambulatory site or veterinary hospital, diagnose and treat the emergency, write up the record, and collect payment. Eventually, they return home to try to catch some sleep, exhausted. Worst of all, approximately 10% of the time small animal clients fail to show up at the hospital or get lost en route, leaving the doctors waiting around for an hour getting nothing more than a headache and several hours of lost sleep for the effort.

New associates do benefit from emergency calls in that they have the opportunity to hone their emergency skills and bond with appreciative animal owners much more quickly than they can during the provision of routine care. This helps to grow the clientele and build one's reputation in the community more rapidly than almost any other method. Nevertheless, employers still are the primary beneficiaries because most of their associates will come and go, while their practices inherit the long-term bonding benefits with minimal costs to acquire these new clients. Without adequate compensation, though, the experience they gain comes with insufficient personal financial reward to offset the stresses caused by the provision of such medical care.

In sum, when the provision of emergency care is a required element of employment, compensation packages should be motivational for employees and fair to clients and employers. With proper thought and planning, everyone wins. Animals receive better care, on-call associates benefit from emergency care experiences and increased pay, clients will not be overcharged by overly eager associates motivated more by money than medicine, and employers will be able to build the reputations of their practices. Ultimately, well-paid emergency doctors are more likely to provide the compassion, enthusiasm, empathy, and quality of medical care desired by all the players.

Paying Doctors and Establishing Emergency Fees

Most employers pay additional emergency service compensation to employed veterinarians only in those circumstances where clients have paid at least 75% of their bills for such services. For young doctors who believe they earned this additional money regardless of whether clients have paid their bills, this seems like a harsh dose of reality. However, many employers feel it is critical that their employees

- learn not to give away services to insolvent or deadbeat animal owners even under emergency circumstances,

- learn to discuss money as well as medicine before attending cases or running up big bills, and

- understand that without payment by clients for these services, they cannot afford to pay their staff and make ends meet.

How should practices establish emergency after-hours examination fees? The most appropriate way is to query another trade group. In Yardley, PA in 2009, plumbers charge one and a half their $110/hour rate, portal to portal, with a minimum fee of $165. They do not charge flat, add-on emergency fees. Instead, they increase their hourly rates, including double time for holidays. Since it is difficult to determine how long it takes to treat emergency plumbing disorders, conducting their business is a lot like offering veterinary services. The author's experience is that add-on emergency fees range from $50 to $100 for evenings and $90 to $125 after 11 p.m. and on holidays. Table 3.10 shows two different forms of emergency duty pay.

Percentage-Based Compensation as a Benefit

The subject of commission-based or percentage-based compensation is discussed in detail later in this chapter. Because of its importance in adequate budget preparations prior to contract negotiations, however, a brief synopsis and two hypothetical examples of its effect are included here.

Table 3.10. Two Common Plans for Emergency Duty Compensation

Emergency duty pay varies widely, with some practices offering no additional compensation. Also, don't forget that seeing all these patients and taking the calls that generated them takes a great deal of time and creates significant disruptions in one's home life.

1. Flat Rate Per Call ($60 is still common in addition to the office call fee	
3 DVMs (including practice owner) share weeknights - on call twice/week	
Average 1 emergency every other shift	
= 88 weeknights x 0.5 call @ $60 each	$2,640
2 DVMs (excluding owner) share weekends - on call every other weekend	
Average 2 calls/weekend	
= 26 weekends x 2 calls @ $60 each	$3,120
Total Emergency Income with No Additional Production Compensation (96 calls @ $60/call)	**$5,760**
2. Percent of Gross Income Per Call (100% of the emergency fee plus 25-50% of revenue generated until the practice reopens for business)	
Example: Average transaction per case for fees in excess of the emergency call fee: $180	
100% of $60 emergency call x 96 calls	$5,760
30% of additional $180/call x 96 calls	$5,184
Total: (96 calls @ $60/call + 30% revenue generated)	**$10,944**

The most common method of compensation in veterinary medicine is to provide associates with base salaries or percentages of income generated by their medical efforts and collected by their employers, whichever is higher. There are many variations on this theme in private practice, but basically they all allow doctors to receive guaranteed monthly salaries as well as production reconciliation compensation in each month or quarter of the year after the conclusion of the base pay period.

Percentage-based pay is not so much a benefit as it is a business philosophy. Some employers have tried it and found that it creates too much competition between doctors. Others have tested the waters and concluded that, with good leadership, it generates considerable growth in their practices while helping their doctors earn higher salaries. A New England study found that associates paid on a percentage of productivity generate 14% more revenue than their flat-salary based counterparts, and practices that base compensation on productivity earn 26% more than practices that do not.[41]

For doctors with expensive lifestyles or massive debts, this type of compensation gives them some control over their earnings. Although they may not be able to control their patient loads or the fee schedule for the practices, they can effectively increase their personal income by becoming outstanding communicators, providing optimal veterinary care for patients, charging for all services performed, and managing their time effectively. Systems for calculating percentage-based compensation are illustrated in Tables 3.11 & 3.12.

COMPARING JOB OFFERS

The goal of this budget exercise has been to place approximate dollar amounts on various employee benefits, compare them in hypothetical job offers, and calculate the total value of each job offer before and after the tax consequences of the benefits.

Table 3.13 illustrates the remarkable variation in two employment contract offers. The first practice, Lakeview, starts with a fairly low salary, adds many desirable employee benefits to it, and offers the opportunity for considerable income generation via the provision of emergency care. The

Table 3.11. An Example of Percentage-Based Compensation and Common Percentages for Various Specialties in the Profession

Productivity Pay/"Pro Sal" - 2009
See Figure 4.1, p.162 for the most accurate way to value an entire compensation package

Productivity pay is extremely variable — there are probably as many formulas as there are practices! Needs good definition of income produced to work. Here are two common plans:

1. Percent of productivity above base salary

Example: Base salary of $70,000 for up to $350,000/year of income production (equal to 20% of $350,000) plus 10% of income production above that

Base salary		$70,000
Associate's hypothetical annual gross income production	$390,000	
Required base income production prior to 10% commission	-$350,000	
Production above base	$40,000	
Additional percentage for excess production	x 10%	
Compensation bonus		$4,000
Total veterinary compensation for year		$74,000
Benefits (average for first job immediately post graduation)		
Health, disability, and life insurance Table 3.7 (could rise to $6,299 next year)		$4,151
Continuing education - Table 3.8		$750
Dues, licenses, liability insurance (average small animal) Table 3.9		$1,374
Total average fringe benefits		$6,275
Total compensation for year including benefits		**$80,275**

2. Straight Percent of Productivity

Example: 20% of income produced, plus benefits

Gross income produced	$390,000	
	x 20%	
Total veterinary compensation for year	$78,000	
Total average fringe benefits		$6,275
Total compensation for year including benefits		**$84,275**

Common % numbers among general practices:

Small animal general practice	18-22% + benefits
Large animal general practice	22-25% + benefits
Small animal % with payroll taxes & benefits deducted	25-26%
Emergency practices	20-30% + benefits

Common % numbers among specialty practices:

Animal behaviorists	33-50% + benefits
Cardiologists	28-32% + benefits
Dermatologists	35-50% + benefits
Internal medicine & oncology	23-27% + benefits
Soft tissue surgeons	23-28% + benefits
Opthalmologists & neurologists	26-30% + benefits
Orthopedic surgeons	23-25% + benefits

Table 3.12. Comparing Job Offers

1. **Lakeview Veterinary Clinic**

   Suburban practice, sole proprietor, 3 doctors (you are replacing associate who is moving to Alaska)
   Busy practice, 3 doctors share weeknight emergency duty, 2 doctors share weekend duty

Base pay	$72,000
Emergency duty	$60 per case seen
Insurance benefits (health, dis, life)	AVMA
Continuing education	Yes
Dues, licenses, DEA	Yes
Professional liability and license defense	AVMA

   Or...

2. **Central Animal Hospital**

   Urban/suburban practice, incorporated, 4 DVMs expanding to 5 (you). Busy; appears to be growing. All emergency work sent to a cooperative emergency clinic (no emergency pay).

Base pay	$78,000
Incentive pay	10% of gross over $390,000
Insurance benefits	None
Continuing education	None
Dues , licenses, DEA	None
Professional liability and license defense	None

second practice, Central, offers a salary that is $6,000 higher than Lakeview, sends all of its emergencies to an emergency hospital nearby, and provides almost no employee benefits. On first blush, the latter of these two looks like a very attractive offer, especially for someone who does not wish to tolerate the disruptions inherent in the provision of emergency care.

When asked, "Which job do you want?" the answer could easily be, "The job with no emergencies!" However, the more important question to ask is, "Which job will I need to balance my budget?"

As discussed earlier, the question regarding which offer will fit one's budgetary needs cannot be readily answered until applicants have completed their personal budgets.

On one hand, it may be that neither of the offers is satisfactory because of personal budgetary requirements in the $70,000 to $80,000 range. On the other hand, assuming either job offer will cover an applicant's budget, all those benefits at Lakeview, despite the volume of emergency cases attended, may look more enticing to applicants than the insecurity of generating $390,000 of collectible income at Central. This is especially true if the owner's spouse is the practice manager and/or receptionist at Central, i.e., someone who has considerable control over the distribution of clients among the practice's doctors and a bias in favor of the practice owner.

Table 3.13. A Comparison of the Monetary Values of Two Employment Offers

	Income	
	Lakeview	Central
Base pay	$72,000	$78,000
Medical insurance	Paid by employer	None
Continuing education – $500/yr.	Paid by employer	None
Dues, licenses, DEA	Paid by employer	None
Professional liability & Lic def rider	Paid by employer	None
Retirement	N/A	N/A
Emergency pay	$5,000	None
Productivity pay	None	10% of production over $390,000
Total compensation	$77,000	$78,000

	Effect on Budget			
	Lakeview		Central	
Individual expenses	W/Car Loan	W/O Car Loan	W/Car Loan	W/O Car Loan
Cost of living	$48,360	$42,360	$48,360	$42,360
Med/dis/life insurance	$0	$0	$4,032	$4,032
Continuing education	$0	$0	$1,000	$1,000
Dues	$0	$0	$750	$750
Professional liability & Lic def rider	$0	$0	$315	$315
Debt management (assumes $119,820 nat'l average 2008 for 25 years)	$9,960	$9,960	$9,960	$9,960
Savings	$1,200	$1,200	$1,200	$1,200
Total expenses	$59,520	$53,520	$65,617	$59,617
Less interest tax deduction on student loan	$2,500	$2,500	$2,500	$2,500
Adjusted total expenses	$57,020	$51,020	$63,117	$57,117
x Tax Multiplier from Table 3.5	1.457	1.439	1.475	1.460
Needed gross income	$83,078	$73,418	$93,098	$83,219
Actual gross income	$77,000	$77,000	$78,000	$78,000
Extra/(short)	($6,078)	$3,582	($15,098)	($5,219)
Difference: Without a car loan, Lakeview is better by: $3,582 – ($5,219) =$8,802				

Table 3.14. Determining the Income Production Needed to Equate the Offer from Lakeview

In Summation:			
To receive income comparable to the doctor at Lakeview, the doctor at Central must generate:			
$478,020	Total income production		$88,020 of income in excess of the $390,000 upon which his/her initial salary was based
($390,000)	Income production upon which base salary was predicated	x	$88,020 x 10%
$88,020	Additional income production above base level		$8,802 additional salary needed to equal Central
		+	Plus base salary of $78,000
			Total compensation $86,802 to equal Central's package with benefits

Note: While the offer at Central initially appeared to be more desirable because it included a higher base salary, no emergency calls, and the potential for incentive pay, Lakeview may prove to have been a better offer!!!

TODAY'S NORMS IN BASE SALARIES AND BENEFITS

A key component of any job offer, and the one on which new graduates tend to focus, is base salary. The mean starting salary for new graduates entering private practice in 2008 was $61,518, with small animal exclusive practices paying the highest salaries at $64,744 and equine practices paying the lowest at $41,636.[42] This reflects an increase of 5.9% over starting salaries for new graduates in 2007, as compared to a similar 5.7% jump over 2006.[42]

Geographic location certainly affects salaries. Historically, associates in the northeastern United States and West Coast have had higher base salaries than those in the southeastern, Great Lakes, and central regions.[43] Contributing factors may include differences in the cost of living, depth of the human-animal bond, and supply and demand for veterinarians in these locations. It appears to be more than coincidental that 15 of the 27 veterinary schools are located in the least populous mid-section of the country. Perhaps this has led to an oversupply of veterinarians in those regions and, subse-

quently, lower salaries than in the populous, undersupplied coastal regions of the United States. A study performed by AAHA shows salaries in low, medium, and high cost of living regions of the country. Surprisingly, it reveals that salaries do not necessarily correspond to the cost of living index.[44]

In addition to geographic location and years of experience, a practitioner's sex also appears to impact salary. In recent years, several studies have addressed the salary difference between male and female veterinarians. Unfortunately, the conclusions that can be drawn are limited by the data collection and methods of analysis employed. However, a study of income data by *Veterinary Economics* revealed that the average net income for female veterinarians in 1990 was only 60% of that for male veterinarians.[45] A follow-up article detailed the differences in demographics between male and female survey respondents. Productivity did not appear to be a contributing factor, because reported data on average client transaction fees, number of client visits per week, and numbers of hours devoted to practice per week were remarkably similar.[46] However, nearly 80% of the men surveyed were practice owners, whereas only 45% of women respondents were owners.[46]

This fact alone could account for a considerable amount of the reported difference in net income. Unfortunately, net incomes broken into four categories based on ownership status and sex were not available in this study. Likewise, the data did not reveal the effects of private practice type on the salaries of male versus female veterinarians. Furthermore, no study has evaluated the impact of nonveterinary female spouses working in their husbands' veterinary practices and receiving either no salary or an understated salary as a means of avoiding the payment of FICA and Medicare taxes on their income. If this situation occurs as often as suspected, especially with older practitioners, it could account for a considerable portion of the disparity.

Nonetheless, the most recent AVMA survey of veterinary compensation reaffirms the differences reported earlier in the *Veterinary Economics* study. This 2007 study found that female practice owners earned $115,768 compared to male owners earning $158,910 — a difference of $43,142 more per year.[4] While it is true that male practice owners worked nearly five hours more per week than female owners, they also earned approximately $8.50 more per hour than did their female counterparts.[5] Additionally, while the average male associate earned $102,672 and worked 44.75 hours per week, the average female associate earned $83,106 working 38.88 hours per week, a difference of $19,566 per year and 5.9 hours per week.[4] When income was compared on an hourly basis, male owners earned $65.57 per hour while females earned $54.03, a difference of $11.54 per hour and male associates earned $44.75 per hour versus females at $38.88, a difference of $9.28 per hour.[5]

While ownership and years in practice have been cited to explain some income discrepancies between men and women veterinarians in previous studies, these factors fail to substantiate the discrepancies in the 2007 AVMA data. Median salaries for male owners

of equine practices were $60,000 higher than females, $48,000 in companion animal, and $36,000 in food and mixed animal. Medians for male associates in equine practices were $22,000 higher, $18,000 higher in companion and food animal exclusive, and $6,000 in mixed animal.[48]

An analysis of mean starting salaries of new graduates from 2006 to 2008 showed that starting salaries for male graduates were slightly higher than for female graduates in all six of the private practice types identified in the survey (large animal exclusive, large animal predominant, mixed animal, small animal predominant, small animal exclusive, and equine).[49]

It could be argued that veterinary employers consciously or subconsciously offer male associates higher salaries because they have been such a minority among the professional and lay veterinary staff for the past 15 years. It is not uncommon for practices to seek out male associates to help provide balance to an otherwise female-dominated profession, especially when one considers the prevalence of females in the profession as support staff. In their desire to hire male graduates, practices may try to entice them by offering higher salaries, much as they would to any highly desirable new associate. While this type of potential hiring bias merits further investigation, designing and conducting a study to explore its ramifications on salary would be a tall task.

A data collection quirk inherent in the previously cited compensation studies is that the salaries are self-reported by veterinarians. No system exists for confirming the accuracy of the data. When interpreting any data from these surveys, researchers are forced to assume that male and female veterinarians report their salaries with equal honesty and accuracy. As reported in Carin Smith DVM's excellent article on gender and work, this could be an erroneous assumption. (JAVMA 220(9) 1304-1311, 2002.

It also is problematic that both new graduates and employed veterinarians could choose not to submit the salary surveys that they received from the AVMA or *Veterinary Economics*. Arguably, men receiving generous compensation may be more inclined to submit their salary surveys than men receiving below average salaries. This type of self-selection bias could lead to errors in calculating the true mean salaries of veterinarians employed in private practice. While several of the studies cited above conclude that more research is needed on salary discrepancies based on sex, it is important that these new studies be designed and analyzed in a manner that allows these issues to be addressed with accuracy.

Another important aspect to consider is noncash benefits. According to AVMA data, approximately half of all new graduates entering private practice received noncash benefits.[48] These packages commonly included health care plans; payments for continuing education expenses; liability insurance; licenses; association dues; and leave granted for annual vacations, sick time, and continuing education. Less than 20% of benefits packages included pension plans, profit sharing, or dental plans.[48] Unlike base salaries, there were no significant differences in benefit packages offered to male versus female graduates in 1997.

POTENTIAL UNDERREPORTING OF NEW GRADUATE SALARIES

In view of the increasing popularity of percentage-based or commission-based salaries in the profession, it is likely that starting salaries for new graduates are deceiving. Since these individuals complete their AVMA salary questionnaires at the time they graduate, they have no choice but to report their base salary as the salary for their first year. The authors have found, however, that many new graduates generate over $350,000 and in some cases greater than $500,000 of income their first year. Those

who received percentage-based compensation often reported that they were paid $70,000 to as high as $95,000 during their first few years of practice even though their base salaries were in the mid $60,000 to mid $80,000 range.

In fact, the authors are aware of several recent University of Pennsylvania graduates plagued with massive debts (over $180,000) who have found ways to earn $90,000 to $200,000 by working two jobs or being employed at busy practices that provide salaries of 20% of income paid by clients or higher. When push comes to shove, it is amazing what effect the fear of financial failure can have on the earning power of highly indebted young veterinarians.

COMPENSATION SYSTEMS FOR ASSOCIATE VETERINARIANS

Previous materials have examined salaries for new graduates, associate veterinarians, and practice owners. These change from year to year and, thus, for the most current information, readers should review the annual salary reports in *JAVMA* or reports generated by the AAHA. However, as introduced earlier in the chapter, a growing method for compensating veterinarians involves paying them based on predetermined percentages of or commissions on their collected gross incomes.[50,51] Although further refinement in the percentages paid to associates can be expected as the veterinary business climate changes, most of the percentage figures discussed in this chapter have been in vogue for many years and are unlikely to change remarkably in the years ahead.

COMPENSATION FOR ROUTINE DAYTIME CARE

There are three principal methods for paying associates for daytime (nonemergency) veterinary services. These are (1) flat salaries plus benefit packages, (2) straight commission-based salaries with or without benefits, and (3) production reconciliation hybrids, with or without benefits, that guarantee monthly or quarterly base salaries but then reconcile that base with preestablished percentages of collected revenues during specified time periods and, ultimately, pay the higher of the two at the end of the time period.

FLAT SALARIES PLUS BENEFITS

Under the most commonly used compensation system, employees receive compensation established at a set dollar rate per day, month, or year (the base salary). This is the time-tested, "warm-body" method of payment whereby salaries are fixed until raises are given, usually at the beginning of each new year. Under this traditional system of compensation, employees expect annual raises merely because of their time in service.

This is commonly referred to as the "entitlement" theory of employment, wherein employees conclude they are entitled to compensation based on their educational degree and years of service, rather than productivity, acceptance by clients and staff, time management skills, compliance with hospital policies, professional growth, and contributions to the business.[52]

As of 2009, salaries for generalists ranged from $35 to $75 per hour depending on the level of experience, region of country, schedules worked, and type of veterinary medicine practiced, i.e., small vs. large vs. emergency medicine. Yearly salaries for full-time associates vary from as low as $45,000 in some equine practices to as high as $190,000 for experienced small animal clinicians in large urban settings. Meager, moderate, or major benefit packages generally accompany these flat salaries.

STRAIGHT COMMISSION-BASED PAY

The second system of associate compensation is derived from commissions equal to 18% to 25% of the gross billable income generated by the employees' efforts and paid by clients to small animal practice owners[50,52,53,54,55] and 25% to 30% for large animal practices. In this system, associates depend on receptionists to fill their schedules and help them generate their salaries. Their financial picture improves with hard work and pleasing clients with their punctuality, quality of medical care, compassion, and communications. The more these qualities are in place, the more is charged for all the services they perform and products they prescribe; and the more often their employers raise their fees the better off they are. Under this system, associates have an opportunity to control their own financial destiny, a quality that is not possible with flat salary compensation.

A problem with this system is that it often stimulates acrimonious competition between doctors for the largest volume of or most economically advantageous cases. Thus, it is not among the favored forms of compensation for employees, unless it is accompanied by a base salary as discussed in the third system of compensation, the hybrid.

Although commissions as low as 18% of income collected, plus benefits, may be acceptable starting points in some practices, this level is on the low end of the scale. Nonetheless, occasional practices exist where the fee schedules, quality and quantity of staff, time management skills of the doctors and client volume are sufficient to generate above-average income per doctor even at this low percentage. For most practices, the 19% to 21% range, plus benefits, is a more appropriate starting point for small animal practices, with 20% the accepted norm. Because of lower staff overhead costs and lost work time traveling between ambulatory calls, large animal practices usually pay commissions in the 25% to 27% of income collected range.

Commissions of 21% to 22% are sometimes used for exceptionally good, community-service-oriented, more senior, staff mentor types of veterinarians. In general, this factor can raise or lower pay 1% to 2% to compensate for the goodwill–building activities of key associates.[54] This higher percentage range also may be essential in understaffed practices where veterinary associates spend considerable time completing routine animal nursing, patient treatments, and diagnostic tasks.[51,52] Commissions as high as 23% plus benefits generally are reserved for small animal practice owners and key associates who have excellent medical, surgical, communication, teamwork, and leadership skills to accompany their long-term familiarity with the clients and the community.

In sum, percentages paid under commission-based systems must vary. In a September 1992 Veterinary Economics article, Dr. Ross Clark outlines many key management and practice expense issues that affect these numbers.[54] They include:

- the quantity, quality, training, and salaries of support staff,

- the definition of and method used to calculate the doctors' production,

- the amount of capital the practice has invested in sophisticated equipment and the physical plant,

- the volume of advertising and marketing expenses experienced by the practice,

- the mix of services provided (high vs. low product and service sales),

- nonrevenue associate activities that contribute to the practice's financial success (such as community leadership and service and speaking at local schools, service organizations, or youth organizations),

Additional issues beyond those observed by Dr. Clark include:

- the practice's fee schedule and the frequency with which it is upgraded,

- the size and age of the practice,

- the floor plan of the physical plant in which the practice operates (older facilities tend to have multiple small rooms with many doors and windows, making it difficult to locate and use staff efficiently; newer ones tend to have central treatment areas without hallways, and windows instead of walls between rooms),

- unique overhead problems experienced by employers such as the extremely high rent often experienced by young practices, and

- the time management efficiencies, teamwork qualities, and moral, ethical, and competitive values of each employed veterinarian.

It is because of all these factors that percentage-based compensations packages will continue to vary throughout the industry.

PRODUCTION RECONCILIATION HYBRIDS

This method of compensation combines the previous two. Under this system, employees are guaranteed specified base salaries but are paid a percentage of their gross income collected by their employers when this yields a higher take-home pay than they would earn from a flat salary.[50,56] This compensation system has also been called the ProSal formula.[51] With production reconciliation methods, base salaries are set either by (1) selecting salary numbers approximating that paid equally qualified and skilled veterinarians in the city, county, or region of the country; (2) deciding on the specified percentage of an estimated income production figure the employee is likely to generate and using that number as the base, or (3) pulling a number out of a hat in hopes that it will be approximately 20% lower than the salary employees are likely to earn under their percentage-based compensation formulas.

With this system, production reconciliation bonuses are used to augment employees' salaries either monthly or quarterly when their percentage-based production exceeds their base salaries. However, when employees fail to meet their income production goals and have been overpaid during the previous time periods, well-conceived plans require that the shortfall be carried over to the next financial time period and subtracted from that period's production reconciliation calculation before any additional compensation is due. If at the end of the fiscal year employees have not been as productive as anticipated and carry negative reconciliation balances, they are not financially responsible for the differences but will either be terminated or have their estimated gross income production and bases salaries adjusted downward for the following contract year. This concept and contract language to deal with its nuances will be discussed again later in the chapter.

Guaranteeing base salaries affords constant income and security to associates, especially those who are anxious about their educational or other debts. Providing associates the option of commission-based salaries affords them the benefit of financial rewards for the possession and development of important technical and communication skills, the development of successful sales skills, good time management techniques, and hard work.

A pitfall encountered frequently by employers is the risk of establishing base salaries that are very close to the salaries their associates will earn under their percentage-based calculations. For example, an employer offers a base salary of $70,000 or 20% of income collected, whichever is higher. As the year progresses, it becomes apparent that the employee is unlikely to exceed $350,000 of collected income. When this occurs, there are no or very limited financial incentives for associates to increase their production.

However, when practices are well managed and base salaries sufficiently below the associate's percentage-based earning capacity, e.g., $70,000 in the above example, both employers and employees can do well. The result is that employees are able to exert considerable control over their own income and raises, while employers should be able to receive 10% to 15% profit returns on their investments in the business and on their employees' time.

PERCENTAGES PAID TO LARGE ANIMAL ASSOCIATES, EMERGENCY CLINICIANS, AND SPECIALISTS

All of the prior discussion has focused on percentage-based compensation for generalists in small animal practice. The subject becomes even more complicated when practice owners need to determine what to pay equine practitioners, bovine and porcine food-animal associates, mixed-animal employees, emergency clinicians, and veterinary specialists.

Emergency Medicine

Because of the disagreeable hours, higher fees for emergency services, long shifts, and shortage of qualified and enthusiastic emergency clinicians, veterinarians in this medical specialty generally receive higher percentages of income collected than generalists. In the 1970s and early 80s, emergency clinics often paid as high as 32% of income collected. However, as competition among emergency clinics has increased and overhead costs for the treatment and monitoring of critically ill patients have risen, salaries available for emergency doctors have dropped somewhat. Currently, most emergency clinics offer percentages in the 22% to 25% range depending on the volume of cases seen and overhead of the facility.[57,58] The key to finding and keeping quality emergency clinicians is to pay them as highly as possible after paying good salaries for support staff and allowing owners to make a reasonable profit.

Boarded Specialists

Specialists are compensated in one of three ways: (1) as employees of general, emergency care, or specialty practices; (2) as independent contractors responsible for their own staff, appointments, medical records, and collections; or (3) as tenants or subtenants of facilities wherein they operate their own businesses but share overhead with other separate specialty businesses in the facility. Salaries for employees and percentages of income production for employees and independent contractors vary extensively because of differences in expenses for equipment, hospital floor space required, leasehold improvements, drugs, and staff.

Examples of specialties with heavy overhead costs include orthopedic surgery (surgical equipment and implant hardware), critical care (floor space, respirators, oxygen cages, blood gas machines, infusion pumps, monitoring devices, and highly trained staff), internal medicine (endoscopy, ultrasonography, expensive drugs, and a large staff), oncology (increased staffing costs for seriously ill and hospitalized cases, and inventories of expensive drugs), ophthalmology (a darkened exam room, electroretinograpy and tonotometry equipment, and an array of surgical instruments), and radiology (fluoroscopy, ultrasound, and excellent x-ray equipment and film processors).

Specialties with moderate overhead costs include cardiology (ultrasonography and electrocardiography but limited drugs and staff) and neurology (electromyography and access to good imaging equipment). Those with light overhead costs include dermatology (a technician, an exam room, and an inventory of hyposensitization vaccines), clinical nutrition (a computer, a kitchen, and some specialized food), and animal behavior (an exam room and a phone).

Because of limited numbers of residency programs in dermatology, ophthalmology, animal behavior, radiology, neurology, cardiology, oncology, and dentistry, competition for specialists in these areas has driven salaries and percentage-based compensation up in recent years. It is unlikely that the numbers of these residencies will increase signifi-

cantly in the near future.[59] Hence, shortages of clinicians in some of these specialties probably will continue to grow, while surpluses may occur on a regional basis in surgery and internal medicine.

According to Owen McCafferty, CPA, "The good news is that by the year 2000, there will be so many more people graduating with specialist designations, there will be wonderful opportunities for existing practitioners in the marketplace." The result is that "doctors [generalists] will be using specialists to build and create new profit-centers in their practices."[60]

Specialists usually are offered between 23% and 40% of income collected plus benefits.[61] The agreed-upon percentages (set forth in more detail on page 107) depend on the

- employers' overhead and start-up costs for the particular specialty,

- individual specialty and amount of competition in the region among similarly qualified specialists,

- specialist's level of experience and status as a board-qualified vs. board-certified doctor,

- perceived market value of the specialty to referring veterinarians and animal owners,

- employer's desires to add a particular specialty or charismatic specialist to the practice, and

- bargaining powers and communication skills of the applicants.

Large Animal Practices

Reports on compensation in large animal practice are few, but according to one author, using "the commission system [of compensation] has eliminated much of the complaining that occurred in our practice as individual veterinarians developed new programs.[62] Now all veterinarians are fairly compensated so if one works harder, they [sic] are paid more for their [sic] efforts." In the system employed by this Wisconsin dairy practitioner, commissions were 50% on professional services and 15% on lab fees, feed testing, feed sales, drugs used or dispensed, and other services.[62-66]

In a Pennsylvania large animal practice where percentage-based compensation has been used for 12 years, associates receive 15% of all drug and supply sales and 30% to 38% of the fees for professional services billed by the practice. Newly hired inexperienced veterinarians ride with experienced veterinarians at the practice for the first three to four months of their employment, during which time they are paid $100 per day. Thereafter, they start on the practice's commission-based compensation system, gradually migrating from 30% of income billed to clients to 38% as they mature in the practice.

Most associates at this practice earn gross personal incomes of approximately $50,000. In addition to this monetary compensation, associates are provided with health and professional liability insurance, vehicles, license fees, emergency phone expenses, and AVMA, PVMA, local VMA dues, and a choice of AAEP or AABP dues, depending on the doctor's specialty.[67,68]

Equine Practices

As reported in *Veterinary Economics*[69], half of all equine practices pay associates fixed salaries, and those that pay a percentage do so based on either total production or collected revenues. According to the in-depth 2008 AAEP Lifestyles and Salary Survey, the average salary for an equine associate was $75,940. Of note with respect to equine practice is the fact that that already small segment of the veterinary profession is broken down further into general practice, track, hospital, broodmare, and mixed equine practices. Hours worked per week vary among these subspecialties from 45 to 47 hours for general, broodmare, and mixed practices to 53 to 54 for track and hospital practices.

PERCENTAGE-BASED COMPENSATION WITH OR WITHOUT BENEFITS

Comparing percentage-based compensation contracts with or without benefits for associate veterinarians can be tremendously confusing. This is because percentage-based compensation systems are often discussed without addressing the sizable variations in benefits among practices. Because the scope and value of employers' benefits differ so greatly from one practice to another, comparing total compensation packages becomes even more bewildering when employers and consultants add different types of percentage-based systems of compensation to the mix.

BASE SALARIES OR PERCENTAGE-BASED COMPENSATION

There are three basic ways that combinations of percentage-based compensation and benefits can be determined and assessed. The first method is for employers to pay either a fixed monthly, quarterly, or yearly guaranteed base salary or a percentage-based salary, whichever is highest, plus benefit packages for their associates.

The second method is to pay small animal associates based entirely on a commission of 25% of income collected from clients (or large animal associates at the 30% level), without a guaranteed base salary, and deduct the costs of all employee benefits from their gross earnings. This method of compensation came into vogue in the early 1980s, at which time practice owners allowed employees to select which benefits they wanted to receive and then deducted the value of those benefits from their employees' 25% of income-collected paychecks. In the

- employers' and employee's share of FICA and Medicare;
- costs of federal, and sometimes state, unemployment insurance costs;
- employers' costs of workers compensation coverage for the employee;
- costs of the employees' health coverage; and
- cost or value of any other benefits desired by employees such as vacation, continuing education, professional liability insurance, disability insurance, and pension plan contributions.

As one might guess, all of this confusion led to employment disputes, distrust between employers and employees, resignations, terminations and, in some cases, lawsuits.

The third method of percentage-based compensation is a blend of the first two, wherein employers' percentage commissions are somewhere between those offered in Categories 1 and 2. In these examples, some employers pay their required share of FICA, Medicare, and workers compensation instead of deducting that amount from the associates' earnings, but deduct all other benefits. Other employers do the same but pay for some additional benefits and charge employees for others.

The example shown in Figure 3.2 was created by the authors and Ms. Marty Bezner, practice manager for Boulevard Animal Hospital in Syracuse, New York, in response to disagreements and confusion with veterinary associates who worked in the practice she managed. As seen in the last line of the spreadsheet, associate compensation for generalists based on 20% of income collected plus benefits paid by employers is identical to 25% of what is termed in the industry *no benefits*. In this context, and as shown throughout the details of Figure 3.2, no benefits means that all employer-related payroll taxes and all costs of employees' benefits are deducted from the 25%-income-collected compensation figure. One of the principal reasons for

including Figure 3.2 is to illustrate that employers' costs for payroll taxes and standard benefits packages consume 5% of income paid by clients to employers. Thus, 20% with benefits generally is equal to 25% with no benefits.

The 25% of income collected minus benefits method of compensation makes life easy for employers, who simply deduct all employer payroll taxes and whatever benefits their employees would like from their percentage-based earnings. It also brings with it serious detriments, though. For example, associates who are not good at budgeting tend to adjust their expenses to fit the salaries to which they have grown accustomed under their percentage-based salaries. When this occurs, they often do not have any money left over to pay their association dues or register for and attend continuing education seminars because they already have used their income to pay other expenses.

Even more problematic, some associates discover that they have spent all their income on day-to-day living costs and cannot afford to take any time off for sick days or vacation. This can negatively affect their mental attitudes and productivity. Thus, they end up working many more days per year than they had planned because they fear the financial consequences of not working every possible day.

For several complicated tax reasons, including the potential disqualification of employers' pension plan contributions, to avoid employer-employee distrust, and for simplicity, the "percent of income collected plus benefits" plan is a better system for employees and employers than the alternative. Consequently, its use is encouraged over the "25% of income collected with no benefits" system of compensation.

Conflicts Regarding the Provision of Benefits

Conflicts regarding the provision of benefits often arise between employers and

Incentive Compensation for Employed DVMs		
Plan A: 25% -- No benefits, employer's and employee's payroll taxes deducted from salary Plan B: 20% -- With benefits provided by employer, employer's payroll taxes paid by employer		
	Base Salary = $60,000	
Comparing Plan A with Plan B	**Plan A = 25%**	**Plan B = 20%**
Dr. gross income billed Dr. gross revenues received by employer	$315,000.00 $300,000.00	$315,000.00 $300,000.00
Compensation owed based on % plan	**$75,000.00**	**$60,000.00**
Employer expenses Base salary during year Employer's share of FICA and Medicare 6.2% & 1.45% Health insurance State unemployment .03/$7,000 Fed unemployment .062/$7,000 Employer's worker's compensation costs 3.99% Disability insurance $2.73/wk AVMA professional liability insurance - $1,000,000 Other reimbursable professional expenses Vacation/personal/sick leave/2.5 wks Continuing education - registration, travel, lodging **Total employer expenses before bonus**	$60,000.00 $4,590.00 $1,620.00 $210.00 $434.00 $2,394.00 $141.96 $247.00 $0.00 $0.00 $1,250.00 **$70,886.96**	$60,000.00 $4,590.00 $1,620.00 $210.00 $434.00 $2,394.00 $141.96 $247.00 $0.00 $2,884.62 $1,250.00 **$73,771.58**
Dr. bonus before employer's expenses $75,000 - $70,886.96 = $4,113.04	**$4,113.04**	0
Less employer expenses (paid by employee) Employer share of FICA 6.2% of first $68,400 + 1.45% Medicare Worker's compensation .0399 **Adjust for employer's expenses**	$314.65 $164.11 **$478.76**	$0.00 $0.00 **$0.00**
Dr. bonus after employer's expenses $2,109.04 - $245.49 = $1,863.55	**$3,634.28**	**$0.00**
Dr. base salary/bonus before tax Base salary during year Bonus after employer expenses	$60,000.00 $3,634.28	$60,000.00 $0.00
Base salary/bonus before tax Base salary/bonus as a % of gross received	**$63,634.28** 21.211%	**$60,000.00** 20.000%
Less employee taxes on base salary/bonus Employer share of FICA 6.2% of first $68,400 + 1.45% Medicare Federal withholding tax approx. 20% State withholding tax approx. 10%	$4,590.00 $12,726.86 $6,363.43	$4,590.00 $12,000.00 $6,000.00
Dr.'s take-home salary after taxes Dr's take-home % of gross received	**$39,954.00** 13.318%	**$37,410.00** 12.470%
Dr. salary/bonus & benefit package Base salary/bonus before tax Vacation/personal/sick leave/2.5 weeks AVMA professional liability insurance Health insurance Continuing education - registration, travel, lodging	$63,634.28 $0.00 $247.00 $1,620.00 $1,250.00	$60,000.00 $2,884.62 $247.00 $1,620.00 $1,250.00
Dr. package comparison Dr. package % of gross received	**$66,751.28** 22.250%	**$66,001.62** 22.001%
Employer expenses for Dr. Employer expenses % of gross received	**$75,000.00** 25.000%	**$60,000.00** 20.000%

Figure 3.2. An incentive compensation spreadsheet created by the authors and Ms. Marty Bezner, Practice Manager at Boulevard Animal Hospital, Syracuse, New York.

employees when employers are forced to explain why they cannot afford all the benefits their associates would like. Disputes are even more likely to occur when employers are asked to provide disparate benefit packages to accommodate the desires of different employees. For example, some doctors who are married receive health insurance through their spouses' jobs and, thus, prefer receiving higher salaries rather than a duplicative benefit. Others would rather receive their compensation in the form of cash than association dues and continuing education stipends.

Because of the difficulties encountered satisfying the desires of their associates, some employers have elected to allocate one lump compensation sum to employed associates (25% of income collected for small animal or 30% for large) and let individuals pick their desired benefits from that pool of money. This places the responsibility for choosing benefits with employees, leaving employers uninvolved in their choices or the cost. It all comes out of the 25%.

Unfortunately, the obstacles related to this method of compensation have led the authors to discourage such systems and, instead, encourage the adoption of cafeteria benefit plans like those discussed in Chapter 4 or the use of percentage compensation plus benefits packages. In sum, the additional time required when associates are first hired to discuss and agree upon a benefit package to accompany the 20% plus benefits system more than offsets the turmoil, distrust, and frustration experienced later in the employment terms of employees hired under a 25%, no benefits contract.

Pros and Cons of Percentage-Based Compensation

To set the stage for the subsequent material on percentage-based compensation, readers need to recognize that salaries based on income collected by practices present many benefits and an equal number of detriments.

Advantages of Percentage-Based Compensation

- Motivates doctors to work hard and produce income because they know the harder they work the more money they will make.

- Emphasizes both the business and medical aspects of veterinary practice.

- Compensates doctors' successful efforts and skills selling high-quality veterinary services (after all, if quality medicine and surgery cannot be sold, neither can it be practiced).

- Increases the need and desire for associates to comprehend and understand the practice's fee schedule.

- Improves doctors' motivation to give estimates with accurate ranges so that clients are able and willing to pay the bills that pay their doctors' salaries.

- Stimulates veterinarians to obtain assurances from clients that they have sufficient financial resources to pay for the care they authorize before such services are rendered. (Since most employers using this system of compensation do not pay employees for income produced but not collected within 90 days of the billing date, there is a strong incentive to collect for services provided at the time they are rendered and not to approve easy credit.)

- Allows doctors who work hard and generate above-average income for the practice to control (and increase) their salaries as employed veterinarians.

- Produces extra income for employed veterinarians at the "20% + benefits" or "25% without benefits" compensation level while leaving approximately 75% of the practice's income for the owners.

Allows both parties to become financial winners (Figure 3.2 on page 119).

- Provides a constant measure of each doctor's productivity. Goals that get measured get completed.

- Helps relieve employers of the undesirable "9 to 5" behavior related to old-fashioned employment procedures.

- Challenges associates to monitor the status of their accounts receivable and call owners who have failed to fulfill their agreed-upon payment schedule. This makes them think about the financial side of the business as if they were owners.

- Eliminates opportunities for and claims of sex discrimination because compensation is based on time management skills and production, not gender.

- Treats associate veterinarians like owners in that both parties now are working to achieve a reasonable percentage of the income they generate from the practice to pay their salaries. Of course, as discussed previously under the five tiers of owner compensation, owners have the advantage of receiving distributions of profits in addition to their salaries.

If one merely reviewed this positive group of reasons why percentage-based compensation is so good, the entire profession would be using and endorsing it. That is not the case. This is because for every reason to compensate veterinarians using this technique, there also is a reason not to.

DISADVANTAGES OF PRODUCTION-BASED SALARIES

- Stimulates unhealthy competition between veterinarians in the practice for high volumes of clients and big cases belonging to wealthy clients or owners deeply bonded with their pets, which can lead to excessive individualism (or greed) at the expense of team harmony.

- Tends to overemphasize the business and financial side of practice; can lead to claims that doctors are gouging clients.[70]

- Discourages percentage-based employees from engaging in any practice activities that do not generate income (such as veterinary services for animals belonging to the practice's support staff and free exams for new dogs, cats, puppies, and kittens from humane societies, animal control, and pet stores with which the practice works.

- Harms employees at understaffed businesses or practices with poorly trained staff because doctors will be required to work harder and put in longer hours or suffer considerable loss of productivity and, thus, personal income. Moreover, because associates usually have little or no control over the staffing policies at the practices in which they work, they tend to become disenchanted with management.[70]

- If the percentage-based-compensation package provides no employee benefits, it discourages doctors from taking time off for vacations or sick leave, spending money on association dues, or investing money in and attending continuing education seminars.

- Creates an atmosphere for doctor distrust of receptionists based on claims of favoritism. Because of this, associates often ask questions such as "How come Dr. 'X' gets all the big or difficult cases?" or "Why do I get stuck with all the 'freebie humane society' initial examination cases" or all the "boss's Rotary friends who receive discounts."

- Demotivates doctors at practices that lack a clear definition of "income production." Doctors become skeptical when they discover inconsistencies or alterations in how their income production is calculated. This disadvantage is exacerbated when contracts do not provide for mechanisms by which associates can review their employers' calculations and appeal financial allocations that negatively impact their compensation.

- Produces income losses for associates who work for practices that lack a well-conceived credit application process or provide clients with liberal credit.

- Leads to decreased earnings for employees working for employers who routinely give discounts to friends, family, staff, business acquaintances, and/or owners of animals adopted from pet stores, humane societies or animal control shelters because, though employees have no control over these policies, their personal income generated from such cases has been decreased.

- Produces hard feelings in situations where employers provide credit and clients are making the agreed-upon monthly payments, but where the employers' income collected time period for which employees receive their percentages terminates 60, 90, or 120 days after the services were rendered.

- Creates time-consuming bookkeeping nightmares when determining if payments on accounts receivable are applied to the oldest invoice first, the most recent first, or equally to all. Also requires time and effort calculating which doctor provided the care on each separate account receivable invoice.

- Requires considerable staff time to track accounts receivable that are past the agreed-upon deadline wherein associates receive credit for income productivity. Such effort is required, however, so that management can deduct the bad debts from employees' monthly or quarterly income production figures or add the amounts where payments have occurred to their daily income collected calculations.

Employers need to realize that not all employed veterinarians will be motivated, or in some cases be properly motivated, by percentage-based compensation. It is true that some associates may oversell the volume of services and products needed by patients, leading to claims of gouging. But many others may not be motivated by percentage-based compensation at all or may actually be demotivated because they believe they should be recommending and doing what is best for their patients regardless of the amount of income generated from their efforts.

Employers Roles as Coaches

For percentage-based compensation to be most effective, employers need to understand the magnitude of the role they play as coaches and the value they impart by helping employees become productive as quickly as possible.[68] During this process, employers constantly must remind themselves that their relationships with their associates under this compensation system are intended to create a win/win situation. In other words, the more productive the associates are, the more they will earn and the more likely they will become long-term, highly productive and satisfied employees, helping to fuel the practice's net profits.

At the same time, employers must stop thinking, "I can't afford these 'production-based' employees because they are making more money than I do or than I did at the same point in my career." Instead, they need to replace those thoughts with coaching and mentoring philosophies based upon the rationale that "the better our associates do, the more our revenues and profits will grow and the more valuable the practice will be at the time it is sold."

Among the directions employers can take are

- listening carefully to the feelings and thoughts of their employees before assuming that they as the coaches have all the answers,

- creating game plans for actions desired by employees and efforts required by employers to bring those plans to fruition,[69]

- explaining to associates why expectations are necessary,

- agreeing on the expectations and methods for measuring compliance,

- identifying the resources that are needed and will be provided to help associates succeed,

- following through on all promises,

- agreeing on positive and negative consequences of performance,[70] and

- keeping avenues of communication open via weekly or bi-weekly meetings with newly hired associates.

Employee Duties for All New Team Members

Important directions that employees can take to insure their success at any job, maintain staff harmony, and enhance their productivity under percentage-based compensation systems include determining how they will

- elude the political whiplash associated with upsetting the pecking order before earning the respect of existing staff members;

- show compassion for the feelings of support staff and other associates in the practice;

- avoid threatening the job security of anyone on the team;

- adapt to the practice's routine rather than expect the practice to adapt to the theirs;

- avert the difficulties inherent in replacing an extremely well-liked doctor;

- remain neutral when conflicts arise, rather than confronting one faction

head on or siding with one individual against another;

- evade the troubles created by staff members who stir it up through their gossip, exaggerated story telling, or backstabbing of others;

- determine which employees are trustworthy and turn to them for information and advice;

- learn to ask staff to help rather than telling them to do so ("Sarah, could you please clean this cage while I take a look at this blood smear?" rather than, "Sarah, this cat's cage needs to be cleaned.");

- work as a team player (clean up one's messes, help others with heavy workloads, and share all lifting of heavy animals);

- develop methods of asking owners and staff members for their opinions about handling tasks so that staff members feel they have been asked to share in the decision-making process while new associates learn new options in the process.[71]

Defining Income Production

A Simple Definition

A commonly occurring dispute between employers and commission-based employees focuses on the employer's definition of income production. To avoid disagreements regarding how production is derived, the following definition for gross billable income is suggested.

Gross income produced by efforts of Employee and paid by clients to Employer is defined as the gross billable income paid by clients to Employer and generated by the performance of Employee's services or sale of products in conjunction with patient visits, including all office and ambulatory calls, examination fees, laboratory fees, radiographs and other in-house imaging pro-

cedures, anesthesia, surgery, hospitalization, treatments, immunizations, refills of prescriptions, dental extractions and prophylactic procedures, consultation fees, medicated baths prescribed by the doctor, medical treatments for animals being boarded, and (1) prescription drugs, (2) prescription diet pet foods, and (3) over-the-counter products dispensed at the time of the visit wherein Employee is involved in rendering medical care for a client's animal.[72]

Where definitions of income production exist, they vary somewhat from this standard depending on how well organized the practice manager is and how many disputes associates and practice owners have had on this subject. The reasons for including definitions of income produced in all employment agreements are (1) to enhance the trust between employers and employees, (2) to prevent discrimination in the allocation of income between doctors, and (3) to create a standard that does not change over time because of errant recollections of the parties.

While many practices have defined which services are included in associate commissions, definitions also should contain listings of services for which associate income production will not be attributed. The rationale for this is due to (1) the lack of profitability of certain services identified in the group or (2) the minimal impact employees are likely to have on animal owners' decisions to request or proceed with the services specified in this group.

Situations where income production is not attributed to doctors:

No compensation will be granted for boarding, grooming, or routine bathing; prescription diets (some employers put prescription diet pet foods in this "no compensation" section - others prefer to include them at the time of the first sale but not subsequent sales); prescription refills (employers who include the initial dispensing of prescription foods as income generated usually omit commissions on refills; those who include refills generally do not include prescription foods); vaccinations administered by associates to animals admitted to the hospital primarily

for boarding, grooming, or bathing services; over-the-counter products, laboratory procedures or follow-up visits where no fee is charged for Employee's examination time; or laboratory work not associated with an office visit where Employee is not involved with the test, e.g., routine fecal analyses, analysis of urine specimens submitted by owners, and heartworm tests.

A More Complex Definition

Although these definitions of income produced and income excluded seem complete, some practices have established considerably more detailed listings of categories than these. One such practice is Dr. Lloyd Meisel's multi-doctor general and specialty practice in South Florida. Because of the size of this practice and the owner's attention to detail, the definitions of income produced and excluded are more specific.

In this case, the owner attempted to determine the amount of time and effort needed for doctors to sell and perform specific services. He then evaluated the practice's margin of profit on each service. Services with higher time requirements and profit margins were placed in Category 1, wherein associates received commissions for their efforts. Services with lower time and profit margins were placed in Category 2, where no commissions were granted. Under this more precise determination of income generated by the efforts of doctors, the following definition is used:

"Gross income produced by efforts of Employee" is defined as the gross billable income generated by the performance of Employee's services or sale of products in conjunction with patients' visits and collected by Employer including all:

1. *Office calls*

2. *Examination fees*

3. *Laboratory fees*

4. *Radiographs*

5. *Ultrasound, endoscopy or other imaging procedures performed by the attending doctor*

6. *Anesthesia*

7. *Surgery*

8. *Hospitalization*

9. *Treatments*

10. *Immunizations*

11. *Dental extractions and prophylactic procedures where the doctor directs and/or oversees the procedures*

12. *Consultation fees*

13. *Medicated baths prescribed by the doctor*

14. *Veterinary examinations and medical care provided for animals which become ill, are suspected of becoming ill, or are diagnosed as being sick while being boarded or groomed. (See also number 12 under the "no compensation" section below.)*

15. *Prescription drugs, but only where active veterinary oversight of a prescription is required to satisfy the valid veterinary-client-patient relationship regulations required by the FDA (Note: when the practice is merely acting as a pharmacy and refilling prescriptions where valid V-C-P-Rs already exist, employees will not receive credit for income production)*

16. *Over-the-counter products recommended by the employee, highlighted on the client "travel sheet," and dispensed at the time of a patient's office or consultation visit wherein Employee is involved in rendering medical care or providing medical recommendations for a client's animal*

17. *Sales of prescription diet pet foods, but only those prescription diets sold during the course of an office visit or consultation that are directly related to a nutritional need of the pet being examined or evaluated, and then only (5%?, 10%?) of the retail price of the food sold*

18. *Medical work-ups and care provided for personal pets belonging to employer's support staff*

19. *Euthanasia and routine cremations*

No compensation will be granted for:

1. *Routine boarding, grooming, and bathing*

2. *Rabies tags*

3. *Verifying vaccinations*

4. *Express mail, postage and handling of drugs and products sent to clients*

5. *Interstate and international health certificates*

6. *Cremations - special handling (any services or products sold above and beyond routine euthanasia and cremation)*

7. *Ultrasound examinations or other imaging procedures including ultrasound guided per cutaneous and needle biopsies performed by outside generalists or specialists engaged in diagnostic efforts and/or consultations at employer's place(s) of business*

8. *Copying of radiographs and/or medical records*

9. *Sales tax*

10. *Biohazardous waste fee*

11. *Medical work-ups and care for doctors' personal pets*

12. *Vaccinations, heartworm, urine, and fecal examinations provided for boarders where there is no physical examination performed by nor charged for employee's time (Note: when animals being boarded become ill, requiring a doctor's examination and oversight, employee will receive credit for income generated from heartworm tests, vaccinations, fecal examinations, diagnostic tests, and any medical examinations and services and products directly related to the illness for which the animal is being treated)*

13. *Follow-up visits where no fee is charged for the employee's examination time*

14. *Laboratory work not associated with office visits, where employee is not involved with the test, e.g., routine fecal analyses, urinalyses, and heartworm tests*

15. *Products or services provided by support staff after employees have completed their travel or billing sheets*

16. *Items purchased upon the initiative of clients after the conclusion of doctor-client visits or consultations*

17. *Cardiopet EKG and other telephonic image transmissions and consultations with specialists.*

Some New Twists on Percentage-Based Compensation

Variable Percentages for Various Professional Services

Traditionally, employers who compensated employees using one of the previous percentage-based or commission-driven methods of compensation have multiplied the fee for all professional services performed, administered, or prescribed and all products sold in conjunction with an office visit or ambulatory call by a specified percentage, e.g., 20%. However, as practitioners have looked at the relative profitability of various professional services and products, some of them have begun to provide different percentage compensation for different services and products. Table 3.15 reflects a Pennsylvania equine practitioner's attempt to compensate his associates appropriately for professional services based upon his perceptions of the profitability of those services.

In addition to paying different percentages for various types of services, in Table 3.16 this practitioner also has attempted to account for the increasing profitability of his practice as the productivity of the associate veterinarians rises and after his fixed costs are paid. The multipliers for the associates' percentage-based compensation calculations from Table 3.15 are reflected in the variations of yearly income production for the associate as shown in Table 3.16.

Table 3.15. Sample Percentage Compensation by Service Type for a Large Animal Practice

Service Category	Percentage
Professional services	45%
Reproductive exams	45%
Musculoskeletal exams	45%
Surgery	45%
Medicines administered	30%
Medicines dispensed	15%
Travel expense & billing fee	30%
Radiology	30%
Programmed health	30%
Laboratory	30%
Medical supplies used	25%

Not to be outdone, one of the small animal corporate consolidators in the United States also has been experimenting with a complex commission formula. The system employed by that organization is shown in Table 3.17. This model not only considers variations in the profit margins of each professional service, it also takes fixed costs of the practice into account by allocating increasing percentages of income collected to its associates as their monthly productivity rises, much as occurred in the large animal example above.

With this template, all of the services rendered, procedures performed, and products sold or dispensed at the direction of the doctors are organized such that they fit into one of the categories in the table. Calculations are then tabulated by the practice's computer in accordance with the data entries made by doctors or staff at the hospital to come up with a monthly income production figure and, ultimately, a monthly salary.

As in all professions, increasingly fast and sophisticated computers and computer software programs are becoming available. Additionally, as veterinary practices expand the numbers of doctors, increase revenues, and/or consolidate, they tend to have and allocate resources to establish and monitor profit margins for assorted profit centers within the

Table 3.16. Use of a Multiplier Based on Income Production of an Associate*

Gross Income Paid by Clients	$270,000 - $299,999	$300,0000 - $329,999	$330,000 - $359,999	$360,000 - $389,999	$390,000- $419,999	> $420,000
Multiplier	1.1 - 1.14	1.15-1.19	1.20 - 1.24	1.25-1.29	1.30-1.34	1.35

*This accounts for higher profitability of the practice after payment of fixed expenses and enhances earnings of the employee.

practice. In part, this micro-management allows them to better monitor their doctors' income production and collection data to provide for more appropriate compensation. In the process they undoubtedly will discover more effective ways to price their products and services. A side effect of human nature and that process is that motivated doctors will learn how to work within an incentive-based compensation system to practice good medicine and generate salaries sufficient to pay their debts, make a good living, and save for the future.

ANOTHER SIMPLER APPROACH - VARIABLE COMMISSIONS ON SALES OF PRODUCTS

As more and more "big ticket," long-term care products have become available in small animal medicine, price competition among practice owners and price sensitivity among consumers is taking its toll. Products that fit in this category include Heartguard-Plus® and Interceptor® among the small animal heartworm preventatives; Advantage™, Front-Line™, Program®, and Sentinel™ among the flea control products; and Rimadyl® for chronic arthritis. Whereas office calls and examinations often are charged at $44 in many small animal practices ($1 times the price of a postage stamp), sales of the above preventive medicine products can add $50 to $120 to the fees for routine visits.

As a result of these fees, price competition for these expensive, long-term drugs is driving consumers to look for alternative suppliers.[73] Among the suppliers are catalog and internet-based veterinary product pharmacies. When clinicians multiply their 20% commissions by the fees for these expensive

and effective well-care products, they quickly realize how easily they can enhance their personal income production from such sales. But as competition among practices and other suppliers in the market increases, the margins on these big-ticket products continue to deteriorate to the point where practice owners are discovering they no longer can offer their doctors such attractive percentages of these products sales.

A few astute practice owners have retained the standard 20% commission for all services and pharmaceuticals except the big-ticket items mentioned above. To help retain profit margins sufficient to generate acceptable net incomes, these practitioners have dropped the commissions on these products from the standard 18% to 22% level to a more conservative range of 5% to 10%. At the same time, to encourage their doctors to provide increasing volumes of higher-profit professional service types of workups, they have raised the commission on doctor-generated professional services 3% to 4% over prior levels.

These changes reflect what some of the other employers mentioned in this chapter have tried to do (Tables 3.15-3.17). Big-ticket products are priced competitively, and doctor salaries are sustained by motivating doctors to provide higher volumes of more complete medical workups and treatments, rather than by selling more products.

STAFF TRAINING AND EFFORTS REQUIRED TO MAKE THESE SYSTEMS WORK

Considerable management effort is required in any version of percentage-based compensation to ensure that receptionists,

Table 3.17. The Most Complex Type of Percentage Compensation Formula Seen to Date

Employee Percentage-Based Compensation

An employee's compensation shall be calculated by (1) determining the doctor's gross monthly income produced; (2) selecting the applicable rate category from the table below; (3) applying the percentages associated with that rate to all gross monthly income production as categorized below; and (4) totaling the amounts calculated by this process.

Gross Monthly Income Production From:	$0	$10,000	$18,000	$22,000	$28,000	$34,000
To:	$9,999	17,999	$21,999	$27,999	$33,999	Higher
Category	Rate 1	Rate 2	Rate 3	Rate 4	Rate 5	Rate 6
Administration	15%	15%	15%	15%	15%	15%
Office Visits	24.75%	25.5%	26.25%	27%	27.75%	28.5%
Vaccinations	24.75%	25.5%	26.25%	27%	27.75%	28.5%
Injections	24.75%	25.5%	26.25%	27%	27.75%	28.5%
Surgery	24.75%	25.5%	26.25%	27%	27.75%	28.5%
Dentistry	24.75%	25.5%	26.25%	27%	27.75%	28.5%
Prof'l Services	20.75%	21.5%	22.25%	23%	23.75%	24.5%
Hospitalization	20.75%	21.5%	22.25%	23%	23.75%	24.5%
Anesthesia	18.75%	19.5%	20.25%	21%	21.75%	22.5%
Radiology	18.75%	19.5%	20.25%	21%	21.75%	22.5%
Euthanasia	15.75%	16.5%	17.25%	18%	18.75%	19.5%
Lab - In-house	12.75%	13.5%	14.25%	15%	15.75%	16.5%
Lab - Outside	10.75%	11.5%	12.25%	13%	13.75%	14.5%
Pharmacy	10.75%	11.5%	12.25%	13%	13.75%	14.5%
Flea/Skin/Shampoo	10%	10%	10%	10%	10%	10%
Rx Diets	5%	5%	5%	5%	5%	5%
Premium Diets	5%	5%	5%	5%	5%	5%
Supplies	5%	5%	5%	5%	5%	5%
Boarding	0%	0%	0%	0%	0%	0%
Grooming	0%	0%	0%	0%	0%	0%

hospital managers, doctors, and other support staff identify income production by their doctors and enter data properly into hospital computers. Even the most accurately designed commission-based compensation systems will fail unless the practices' doctors believe that their income production efforts are being properly calculated. Moreover, for the calculation of these numbers to be motivational, associates must be apprised of their income production figures on a daily, weekly, monthly, quarterly, and annual basis. To require that employers perform this task, one of the following options should be included in employment contracts:

Employer will provide Employee with (daily?, weekly?, monthly?, quarterly?) "gross income produced by efforts of Employee" production reports, enabling Employee to review them for accuracy and to be kept current on progress toward eligibility for (monthly? quarterly?) production reconciliation compensation. At the end of each (contract? fiscal?) year, if Employee's (18%?, 19%?, 20%?, 21%?, 22%?, 23%?) production reconciliation calculation for the entire year is less than Employee's base salary, Employer will either (a) lower the base salary for the subsequent year to reflect Employee's actual production for the year or (b) reconsider whether or not the Employer/Employee relationship should be extended.

A harsher alternative in use by a few employers, but not recommended, is as follows:

If at the end of a full year of employment, Employee has not produced sufficient income to be entitled to any reconciliation compensation above the base salary for the entire year, sufficient money will be withheld from Employee's final paycheck, or if the contract term is extended, equally from the first two month's pay periods of such extended contract term, so that Employee receives a salary equal to the base salary for the previous contract year.

CREDITING INCOME
TO DOCTORS

An issue that often surfaces regarding percentage-based compensation focuses on which doctor receives credit for income production for professional services. There are two trains of thought on this subject: (1) the income is attributed to the doctor who recommended and "sold" the products and services to the client, or (2) it is credited to the doctor who performed, dispensed, or provided the services. The key differences in the two are that one rewards the development of terrific exam room or ambulatory call client communications and sales skills, while the other inspires hard work, delegational success, and the provision of personalized, high-quality medical and surgical care.

Although both methods of income tracking occur in the field, it appears that most practices have elected to credit income to the doctor who performed the work. The rationale for this is that doctors and practice owners tend to prefer rewarding hard work rather than extraordinary sales skills. Also, this approach seems to decrease competition among doctors and reduce the bickering about who really convinced a client to proceed with diagnostic care and treatments.

To properly track doctors' production of income, practices must devise ways of accurately crediting and recording their income generation efforts. In the age of computerization, this task is easily accomplished using the following process. First, practices must create "travel sheets." These are lists of all common professional services rendered and medications administered or dispensed, each with an identifying computer code number (see Figure 3.3 for an example).

As clients arrive at the practice or before ambulatory clinicians leave their home bases, receptionists check the services requested by the clients and/or recommended by personnel at the front desk. This travel sheet then accompanies the patient's medical record to the exam room or on the ambulatory call. During the course of or at the conclusion of a clinician's physical examination and treatment of the patient, the attending doctor highlights the procedures performed and products administered or dispensed.

For ease in tracking, each doctor can use a different colored highlighter. When these travel sheets are returned to the receptionist's or bookkeeper's desk, assigned staff members enter the procedure and doctor codes into the computer. Practices that are not yet computerized can record information by doctor in the breakout columns of their one-write daily bookkeeping systems. At the end of each day, the doctors' production totals can be tallied and either provided to them the next day, upon request, or cumulated for the week, month, or quarter, and provided at a that time.

Over-the-counter products recommended by doctors and purchased by clients at the time of the visit either can be credited to the doctor or the practice, at the discretion of and as negotiated between the prac-

Newtown Veterinary Hospital – Outpatient Checklist

Client ID_____ Patient ID_____ Dr. ID_____ Date_____ Pt. Weight_____

Examination & Visit

103	Exam or visit-regular (E) emergency, (W) walk-in, no-appointment (I) in-house
103A	annual comprehensive physical
103M	mature pet comprehensive physical
1032	office visit/exam – 2nd pet
1033	office visit/exam – 3rd pet
101	exam or visit-brief ® recheck < 30 days (X) tech visit, no exam
102	exam or visit – extended
104	exam or visit – courtesy (S) sut (D) drain (B) band
100	emergency-including OV-after hrs before 11PM
106	emergency-including OV-after hrs after 11PM
105	(C) health certificate-menu 252 HCC, HCF
289	(C) write RX (Courtesy)

Vaccination Services

556	**DHLPPC**-annual canine vac
553	DHLPPC-puppy 6-7 weeks
554	DHLPPC-puppy 8-10 weeks
555	DHLPPC-puppy 11-14 weeks
554C	**DHLPP**-annual canine vac
553C	DHLPP-puppy 6-7 weeks
555C	DHLPP-puppy 8-10 weeks
556C	DHLPP-puppy 11-14 weeks
556A	**DHPPC**-annual canine vac
553A	DHPPC-puppy 6-7 weeks
554A	DHPPC-puppy 8-10 weeks
555A	DHPPC-puppy 11-14 weeks
556B	**DHPP**-annual canine vac
553B	DHPP-puppy 6-7 weeks
554B	DHPP-puppy 8-10 weeks
555B	DHPP-puppy 11-14 weeks
560	(A) Lyme vac (1st)
301	(A) Corona vac (1st)
300	(A) Bordetella Annual (1st or Puppy)
300N	Bordetella – Intranasal

557	DISTEMPER – small exotic animal
317	Rabies-canine 1 year tag#
318	Rabies-canine 3 year tag#
317F	Rabies-ferret, raccoon, skunk 1 yr tag#
338	(A) Porcine vac (1st)
311	FVRCP/C-annual feline vac
311C	FVRCP/C-Leukemia Virus Combo-annual
308	FVRCP/C-kitten 6-8 weeks
309	FVRCP/C-kitten 9-11 weeks
310	FVRCP/C-adult (1st)
310C	FVRCP/C + leukemia combo (1st)
311S	FVRCP/C-leukemia separate
313P	(A) FIP Vaccination annual fel (1st)
319	Rabies – feline 1 year tag#
320	Rabies- feline 3 year tag#

Radiology/Cardiology Services

505	(S) radiology-1st plate large (small)
500	(S) radiology-extra film large (small)
400	cardiology-routine
401	cardiology-STAT
403	cardiology- pre op
400R	cardiology – repeat ECG <6 days

Office Sedation/Light Anesthesia

Charge by inventory items used.

Professional Services/Procedures

200	abscess – clean/medicate/5 minutes
600	abscess – surgical drainage/5 minutes
714	drain for abscess (umbilical tape)
201	(C) anal sac expression (Courtesy)
202	(#_____) anal sac infusion (each)
203	bandage application - routine
203T	bandage application - tubegauze
204RC	bandage/dressing-remove/reapply
204	bandage removal (204C-courtesy removal)
616	biopsy – cutaneous punch

Figure 3.3. A sample outpatient travel sheet or checklist
Provided by Dr. Tim Ireland of Newtown Veterinary Hospital, Newtown, PA

Professional Services/Procedures (cont.)

620	casting – metasplint (charge_____) minimum charge $20
213	(C) ear/s cleansing (courtesy)
213R	ear-otoscopic exam (C) courtesy
216	eye-cleansing/medicating
217	eye-corneal staining/tear duct patency
218	eye – tear test (Schirmer)
219	eye – tonometry (eyeball pressure)
238	(C) pedicure (Courtesy) (T) teeth trim (W) wing trim
238F	pedicure – fracture nail
1107A	rabies exam for 10 day quarantine
1107B	rabies release from 10 day quarantine (menu 823 – paragraph RC)
241	(C) Wood's light exam – fungal screening
842	wound/surgical site-clean, medicate/5 minutes
242	wound/primary care/medicate/5 minutes
242H	Hot spot-clip/clean/medicate/5 minutes

Vaccinal Response

523	Distemper
516	Parvo
533	Panleukopenia
522	Corona
RFFIT	Rabies Titer (Kansas State University)
5013	geriatric Screen – Canine
4123	geriatric Screen – Feline

Laboratory Services

424	hema/CBC/Screen
424S	hema – CBC/Super Chem
424M	hema – CBC/mini screen
414	chem-profile (major)
414A	chem-profile (superchem)
415	chem-profile (minor)
425	® hema – CBC (repeat)
429	hema – PCV + total protein
412	chem – glucose paper strip test
485	drug – phenobarb level

484	drug – digoxin level
435	micro – bacterial C + S
437	micro – dermatophyte culture
438A	micro – aspirate/in house cytology
210	centesis – percutaneous aspirate only-no cytology
440	para – fecal
445	para – skin scrape
439	para – ear swab-micro, mite exam
419	fecal – trypsin film test
464	para – Occult Heartworm (blood serum)
459	sero-FeLV test-Elisa (A) floures antibody
491A	sero-combo FeLV/FIV
491	sero – FIV only
458	sero – FIP test
486	sero – Tick Serol-Rocky & Lyme (L) Lyme only
464	sero – Thyroid T4, fT4, TSH, T4AA
464A	sero – T-4 only
456	sero – serum cortisol
1925	sero – free T4/TSH
1929	sero – T4/free T4
494A	sero – VHUP Elisa allergy test
494F	sero – Spectrum primary food
486L	sero – Lyme Disease IgG/IgM
486LW	sero – Lyme Western Blot
448	path – cytology/ (A) vaginal smear
449	path – histopathology
465	urinalysis, complete
465A	urine profile
466	urinalysis, paper strip only
465C	urinalysis, complete cysto
206	catheterization – urinary
208	centesis – urinary

Vettest (Inventory ID)

L301	Profile
L203E	NA/K/Cl
L134a	Albumin
L459	Alk Phos
L750	ALT/SGPT
L400	Ammonia

**Figure 3.3. A sample outpatient travel sheet or checklist (cont.)
Provided by Dr. Tim Ireland of Newtown Veterinary Hospital, Newtown, PA**

Vettest (Inventory ID)(cont.)

L191c Amylase

L211 AST/SGOT

L326 BUN/Urea

L209 Calcium

L200 Cholesterol

L477 Creatinine

L536 Glucose

L250 LDH

L210 Lipase

L853 Phosphorus

L207 Total Bili

L093 T Protein

L208 Triglyceride

Euthanasia Services

	Under 30#	30-60#	Over 60#	100# +
Communal	1308	1309	1310	
Private	1324	1325	1326	
Private (single)	1324S	1325S	1326S	
Hold for pickup	1320	1321	1322	1323
Rabies head prep	252S	252M	252L	252XL

Euthanasia – 1081A   charge by inventory items mls used _____

Telazol – 1099   charge by inventory items mls used _____

Acepromazine - 1001   charge by inventory items mls used _____

Items Dispensed

Item ID	Description	Quantity
716C	Complimentary toothpaste	
_____	_____	
_____	_____	
_____	_____	
_____	_____	
_____	_____	
_____	_____	

Departing Instructions

Schedule next office/hospital appointment_____

(enter suggested date for next appointment & reason for appointment)

Figure 3.3. A sample outpatient travel sheet or checklist (cont.)
Provided by Dr. Tim Ireland of Newtown Veterinary Hospital, Newtown, PA

tice owner and the employed veterinarians. Income from OTC products purchased without any doctor recommendation or after the conclusion of the visit are credited to the practice or, if the practice tracks support staff income production, to the appropriate support staff member.[74]

Income tracking for hospitalized patients is performed in much the same way. With the use of in-house hospitalization tracking sheets accommodating several days' treatments, and different colored pens or highlighters, practices again can identify which doctor should receive credit based on who did the work. It is with hospitalized patients that the system of tracking based on who sold the procedure or product a few days previously breaks down, which is why it is not endorsed by most practice managers.

HANDLING PRODUCTION PEAKS AND VALLEYS

An additional problem with percentage-based compensation occurs as a consequence of busy months vs. slow months. When production is reconciled monthly and associates are having busy months, they may be inclined to increase their hours and efforts because they are assured of producing income sufficient to beat their base salaries. They also may conspire with fellow associates who were sick, on vacation, or attending CE in a particular month and, thus, are unlikely to beat their established income production plateaus, to pass some of their cases on to them.

Conversely, when doctors are having slow months and are unlikely to beat their bases, they can easily slack off and simply accept their base salaries for that month because those will be higher than their percentage-based compensation will be anyway. When this transpires, employers discover they are losing money on their doctors during

the slow months but are forced to provide production reconciliation adjustments above their doctors' base salaries during the busy months. Clearly this is not healthy for a practice's bottom line. To avoid this undesirable consequence of percentage-based compensation, the following language often is included in contracts.

At the conclusion of each (month?, quarter?) of the contract year, commencing _____, 200_, Employer will calculate a (20?)% of the "Gross Income Produced by the Efforts of the Employee and Paid by Clients to Employer" figure. (See pp. 123-124 for income production definition). The amount of the base salary paid for each (month?, quarter?), i.e., $ (base salary), will be subtracted from this (20?)% calculation and Employee then becomes entitled to production reconciliation compensation consisting of any surplus, less standard payroll deductions. In the event (20?)% that Employee's gross income produced figure is insufficient to cover the base salary, any negative dollar amount will be carried over to future (months? quarters?), and such deficit(s) must be made up in subsequent time periods before Employee becomes entitled to receive further production reconciliation compensation.

Employer will provide Employee with monthly "gross income produced by efforts of Employee" production reports, enabling Employee to review them for accuracy and be kept current on progress toward eligibility for (monthly? quarterly?) production reconciliation compensation. At the close of the contract year, if the (20?)% of production calculation for the entire year is less than Employee's current base salary, Employer will either (a) lower the base salary for the subsequent year to reflect Employee's actual production or (b) determine whether the Employer/Employee relationship should be extended.

RULES OF THUMB REGARDING SUPPORT STAFF AND VETERINARY SALARIES

When establishing percentage-based systems for general small animal practices, it is important that the total percentage of expenses for veterinary salaries (including salaries for the veterinary efforts of owners) and support staff compensation not exceed a range of 40% to 44% of the practice's gross annual income. Some practices in more rural settings can retain high-quality support staff by paying wages as low as 15% to 16% of gross income. This low labor cost enables them to either pay their doctors a higher percentage of income collected or simply keep their doctors percentages within the norms of the industry and turn a higher profit. The AAHA study on financial pulse points illustrates that the bottom 25th percentile of practices surveyed pay support staff 16% to 18% of the practice's gross income, while those in the top 25% paid from 20.6% to as high as 26.3%, with a median generally in the 19% to 20% range.[75]

To retain quality support staff in urban and suburban locations, practices often find it necessary to budget 20% to 22% of the practice's gross income for support staff salaries.[76]

Additionally, because of effective training, leadership, loyalty, longevity, pension plans, and an appreciation for harmony in the workplace and effective teamwork, support staff salaries in some practices increase to 22% to 26% of the practice's gross income. When this occurs, veterinarians find that they can delegate more tasks to their staff and, through such desirable staff leveraging, they can increase their income production remarkably. Nonetheless, higher support staff salaries may force practice owners to lower the percentages they pay their doctors to 18% of income collected in order to hit the profit margins needed to support their desired return on investment in the practice. (Note: 18% for doctors and 23% for support staff = 41%, as does 23% for doctors and 18% for support staff.)

STAFF LEVERAGING

For percentage-based compensation to work the way it is intended, practice owners and associates must understand the importance of staff leveraging. According to one outstanding practitioner, staff leveraging consists of hiring the right people, training them appropriately, and learning to delegate as many tasks as possible to someone whose time is less valuable than that of the owners or their associate veterinarians.[77] Under this staff management philosophy, doctors diagnose disease, prescribe medications, outline treatments, perform surgery, and establish prognoses. Except in solo veterinarian practices, where the case load is insufficient to justify multiple support staff, doctors live by the theory that they cannot afford to position and expose radiographs, prepare vaccines, manage the drug and hospital supply inventory, draw blood, fill prescriptions, prepare surgical packs, perform routine laboratory diagnostic procedures, or prepare patients for surgery.

As a result of the Hill's Pet Nutrition "Practice Health Successful Practice Study" of 54 hospitals in the United States, the words *staff leveraging* came into vogue in 1994.[78] Among other comparisons, the study evaluated the ratios of nonowners to owners of highly successful practices vs. those appearing in the 1991 AVMA Economic Report. The authors found that while average practices had 4.8 non-owners per owner, highly successful practices had ratios of 12 to 1. It also compared the ratio of technicians to DVMs in the average practices in the AVMA report, i.e., 0.25 to 1, with the norm of 1 technician to 1 DVM in successful practices.

Staff leveraging requires that veterinarians let go of the care-giving tasks they have traditionally enjoyed performing and, instead, delegate these tasks to their support staff personnel. Veterinary technicians and/or veterinary assistants, not doctors, prepare and perform most laboratory diagnostic tests, weigh patients, take temperatures, and set up exam rooms for special types of exams.[79] They also draw blood, pass catheters, perform cystocenteses and dental prophylaxes, prepare and clean surgery rooms, assist with the provision of client education and, depending on state law, anesthetize patients and prepare them for surgery.

In general, staff leveraging either makes or breaks percentage-based systems of compensation. With the well-trained support staff required to implement it, employed veterinarians can delegate 60% of their work load or more to paraprofessionals and, thus, make their efforts much more time effective, cost effective, and profitable. Without it, they will struggle to generate and collect enough income to produce the salaries they desire.

ESTABLISHING PAYMENTS ON INCOME

COLLECTED VS. INCOME PRODUCED

Practice owners who pay associate salaries based on income production percentages have learned that they cannot pay the agreed-upon commissions unless the income from their efforts has been collected.[72] Employed veterinarians accustomed to being paid base salaries, regardless of whether or not the income they generate is collected, find it hard to accept that they must participate in the collection of bills or run the risk of earning lower salaries. They generally object to this feature of percentage-based compensation but have no choice other than to accept it as the industry standard and the only feasible way employers can afford to compensate them in excess of that which they earn as their base salaries.

Except for those veterinarians who are excessively soft-hearted or who lack effective credit management policies, the vast majority of small animal practitioners run cash and carry businesses wherein clients pay in full for services at the time care is rendered or when patients are discharged. In contrast, and as an example of differences between various sectors of the industry, ambulatory large animal practitioners routinely bill for large volumes of their services, and an analysis of equine practices shows that delinquent accounts receivable are clearly a problem.[80] Consequently, they exert considerable energy managing their accounts receivable.

Since production-based compensation for associates almost always is based on collected revenues, not billings, handling accounts receivable can be time consuming and filled with disputes between employers and employees. With sufficient forethought, management policies and contract language can be developed to minimize these challenges.

IDENTIFYING THE CREDIT MANAGEMENT ISSUES

Among the issues that arise with respect to calculations of income generated vs. income collected are the following:

- At what point after bills have been submitted and clients fail to pay for services should employees no longer receive any credit for their income production efforts? After 30, 60, or 90 days with no activity? Should it be 90, 120, or 180 days after the initial billing? At the time such accounts are turned over to attorneys or collections agencies for further action?

- When clients have past due balances, how should employers handle payments on accounts? By applying current payments to the most recent services rendered or as payments for bills that have the longest delinquencies? Should all payments be applied to one invoice until it is paid in full or spread evenly over the entire group?

• When clients owe money on multiple animals and make payments on their billings, how should those payments be allocated? Should some of each payment be applied to the outstanding balances of each animal? Should the payment be applied to the oldest unpaid bill or to the most recently incurred bill which, in some cases, will be for the care patients received that day? Determining how to answer this question is complicated even more when different doctors at the practice provided care for various animals belonging to one owner and the owner owes money on several patients.

• How long must employers continue to reconcile the practices' accounts receivable and pay commissions to associates after they no longer work at the practice? One month? Two months? Should the answer vary depending on whether the associates resigned or were fired?

• Should employers be required to provide commission-based associates with monthly statements of their past due accounts receivable and expect their doctors to contact these debtors and arrange for payments? Or are such tasks considered to be inappropriate for employed veterinarians, in which case the task of contacting these debtors falls entirely on the bookkeeping staff of the practice owners? Should contacting past due accounts and requesting payment be up to the employer or the employee?

• Since considerable time and expense are incurred tracking and collecting accounts receivable, generating interpersonal disputes in the process, would it make sense for practices to set accept- able levels of bad debt for their doctors and tabulate the amount of bad debt per doctor only once or twice a year? For example, most small animal practices accept that 0.25 to 0.75% of their accounts receivable will be uncollectible and conclude that this is just part of every employer's basic cost of doing business. Could not employers merely decide that anything up to that preestablished volume of unpaid bills is acceptable for the business and, thus, pay their associates as if they had collected all of their accounts receivable as long as they stay below that uncollectible quarterly or semiannual threshold?

There are no established answers for these questions. Instead, practice owners have opted for a variety of policies. The following clauses provide solutions for employers and clarify this thorny issue for associate veterinarians.

1. *The amount of any account receivables attributable to Employee's efforts in excess of (1)* (0.25%? 0.5%? 0.75%?, 1%? - select the level that meets the standards of the practice owners) *of gross income produced by Employee that has been submitted to a collection agency or attorney for action or that remains unpaid (2)* (90?, 120?, 150?, 180?) *days after the initial billing or invoicing date for the services rendered or (3) remains unpaid at the time past due accounts are transferred to collection agencies or sent to small claims courts will not be included in the calculation of Employee's* (monthly?, quarterly?, semiannual?) *gross income production figure.*

2. *Upon termination of employment, payments on income produced by Employee but not collected by employer during Employee's employment shall no longer be due nor payable.*

Alternatively, and less harsh for the employee, this clause could read:

3. *Upon termination of employment, payments on income produced by Employee but not collected prior to Employee's departure shall be limited to a period of (30!, 60!) days post termination.*

LINKING COMPENSATION TO PERFORMANCE APPRAISALS

Many practice owners and associates feel that percentage-based compensation overemphasizes income production at the expense of other important employee attributes. Because of these concerns, some practices implement systems that link additional employee qualities and accomplishments to their associates' compensation packages. This requires identifying performance issues other than income production that are important to the practice and providing appraisals that evaluate them.

Irrespective of percentage-based compensation criteria, one of the most important objectives of effective employer:employee relations is to develop and maintain avenues for open communication between the parties.[81] With that in mind, all contracts should set forth time frames in which employees' performances will be appraised.[82]

The bottom line is that evaluations that measure issues other than income production are essential for employers who wish to convey to their associates that money isn't everything. Equally important, employees need feedback about their overall performances to determine how well they have met their employers' expectations and what could be improved to fulfill those expectations.[83] An example of a contract clause reflecting the importance of performance appraisals follows:

To enhance the Employee's and the practice's productivity, Employer will provide first-year Employees with written and oral performance evaluations 3, 6, and 9 months after the commencement of their employment agreements. During the second year, twice yearly appraisals will be performed and, thereafter, once yearly evaluations will be completed.

DIFFERENTIATING PRODUCTION RECONCILIATION FROM PERFORMANCE BONUSES

Performance reconciliation compensation has been described as an assessment of income production after the completion of specified time periods, such as months or quarters of contract years. The completion of these time periods prompts a reassessment of associates' salaries based on the income produced during the designated times, whether or not employers are satisfied with the overall performances of their associates. In these situations, the only attribute measured and rewarded is income production.

Although some practices mistakenly call these production reconciliation reallocations "performance bonuses," the authors prefer to differentiate the two. When performance or merit bonuses are included in the compensation criteria, qualities other than income production are added to the appraisal equation and measured before distributing supplementary compensation. Additionally, whereas production reconciliation is paid at regular intervals, performance bonuses tend to be intermittent lump sum payments provided by employers to reward desired behavior for employees' nonmonetary contributions to the practice. In either case, however, to be effective motivators, employers' desires must be identified and employees' accomplishments measured. This is the realm of the employee appraisal.

Performance Bonuses

In an ideal system, employees' scores on performance appraisals are linked to production reconciliation percentages, and percentage-based compensation systems are linked to performance appraisals. Under such systems, employees become eligible for enhanced compensation based on the proposition that perfect or "10" employees should earn percentages above the standard 18% to 20% of income production levels. Increases of 1% to 2% in their percentages could be applied to specified time periods, perhaps until the completion of successive performance appraisals, or even retroactively, over previous periods. When appraisals incorporate numeric point values, employers can simplify this process by connecting associate compensation bonuses to high scores on appraisals.

Under this theory of motivation and compensation, high marks need not be scored in all categories to qualify for performance bonuses, provided that no glaring deficits exist (such as professional competence or inability to work harmoniously with staff). Moreover, depending on the formula, exceptional contributions in one category could offset no activity or lower ratings in others.

Performance Evaluation Criteria

Basic items to be considered in employees' performance evaluations should include the following criteria: medical and surgical competence; adherence to hospital policies; client acceptance; income production; ability to work effectively as part of a team; personal and professional growth; practice promotion and community service activities; and education of support staff.

Medical and Surgical Competence

One of the best ways to evaluate medical competence is for senior veterinarians to review the medical records of patients seen by the young associates at the end of every or every other day. Doing this for the first month or two after hiring new veterinarians requires considerable time but helps employers and new employees practice with more similar medical and business philosophies. Additionally, it allows newly hired doctors to educate their employers as to what the most recent standards and trends are at university teaching hospitals or other veterinary practices.

Conversely, it allows employers to explain how they do things and what seems to work best in their practices. Ideally, if this extra time together allows for good dialogue and opens avenues for communication, it will prevent multiple small disagreements from mushrooming into larger job-threatening conflicts as the employment term progresses. Committing the time needed to this goal is by far the hardest part of completing this task.

Surgical competence is often more difficult to evaluate because it depends on employers witnessing the skills of their associates' activities during the performance of surgical procedures and postsurgically as patients return for follow-up visits. Among the surgical skills to evaluate are:

- dexterity and tissue-handling processes;
- selection of suture materials, volumes of suture material used, and suture placement and tension;
- aseptic technique;
- anesthetic inductions, depths, safeguards, and outcomes during the course of surgical or anesthetic procedures;
- the speed and accuracy with which surgical procedures are completed;

- evidence of surgical or postsurgical complications and patient recoveries, outcomes; and

- an ability to properly estimate fees for surgery, anesthesia, and postsurgical care and prevent client complaints by staying within those estimates.

Because of the time and costs of one-on-one observation of surgical techniques, surgical observations and supervision by senior veterinarians in most practices is limited. In order to more accurately assess surgical competence, then, employers may need to confer with veterinary nurses who have assisted and witnessed the surgeries. The inclusion of such comments in veterinarian performance appraisals is illustrated in Figure 3.4.

Adherence to Hospital Policies

In practices with procedure manuals or training materials for new employees, evaluating adherence to the business's policies is relatively easy. However, since most veterinary practices lack such manuals, it can be difficult for newly hired personnel to learn company policies and, consequently, it is inappropriate in such cases to criticize them for failing to adhere to them. Examples of policies that should be written out include:

- client call-back processes and frequency after surgeries or diagnostic laboratory procedures (this is one of the best practice builders available to new hires);

- fee schedule for ambulatory and emergency calls, veterinary services provided, and products administered or sold;

- preventive health protocols including vaccinations, deworming, heartworm, fly, tick, and flea control;

- requirements for the completion of ambulatory invoices and medical records,

including entering information on hospitalized patients in legible form;

- hospital procedures for the drawing and processing of various diagnostic blood and urine tests and diagnostic imaging procedures;

- expectations and requirements for client call-backs and recheck examinations;

- client payment and financial policies; and

- credit application and credit management policies.

Detailed training manuals such as *The Receptionist's Training Manual*, available from AAHA and IDEXX Veterinary Software, make great starting points for the development of such practice policy procedure manuals.[84]

Income Production

The issue of income produced by the efforts of associates and collected by the practice cannot be omitted from the overall performance appraisal. This component and its definition have been discussed in detail previously, precluding the need for further discussion here.

Acceptance by Clients

Most practice owners have learned that not all clients stay loyal through thick and thin. It takes hard work, constant feedback, and perpetual reevaluation of one's interactions with clients by veterinarians and support staff to win their confidence, respect, and loyalty. Each client's time must be regarded as valuable, so punctuality, convenience, and speed are important.

Practitioners need to understand that clients don't care how much veterinarians know until they know how much they care. This is true whether one's patients are food animals with special bonds with their owners (dairy cows, Texas longhorn beef cattle, show-quality Columbia sheep, milking goats, pet poultry, or Yorkshire pigs); reptiles; performance horses; or typical small animals like dogs, cats, birds, and pocket pets. When appropriate, clinicians are encouraged to get down on the floor with pets to examine and address them on their own level.

Humility, integrity, and honesty count, too. Doctors who succeed with client acceptance cast their egos aside and get results, rather than protecting their egos at the expense of the results.[85] Self-confidence is essential, but too much often comes across as insensitivity or arrogance.

To show how veterinarians value animals as members of clients' families, the names and ages of children should be written on the medical record and used appropriately to identify them. Equally important, pets should be called by their names and always identified correctly as a "he" or "she." In the awkward moments when names of owners of companion animals and names and sexes of patients are unknown or cannot be recalled, references to owners as "moms and dads" and to pets as "kids" often suffice and provide a satisfactory level of compassion.

To instill a sense of care, sensitivity, and accuracy, patient histories must be taken without interruptions and verbalized as they are recorded in the medical record, asking clients to verify what is about to be entered before entries are made.[86] Doctors who give clients their undivided attention, schmooze with them, and celebrate the bond they have with their large or small animal(s) will pass the client acceptance test quickly.

Young associates should learn that procrastination can be fatal. Putting off diagnostic work or treatments that should be done immediately only exacerbates patients' problems and raises costs for clients. Unless practices are so busy they need no new clients, recheck examinations are good for client bonding, income production, the delivery of quality medical care and, most importantly, to enhance the learning process. For new associates particularly, client call-backs after surgical or hospital procedures are among the surest ways to instill confidence and gain acceptance.

As illustrated in the veterinarian performance appraisal in Figure 3.4, the input of receptionists may be required to effectively evaluate this important employee attribute.

TEAMWORK

The word team can be created from the acronym 'Together Everyone Accomplishes More." Veterinarians and practice owners who think of themselves as quarterbacks or point guards realize that no matter how talented they are, they need coordinated efforts from the rest of the team to be successful.

Ten years of consultations with practice owners have taught the authors that more employees are terminated because of an inability to work cohesively as members of teams than because of insufficient technical skills. Team members put the importance of patients and practices ahead of their personal needs. They are flexible, pleasant, always willing to help, and have a positive attitude about life and work.

Like client acceptance, opinions of receptionists, technicians, and veterinary assistants are essential to evaluate this trait, and employees must realize that in many practices, prominent scores in this sector of the appraisal are prerequisites for the distribution of performance bonuses as well as ongoing employment.

PERSONAL AND PROFESSIONAL GROWTH

Personal contributions in the form of attendance at state, local, and national continuing education meetings and participation in and, even more important, leadership roles in local and state veterinary medical associations are key accomplishments in this category. Keeping up with veterinary journals and writing articles for local newspapers, client newsletters, and handouts also enhance the value of associates to their employers. Likewise, interactions with vet-

Veterinarian Performance Appraisal Rating Guide

4   EXCEEDS EXPECTATIONS:
All basic job requirements in this section mastered. Exceeds expectations in most areas; requires minimal supervision.

3   MEETS EXPECTATIONS:
Basic job requirements performed satisfactorily; requires normal supervision and encouragement.

2   PARTIALLY MEETS EXPECTATIONS:
Has not achieved all job requirements; requires more than normal amount of supervision. Employee and owner should develop plan to improve performance.

1   UNSATISFACTORY:
Many job requirements have not been achieved; needs unusually high level of supervision. If improvement not made in specified time period, job termination may result.

Job Skills	Rating
PROFESSIONAL COMPETENCE	
PROFESSIONAL KNOWLEDGE -Medicine: Possesses knowledge to perform routine medical examinations, selects appropriate and cost-effective diagnostic procedures, and establishes appropriate therapeutic protocols.	
PROFESSIONAL KNOWLEDGE -Surgery: Possesses knowledge to perform routine and specialized surgeries. Knows when to ask for advice and/or assistance.	
PROFESSIONAL KNOWLEDGE - Laboratory Analysis: Demonstrates ability to recommend and use medically appropriate and cost-effective laboratory testing to assist in establishing diagnoses. Possesses knowledge to interpret these tests properly.	
PROFESSIONAL KNOWLEDGE - Radiology: Demonstrates ability to properly recommend radiographic procedures as an aid in establishing diagnoses. Possesses knowledge to properly interpret radiographs.	
TREATMENT PLANNING: Demonstrates thoroughness and accuracy in planning treatment regimes.	
PROFESSIONAL RESPONSIBILITIES	
PATIENT CARE: Demonstrates humane treatment, compassion, and concern for the well-being of the patients. (Evaluation by hospital technicians)	
RECORD KEEPING: Maintains accurate records. Uses modified SOAP, especially D dx, T dx and plan or recommendations.	
RECORD COMPLETION: Completes case records and associated client charges in a timely fashion.	
CASE FOLLOW-UP: Demonstrates a concern for the welfare of patient through case follow-up communications with the client.	
HOSPITAL POLICIES: Knows, understands, and follows the established rules and policies which govern the normal operation of the hospital.	
CLIENT-RELATED SKILLS	
CLIENT ACCEPTANCE: Perceived as a competent and compassionate veterinarian by the average client; clients happy to make future appointments with this veterinarian. (Evaluation by hospital receptionists)	
CLIENT COMMUNICATIONS: Actively listens. Expresses thoughts clearly so clients understand recommendations. Expresses empathy & compassion.	
CLIENT SERVICE: Maintains client satisfaction. Conveys to clients the impression that they have received an honest value for the cost of services rendered. (Evaluation by hospital receptionists)	
CLIENT ESTIMATES: Makes use of estimates, when appropriate, to inform clients of their projected expenses before services are rendered.	

Figure 3.4. A veterinarian performance appraisal form

Job Skills	Rating
HOSPITAL MANAGEMENT	
LEADERSHIP: Communicates objectives, motivates others, promotes teamwork, builds and maintains morale. Demonstrates take-charge capabilities. Takes an active role in hospital staff meetings.	
INTRA-STAFF RELATIONS: Promotes cooperative working environment. Understands value of teamwork and shows enthusiasm and willingness to perform as needed to help practice function as a unit.	
EMPLOYEE DEVELOPMENT: Performs an active role in the in-hospital training and education of the support staff. Encourages and assists support staff in learning new concepts related to the profession.	
PROFESSIONAL/PRACTICE GROWTH	
PROFESSIONAL GROWTH: Maintains currency in professional literature; attends local, state and/or national continuing education meetings.	
INTERNAL PRACTICE PROMOTION: Promotes to clients the role that quality veterinary care can play in the health of their pets; keeps clients informed of new advances in the profession; takes an active role in developing and encouraging projects which promote the practice; assists in the production of client information handouts.	
COMMUNITY ACTIVITIES: Involved in community activities which directly or indirectly promote the practice, i.e., service organizations, Scouting, 4-H, community educational system, etc.	
PERSONAL QUALITIES	
INITIATIVE: Seeks out new assignments and responsibilities.	
JUDGMENT: Identifies essential facts and evaluates alternatives.	
APPEARANCE: Maintains neatness and dresses in accordance with the professional nature of the position.	

This individual has demonstrated positive performance, growth, and development in the following areas:

Areas where improvement in performance and effectiveness can be shown by this individual:

PLAN OF ACTION / GOALS TO ATTAIN

_____   _____
Employee Signature(Acknowledgment of appraisal only)   Date

_____   _____
Employer Signature (Appraisal interview was conducted)   Date

_____
Date of Next Appraisal

Figure 3.4. A veterinarian performance appraisal form (cont.)

erinary colleagues using electronic diagnostic and therapeutic media such as the Veterinary Information Network (VIN) and the completion of VIN continuing education courses, studying for and seeking board certification in practitioner specialties such as the American Board of Veterinary Practice, and attending courses or reading personal development books like Stephen Covey's *The 7 Habits of Highly Effective People* all fall into this category.[87]

PRACTICE PROMOTION AND COMMUNITY SERVICE ACTIVITIES

This section of the appraisal evaluates associates' efforts in promoting their practices and serving their communities. First and foremost for new associates are efforts spent meeting colleagues in the neighborhood. Knowing the names and faces of these people paves the way for a more cordial reception if disgruntled clients seek second opinions at neighboring practices. Friendships and acquaintances with these colleagues also minimizes the "Gosh, I've never met him or her" opportunities that precipitate disparaging comments. Unfortunately, not all employers value this effort nor provide time for new associates to pursue this idealistic goal. However, associates who sow these grains of collegiality will see them produce marvelous crops.

Other community activities worth pursuing include providing leadership or educational seminars for 4-H or scout activities or elementary, intermediate, or high schools; serving on advisory boards for local veterinary technician training programs; writing newspaper columns; working with local humane organizations or animal control facilities; joining local service organizations (Rotary, Kiwanis, Jaycees, parent teacher organizations, and churches); and assisting with local veterinary technician teaching programs.

STAFF EDUCATION AND TRAINING

A time-consuming and often unrecognized and unrewarded task involves assisting with in-house personnel management, teaching, and training for support staff. Because of a nationwide shortage of trained veterinary nurses, technicians, and assistants, most practices are required to train their own paraprofessionals. This means that someone must teach veterinary assistants, receptionists, and stable or kennel staff how to recognize signs of pain, illness, fear, aggression, and emergency crises. Technical support and nursing staff also must learn how to perform cystocenteses, venipunctures, and routine laboratory procedures; safely and effectively restrain animals; position, expose, and process radiographs; prepare vaccines for administration; place and maintain IV and urinary catheters; administer oral and injectable fluids and medications; and read and accurately fill prescriptions. Some veterinary associates excel at teaching these skills, while others lack the tact and sensitivity required to be effective teachers. Still others consider the task to be the practice owner or office manager's job.

Well-conceived performance appraisals recognize the importance of this skill and reward outstanding efforts. Initially, time spent teaching and training staff detracts from time left to generate income. Nonetheless, the more efficient and highly trained a practice's support staff are, the more productive the veterinary associates will be. Thus, efforts expended training support staff can produce big dividends for associates paid on commission.

In practices where staff turnover is rampant, the burden of this training can be overwhelming. When it occurs to the point that it negatively impacts income production, associates who are paid based on income production rightfully feel shortchanged.

If staff education were part of the associate's job description, identified as a valuable contribution, and measured and rewarded via the performance appraisal process, it no doubt would be more palatable. Moreover, if it were a task for which recognition, appreciation, and perhaps even additional compensation or compensatory time off was provided, it could be a motivational component of an associate's job.

In sum, raises and salary adjustments based purely on the traditional yardsticks of time in service or income production breed employee discontent. Such one-sided focus sends messages to support staff and veterinarians in the organization that incompetence, undesirable work habits, lack of teamwork, and/or personality disorders all play second fiddle to the almighty dollar.

The results of carefully defined and conducted performance evaluations, though time consuming to complete, can be used to construct performance or merit bonus systems that reward associate veterinarians who strive for professional excellence. For all parties to thrive, considerable effort needs to be placed on the creation and timing of performance appraisals that maximize employees' personal and professional growth in their contributions to the practice as a whole, not just their contributions to income produced.

Payment Schedules for Bonuses

Choosing the time frame in which to pay performance rewards always is problematic. Reconciling and paying income production adjustments on a monthly basis creates considerable paperwork and may overemphasize its role as a motivator. Consequently, some employers who are concerned about their associates' abilities to achieve additional compensation often prefer to wait until the end of the year, thus ensuring that employed veterinarians have produced sufficient income to justify paying bonuses. However, calculating and paying such adjustments only once annually seriously detracts from the motivational effects of the process.

For simplicity and continuity, most employers provide employees with monthly reconciliation compensation checks within 10 to 15 days of the end of each month without ever evaluating their doctors' overall performances. Employed veterinarians typically prefer to receive their bonuses monthly, but usually this is not in the employers' best interests because the monthly income production figures for veterinary practices can vary widely.

For example, if employees are generating large volumes of income by the middle of a given month, one can theorize that they will tend to work harder for the remainder of the month so they become eligible for a bonus that month. Conversely, if it's a slow month or they have been sick, on vacation, or attending CE meetings, and they are unlikely to achieve bonus status, they may as well take it easy, pass as many cases as they can over to associates who are likely to earn supplemental income that month, and simply accept their base salaries. When the income generated that month multiplied by the percentage they are being paid is less than their base salary, the practice has, in effect, lost money on these associates that month. The following example illustrates this point.

If reconciliations or bonuses were paid monthly, the unprofitable consequences illustrated in Table 3.18 could occur once during the contract year or during as many as 11 months out of the year. Without commensurate numbers of high-income months to offset the low months, practice owners could discover that they have paid some employees more than their base salaries for the year, when the income generated by such associates should have resulted in salaries that were less than the base salaries upon which the parties agreed.

Reconciling production or paying bonuses quarterly rather than monthly seems to achieve a middle-of-the-road result. Furthermore, it

- allows for naturally occurring seasonal or quarterly fluctuations in the practice's income, thus minimizing the need

Table 3.18. Peaks and Valleys with Monthly Statistics for Income Production

Production-Based Percentage	Monthly Income Production	Monthly Base Salary	Production-Based Salary	Monthly Excess or Shortfall
20%	$30,000	$6,000	$6,000	$ 0
20%	$32,000	$6,000	$6,400	+$400
20%	$27,500	$6,000	$5,500	-$500
20%	$28,000	$6,000	$5,600	-$400

to pay bonuses during peak income months while losing money on employed veterinarians during the valleys;

• allows employed veterinarians to receive bonuses during financially successful quarters (rather than having to wait for the completion of full years); and

• reduces the numbers of times employed veterinarians might be financially stimulated to see cases and work them up to the absolute maximum from 12 individual months to four 3-month-long quarters.

Using quarters of the year as baselines, bonuses are paid for high productivity but, hopefully, without the competitive roller coaster of a monthly journey. One of the drawbacks, however, is that paying bonuses quarterly may reduce employees' incentive to work hard, see cases, and produce income because of the relatively long waiting period before the practice's financial figures are calculated. Additionally, employees may believe it is unfair for practice owners to retain the "float," i.e., the interest, on the bonuses for several months each year.

OTHER ISSUES

Employers also must keep in mind that not all employees are motivated by additional money. Because of this, no one formula works for every employer or employee, and employers must recognize that money is not nearly the motivator for some people that it is for others. For many, a new x-ray machine, cassettes, or processor; a new microscope or infusion pump; additional time and money for continuing education; or better trained, higher quality, and more support staff may have greater importance than money. Others will be more receptive to improved fringe benefits, less demanding evening and weekend work schedules, time off, or more praise and positive feedback from their employers.

Additional compensation concerns for employers occur when performance in some of the eight appraisal areas discussed previously, other than income production, are unsatisfactory. To combat this, it may be necessary for employers to withhold portions of production reconciliations or performance bonuses until after employees have completed several months of employment and received an overall performance appraisal.

In sum, there are three cardinal rules to consider when implementing percentage-based compensation with or without performance appraisals:

1. So they walk in the same shoes as their associates, practice owners should pay themselves for their efforts as veterinarians using the same formula used for their associates.

2. Compensation based only on income generation without consideration of other important appraisal criteria probably will result in dissatisfaction and unhappiness for many parties within the business.

3. If initial attempts to implement production-based compensation do not seem to work, employers are urged not to scrap the concept but, rather, troubleshoot it, massage it, consult with others who

have had success and, thus, eventually shape it until it does work. It has and will continue to provide value for employers who believe in and want to implement it. The New England study of veterinary compensation showed that practices that base compensation on productivity produce a whopping 26% more income than practices that do not![88]

VARIATIONS ON THIS THEME

While previous sections of this chapter have described more traditional concepts in associate compensation and outlined basic plans for their implementation, the ideas that follow expand these principles using more complex performance appraisals to control associate compensation. Each was developed by a small animal practice to meet its specific philosophies, needs, and desires. The goal of these systems, as should be the case for all motivational compensation procedures, is to equitably reward associates for their total contributions to the practice. Additionally, these systems motivate associates to achieve their full potential while ensuring a fair return on investment for the practice owners.

THE SHORE VETERINARIANS SYSTEM

The associate compensation system developed by Shore Veterinarians, a five-practice conglomerate doing business as a veterinary partnership in southern New Jersey, blends percentage-based production reconciliation with semiannual merit bonuses based on performance appraisals.[89] As compensation for services rendered to the partnership, employees receive base salaries payable weekly, less standard payroll deductions.

At the start of each contract year, associates choose between two different options for percentage-based compensation and benefits. Option 1 provides them with 19.6% of their gross production and standard benefits (health insurance, professional licenses, association dues, and continuing education), plus a maximum potential merit bonus of 2% of their gross annual production. Under Option 2, associates receive 20.8% of their gross production and the same maximum potential 2% merit bonus, but no fringe benefits except a continuing education stipend identical to that offered under Option 1. Associates selecting Option 2 are responsible for their own license fees, association dues, and professional liability insurance, but they are allowed to purchase their health coverage through the employer's carrier.

Regardless of the option selected for their percentage-based compensation, all associates are eligible for additional monthly production reconciliation compensation calculated within 14 days of the end of each month and disbursed before the 21st day of the subsequent month. Shore Veterinarians provides its associates with monthly income production reports, enabling them to review them for accuracy and keep current on progress toward eligibility for production reconciliation compensation. Compensation for associates who fail to generate sufficient gross collectable income to cover their base salaries for two consecutive months is adjusted downward to prevent the practice from overpaying them for the remainder of the contract year.

The big difference between the systems described previously and in use in most practices, and the one used at Shore is the method by which employees earn what these ingenious employers have termed *merit bonuses*. As seen in Figure 3.5, associates are evaluated twice yearly to determine if they are eligible for merit bonuses.

This practice's performance appraisals set clear standards for acceptable performance and only reward employees who meet or exceed basic criteria. Their evaluation processes utilize a two-part performance appraisal wherein associates are evaluated using a four-point scale. The first part of the performance evaluation appraises

Shore Veterinarian's Veterinarian Performance Appraisal Rating Guide:

4 EXCEEDS EXPECTATIONS:
All basic job requirements in this section mastered. Exceeds expectations in most areas.

3 MEETS EXPECTATIONS:
Basic job requirements performed satisfactorily: requires normal supervision and encouragement.

2 PARTIALLY MEETS EXPECTATIONS:
Has not achieved all job requirements; requires more than normal amount of supervision. Employee and owner should develop plan to improve performance.

1 UNSATISFACTORY:
Many job requirements have not been achieved; needs unusually high level of supervision. If improvement not made in specified time period, job termination may result.

PART I: Adherence to Veterinary Employment Agreement

This section is intended to evaluate Employee's adherence to requirements of the veterinary employment agreement and evaluate Employee's contributions considered to be essential to continued employment with Employer.

Employee must achieve a score of 3 (meets expectations) or 4 (exceeds expectations) in every area to be eligible for semi-annual merit bonuses.

Job Requirements	Rating
ATTENDANCE: Comes to work as scheduled and remains at work during scheduled shift.	
PROMPTNESS: Arrives at work on time and stays until shift ends.	
WORK SCHEDULE: Adheres to work schedule policy and is fair to other staff veterinarians with regard to equitable distribution of shifts.	
DRESS CODE: Adheres to company dress code.	
VACATION/SICK TIME: Complies with vacation and sick time policies.	
CE POLICY: Follows continuing education minimum requirements for continued employment.	
PET CARE POLICY: Adheres to pet care policy.	
MEETINGS: Regularly attends Doctor, Doctor/Manager, and full staff meetings.	
FEE/INVOICING POLICY: Complies with hospital fees and invoicing policies currently in effect.	
PRESCRIPTION REFILLS: Makes decisions about and approves prescription refills in a timely manner.	
ACCOUNTS RECEIVABLE POLICY: Obeys hospital policies concerning estimates, deposits, and financial arrangements with clients.	
EMPLOYMENT POLICY: Complies with paragraph 1 of Veterinary Employment Agreement pertaining to job description and requirements of employment.	
OTHER	

**Figure 3.5. Part I of a two-part performance appraisal establishing eligibility for a merit bonus
Created by Shore Veterinarians, Seaville, NJ**

the associate's performance with regard to basic job requirements. These include compliance with policies addressing work schedules, dress code, vacation and sick time, continuing education, personal pet care, and prescription refills. They also include hospital expectations for punctuality, attendance at staff meetings, accurate invoicing of services rendered, and minimizing accounts receivable. Based on a four-point scale, with four being the highest, associates must score a three or four in each of these categories to be eligible for merit bonuses.

Once Part I of Shore's performance appraisal has been completed and associates have obtained all threes or fours, the amount of the 2% merit bonus is determined using information from the performance appraisal found in Figure 3.6. Whereas Part I assesses fulfillment of basic job requirements established in hospital policy manuals and associates' employment contracts, Part II examines performance of job skills. After scoring associates' accomplishments in all areas, weighted averages are computed.

Assuming employees are eligible for bonuses based on their Part I scores, their percentage scores on Part II are multiplied by the maximum merit bonus percentage (2%) being offered by the employer. The resultant bonus percentage then is multiplied by the individual's gross income collected during the merit bonus time period to arrive at a dollar amount for the merit bonus for that period. Employee appeals regarding unsatisfactory performance evaluations may be made to a committee consisting of one practice owner, one office manager, and an outside professional veterinary consultant selected by the employer.

Careful and accurate assessment of performances of associate veterinarians using the intricate appraisal system set forth herein is time consuming and wrought with subjectivity. Nonetheless, it is more objective than simply basing all compensation on income production and a good example of the process required to inform associates as to what is expected of them and motivate them to pursue the right activities. An even more complex system follows.

THE ROCK ROAD ANIMAL HOSPITAL COMPENSATION PLAN

Rock Road Animal Hospital in St. Louis, MO employs a complex and comprehensive veterinary compensation package utilizing a guaranteed base pay amount, a percentage-based compensation system, and professional bonuses.[90] Under this system, many conditions are set forth and the following terms and calculations are made.

Base Pay for Associates

Associates' base pay is guaranteed exclusive of their production. The base pay is set at 15% of the previous year's collected production (gross collected income). New employees are provided with guaranteed bases commensurate with 15% of the average income production of other first-year veterinarians in preceding years.

This amount is then divided into 24 equal installments and paid twice monthly. Although the base pay provides considerably less compensation than clinicians are likely to earn during the course of the year, it gives them the financial security many of them need at the commencement of their employment.

Percentage-Based Compensation System

The practice's percentage-based compensation system reflects the gross income produced and collected by the practice through the efforts of its individual veterinarians. To calculate the percentage-based compensation production pay for each veterinarian, personal productivity, adjusted production, accounts receivable, cost of production, and production compensation are considered.

PART II: Veterinary Performance for Merit Bonuses

Each area below is given a number in parentheses that refers to its weight or degree of effect on the total score. This number is the percent weight of that area out of 100%. Areas are subdivided into other areas, and these subdivisions receive ratings of 1,2,3 or 4 using the same numerical criteria illustrated in Part I.

Employees' scores in this section determine if they will receive semi-annual merit bonuses.

Job Skills	Rating
PROFESSIONAL COMPETENCE (15%)	
PROFESSIONAL KNOWLEDGE - Medicine: Possesses knowledge to perform routine medical examinations, selects appropriate and cost-effective diagnostic procedures, and establishes appropriate therapeutic protocols.	
PROFESSIONAL KNOWLEDGE - Surgery: Possesses knowledge to perform routine and specialized surgeries. Knows when to ask for advice and/or assistance and does.	
PROFESSIONAL KNOWLEDGE - Laboratory Analysis: Demonstrates ability to recommend and use medically appropriate and cost-effective laboratory testing to assist with diagnoses. Possesses knowledge to interpret these tests properly.	
PROFESSIONAL KNOWLEDGE - Radiology and other diagnostics: Demonstrates ability to properly recommend radiographic, contrast, ECG, ultrasound, and other procedures as aids in establishing diagnoses. Possesses knowledge to properly interpret images and diagnostic reports.	
KNOWLEDGE AND USE OF LEGAL INFORMATION CONCERNING PRACTICE: Understands rabies, health certificate, abandoned pet, controlled drug, medical waste, and OSHA laws. Cooperates and contributes to resolution of legal issues arising from Employer's business operation.	
TREATMENT PLANNING: Demonstrates thoroughness and accuracy when planning treatment regimes.	
PROFESSIONAL RESPONSIBILITIES (20%)	
PATIENT CARE: Demonstrates humane treatment, compassion, and concern for the well-being of patients. (evaluation by hospital nurses or technicians)	
RECORD KEEPING: Maintains accurate records. Uses modified SOAP, especially D dx, T dx and plans or recommendations.	
RECORD COMPLETION: Completes case records and associated client charges in a timely fashion.	
CASE FOLLOW-UP: Demonstrates a concern for the welfare of patient through case follow-up communications with clients. Prepares for and follows up on referred cases.	
HOSPITAL POLICIES: Knows, understands, and follows the established rules and policies governing the normal operation of the hospital.	
CLIENT-RELATED SKILLS (20%)	
CLIENT ACCEPTANCE: Perceived as a competent and compassionate veterinarian by the average client; clients happy to make future appointments with this veterinarian.	
CLIENT COMMUNICATIONS: Actively listens. Able to express thoughts clearly so client understands recommendations. Expresses empathy and compassion.	
CLIENT SERVICE: Maintains client satisfaction. Conveys an impression to clients that they have received an honest value for the cost of services rendered.	
CLIENT ESTIMATES AND CREDIT MANAGEMENT: Makes use of estimates, when appropriate, to inform clients of their projected expenses before services are rendered. Updates estimates, ensures that deposits are obtained and arrangements for payment have been made.	

**Figure 3.6. Part II, merit bonus portion of veterinary performance appraisal
Created by Shore Veterinarians, Seaville, NJ**

HOSPITAL MANAGEMENT (15%)	
LEADERSHIP: Communicates objectives, motivates others, promotes teamwork, builds and maintains morale. Demonstrates take-charge capabilities. Takes an active role in hospital staff meetings.	
INTRA-STAFF RELATIONS: Promotes cooperative working environment. Understands the value of teamwork and shows an enthusiasm and willingness to perform as necessary to help the hospital function as a unit.	
EMPLOYEE DEVELOPMENT: Performs an active role in the in-hospital training and education of support staff. Encourages and assists support staff in learning new concepts related to the profession.	
PROFESSIONAL/PRACTICE GROWTH (20%)	
PROFESSIONAL GROWTH: Maintains currency in professional literature; attends local, state and/or national continuing education meetings.	
INTERNAL PRACTICE PROMOTION: Promotes to clients the role that quality veterinary care can play in the health of their pets; keeps clients informed of advances in the profession; takes an active role in developing and encouraging projects which promote the practice; assists in the production of client information handouts.	
PERSONAL QUALITIES (10%)	
PRODUCTION: Comparison of Employee's production in the following areas to past performance, other staff veterinarians and published norms: Dollars per Transaction: Vaccine Ratio: Diagnostic Ratio: Full-time Equiv. Gross Income	
EMPLOYER & MANAGEMENT COMPATIBILITY: Discretionary assessment by Employer and management staff on ease of managing Employee and Employee's positive or negative contributions in the workplace.	
INITIATIVE: Seeks out new assignments and responsibilities.	
COMMUNITY ACTIVITIES: Involved in community activities that directly or indirectly promote the practice, i.e., service organizations, scouting, 4-H, community educational system, etc.	
JUDGMENT: Identifies essential facts and evaluates alternatives. Makes timely decisions.	
APPEARANCE: Maintains neatness and dresses in accordance with the professional nature of the position.	
OTHER:	

This individual has demonstrated positive performance of growth and development in the following areas:

Areas where improvement in performance and effectiveness can be shown by this individual:

PLAN OF ACTION / GOALS TO ATTAIN

_____   _____

Employee Signature (Acknowledgment of appraisal only)   Date

_____   _____

Employer Signature (Acknowledgment of appraisal only)   Date

_____

Date of next appraisal

Figure 3.6. Part II, merit bonus portion of veterinary performance appraisal (cont.)

Personal productivity consists of the provision of any service that is performed by veterinarians or at their direction and which results in a charge to and payment by a client. These services include but are not limited to examinations, surgery, anesthesia, cast applications, dentistry, radiographs, clinical diagnostic procedures and tests, treatments, immunizations, medications administered and dispensed, and injections. Pet foods and toys are also included if purchased at the time of and in conjunction with a doctor's appointment.

Adjusted production is determined by starting with the doctor's personal productivity and subtracting the value of fees for rabies tags and dog licenses, items purchased in the retail area of the practice by pet owners, and accounts receivable.

Accounts receivable related to the provision of services and products that are owed to the company 30 days after services have been rendered are deducted from veterinarians' adjusted production. For ease of calculation, and until proven otherwise, accounts receivable are estimated at 2.5% of the associate's personal production. Actual accounts receivable are calculated annually, compared to the estimate, and reconciled via a paycheck within 30 days of the end of each contract year.

Cost of production is the employer's costs directly related to the employment of associate veterinarians. It includes each doctor's base salary and costs of health coverage, retirement plans, allocations for business automobile allowances, and other fringe benefits selected by associates.

At the end of each month, that month's production compensation is calculated as 19% of the adjusted production, minus the cost of production. The difference between the guaranteed base salary already paid to the doctor and this dollar amount is paid to associates within 14 days of the end of each month.

Professional Bonuses

In addition to the above forms of compensation, Rock Road Animal Hospital also employs an elaborate performance or merit bonus system for its associate veterinarians. The professional bonus focuses on key aspects of each associate's personal performance beyond income production. Personal performance is evaluated in five areas: service excellence, team leadership and teaching, maintenance of medical records, compliance with policies and contributions to general hospital management, and client satisfaction at the time of the invoice. Performance in each area is tied to a point score. Veterinarians are evaluated on their own merit, regardless of the scores achieved by their colleagues. Bonuses are awarded when veterinarians successfully meet individualized, preestablished performance targets. These targets are set jointly by the hospital director and each veterinarian. Performance targets are set with respect to a 100% benchmark score for each of five evaluation areas. Professional bonus evaluations and their accompanying surveys are administered twice yearly. The five professional bonus evaluation categories are as follows:

1. Service excellence - comprises 40% of the target bonus. Service excellence is based on the results of four different surveys for each associate: client survey at the time of invoice, new client telephone survey, existing client telephone survey, and new client retention survey. Together, these surveys comprise 184 points.

- Client survey at time of invoice (maximum score of 60 points) - This survey is given to clients when they receive their invoices. Issues queried include attitude and courtesy of the veterinarian, quality of doctor's explanation of the pet's condition, level of satisfaction with quality of care, and adequacy of discharge instructions for care of the pet. Doctors encourage clients to complete these because they know if too few are submitted, they will not achieve the requisite number of surveys to qualify for a professional bonus.

- New client telephone survey (maximum score of 32 points) - Within one week of an office visit, new clients receive telephone surveys conducted by an independent telephone survey service under contract with Rock Road. This inquiry includes the client's estimate of wait time required to see the doctor, friendliness and courtesy of the doctor, clarity of the doctor's explanations, and satisfaction with the treatment received.

- Existing client telephone survey (maximum score of 32 points) - The questions on this survey are identical to those on the new client telephone survey. Existing clients are surveyed by the independent survey service within one week of seeing a doctor. Clients are surveyed no more than once every six months.

- New client retention computer search survey (maximum score of 60 points) - This survey determines the percentage of first-time clients seeing a particular doctor who, approximately one year after their initial visit, schedule another appointment with the practice (not necessarily with the original doctor).

2. Team leadership and teacher skills - contribute 15% to the bonus. Employees from various positions evaluate doctors on courtesy and politeness, patience, staff teaching, communication with clients and staff, and service as a team player. Doctors are evaluated only by the employees on their own teams. Each doctor works with a different team approximately every six months, or as allowed by particular scheduling constraints. Surveys from employees are anonymous and are submitted in sealed envelopes.

3. Medical records surveys - evaluate the veterinarians' hospital paper trail for medical and surgical case management and usage and recording of controlled drugs. This evaluation, performed by the hospital manager and practice owner, contributes 15% to the veterinary professional bonus calculation.

4. General hospital management - accounts for 20% of the target bonus. The hospital manager subjectively evaluates each associate on items that do not pertain to direct patient care. These include but are not limited to adherence to the dress code, punctuality, compliance with hospital policies, and unsolicited comments from staff and clients regarding the doctor's performance.

5. Compliance with an ideal invoice - contributes 10% of the points for the bonus evaluation. This survey evaluates the associates' ability to produce an average invoice that meets specified criteria. These include targets for minimum numbers of invoices per month, average invoice charges, the ratio of recheck examinations to office calls, the average fee for rechecks, and the percentage of medical and surgical service items compared to product inventory items.

Using these surveys and evaluations, the hospital director then calculates each doctor's total score and converts it to a percentage. To arrive at the professional bonus amount, each doctor's percentage is multiplied by that doctor's maximum attainable bonus amount. The maximum attainable bonus is calculated as 2% of each doctor's personal productivity during the preceding six-month period.

While administration of this extensive evaluation program is costly and time consuming, the process allows Rock Road to evaluate each veterinarian both objectively and qualitatively. The outcome is then linked to a compensation plan for motivating veterinarians and rewarding those who provide high-quality medical and client service to pet owners and are an asset to the care-giving team concept that is the basis of this hospital's practice philosophy.

CONCLUSION

The more one researches methods for motivating outstanding performance, the more one realizes the complexity of this segment of personnel management. No single formula works for every employer or employee. However, unless employers establish clear criteria, as provided in the examples included herein, and utilize appraisal processes that specify and evaluate the desired performance, they never will achieve the desired results. Excellent performance begins with clear goals.

REFERENCES

1. Mathews J: Employees are getting more money, but not as pay raises. *Philadelphia Inquirer*, July 22, 1995, p D1.

2. Phillips BJ: Merit raises: What raises? *Philadelphia Inquirer*, June 14, 1995, Bus Sect p1.

3. Shepherd AJ: Employment, starting salaries, and educational indebtedness of year 2008 graduates of US Veterinary medical schools and colleges. *JAVMA* 233(7):1067-1070, 2008.

4. Shepherd AJ: Income of US Veterinarians, 2007. *JAVMA* 234(6):754-756, 2009.

5. *AVMA Report on Veterinary Compensation, 2009 Edition* . Schaumberg, IL, AVMA (800-248-2862).

6. *Compensation and Benefits, Fifth Ed.* Lakewood, CO, AAHA Press, 2008, (800-252-AAHA)

7. *2007 Compensation and Benefits Survey.* Alachua, FL, VHMA www.vhma.org.

8. Lynch TA: *Veterinary Compensation in New England - A Descriptive Study.* 340 N. Wood Lane, North Andover, MA 01845 (978-738-9622).

9. Lofflin J: Unhappy associates, associate survey: The statistical response. *Vet Econ* 34(6): 32-33, 1993.

10. Crawford LM: The cost of veterinary medical education. *JAVMA* 209(2):200-201, 1996.

11. Shepherd AJ: Employment, starting salaries, and educational indebtedness of year 2008 graduates of US Veterinary medical schools and colleges. *JAVMA* 233(7):1067-1070, 2008.

12. Graham E: Study now, pay later: Students pile on debt. *Wall Street J*, Aug 11, 1995, p B1.

13. Wilson JF: Inviting the Elephant into the Room: A Dialogue to Co-create a Financially Healthy Veterinary Profession and Student Loans 101 presented at NAVC, 2008 and 2009.

14. Mazzarella D: While costs rise, colleges dance around the reasons. *USA Today*, March 5, 1998, p 14A.

15. http://www.collegeboard.com/student/pay/add-it-up/396.html.

16. Comparative Data Report accumulated from the AAVMC: *Veterinary Medical School Admission Requirements in the US and Canada*, West Lafayette, IN, Purdue University Press, 2009.

17. IRS Code Section 221.

18. Wilson JF: common sense and/or author's experience.

19. Opperman M: Is it time to hire an associate? *Vet Econ* 35(3):66-68, 1994.

20. Sorenson M: Help wanted: desperately seeking anyone. *Vet Prod News* 10(9):1, 1998.

21. Brakeman L: Study of classified advertising reveals high demand for veterinary services. *DVM Mag* 30(2):1, 1999.

22. Heinke ML: Beyond compensation: What to discuss when hiring a new associate. *DVM Mag* (3):51, 1997.

23. Baum FW: Going on a job search? Here's how to detect the right practice. *Vet Econ* 35(5):48-52, 1994.

24. Lofflin J: Unhappy associates. *Vet Econ* 34(6):37, 1993.

25. Becker M: Leave burnout behind: Tips from the superstars. *Vet Econ* 34(10):48-50, 1993.

26. Baum FW: New associates: Finding your fit in the hospital hierarchy. *Vet Econ* 36(2):63-65, 1995.

27. Baum FW: Attention new associates: Find your practice niche. *Vet Econ* 35(3):74-77, 1994.

28. Wood F: To make the most of your staff-and boost profits-do as the dentists do. *Vet Econ* 36(3):65-68, 1995.

29. Rozenberg L: Practice Management Q & A. *Vet Econ* 39(4):32, 1998.

30. IDEXX informatics: Practice Profile Regulation and National Averages. Note: From accumulated data from approximately 500 automated veterinary hospitals throughout the US. This study showed national mean of 2.42 full-time doctors/practice with an average of 63.75 new clients per month, i.e., 26.3 new clients per doctor per month.

31. *Financial and Productivity Pulsepoints, Fifth Ed.,* Lakewood, CO, AAHA Press, 2008. (800-252-2242, www.aahanet.org).

32. Practice Management Q & A, How to tell if an area can support another practice. *Vet Econ* 33(5):16, 1992. (Adjustments need to be made to the example in this reference to account for inflation, but the basic principles still are sound.)

33. *U.S. Pet Ownership & Demographics Sourcebook.* Schaumburg, IL, AVMA 2007. (Note: data is gathered and published by AVMA every two years)

34. *Financial and Productivity Pulsepoints: Vital Statistics For Your Veterinary Practice.* Lakewood, CO, AAHA Press, 2002, p 8-21.

35. A confidential lifestyles and salary survey conducted for the AAEP, 2008, www.aaep.org.

36. *Compensation and Benefits, Fifth Ed.* Lakewood, CO, AAHA Press, 2008, p 17, 36.

37. Ibid., p. 38.

38. *2007 Compensation and Benefits Survey.* Alachua, FL, VHMA www.vhma.org, p.27.

39. McDonald D: Five secrets from a real long-term investor. *Money* 26(13):142, 1998.

40. Osborne B: Research and personal communications. Dean, School of Veterinary Medicine, UC Davis, presenting at the AAVMC meeting of the AVMA Scientific Convention in Baltimore, 1998.

41. Lynch TA: *Veterinary Compensation in New England - A Descriptive Study.* Andover, MA, 1998, p 14.

42. Shepherd AJ: Employment of female and male graduates of US veterinary medical schools and colleges, 2008. JAVMA 233(8):1238-1240, 2008.

43. Tumblin DL, Wutchiett CR: Top practices look for pearls and pay them well: A report on staff compensation. *Vet Econ* 37(6):29-35, 1996.

44. *Compensation and Benefits, Fifth Ed.* Lakewood, CO, AAHA Press, 2008, p. 36.

45. Dooley DR: Earnings are up! *Vet Econ* 32(9):33-35, 1991.

46. Smith C, Dooley DR: Why do women DVMs make less money? *Vet Econ* 33(1):31-33, 1992.

47. Lynch TA: *Veterinary Compensation in New England - A Descriptive Study.* North Andover, MA, 1998, p 16.

48. AVMA Report on Veterinary Compensation, 2009 Edition . Schaumberg, IL, AVMA (800-248-2862).

49. Shepherd AJ: Employment, starting salaries, and educational indebtedness of year 2008 graduates of US Veterinary medical schools and colleges. JAVMA 233(7):1067-1070, 2008.

50. Opperman M: Taking the guesswork out of staff compensation. *Vet Econ* 34(3):65-66, 1993.

51. Opperman M: Associate pay: Combine security with incentive. *Vet Econ* 38(1):48-52, 1997.

52. Wutchiett CR: Associate pay: Which compensation plan is right for your practice? (Part 2). *Vet Econ* 36(3):46-49, 1995.

53. Catanzaro TE: Are you fair with associate compensation? *DVM Newsmag* (10):41, 1997.

54. Clark R: Associate pay: 25 percent may be wrong. *Vet Econ* 33(9):64-67, 1992.

55. *Compensation and Benefits, Fifth Ed.* Lakewood, CO, AAHA Press, 2008, p 38.

56. Opperman M: Making production-based compensation work for everyone in your practice. *Vet Econ* 35(2):38-40, 1994.

57. Practice Management Q & A: How to determine fair compensation for an emergency doctor. *Vet Econ* 34(8):16, 1993.

58. Bohlender E: *Financial and Productivity Pulsepoints: A Comprehensive Survey and Analysis of Performance Benchmarks.* Lakewood, CO, AAHA Press, p 89, 1998.

59. Personal communications: American Association of Veterinary Medical Colleges Symposium AVMA Convention in Baltimore, MD,1998.

60. Lofflin J: Specialist pay: searching for answers. *Vet Econ* 34(8):81, 1993.

61. Lofflin J: Specialist pay: searching for answers. *Vet Econ* 34(8):74-81, 1993.

62. Johnson AP: Commission system: The practice equalizer. *Proc Am Assoc Bovine Pract Conf* 2:196-197, 1992.

63. Gardner CE: Getting paid: How to charge and collect. *Vet Clin North Am: Food Anim Pract* 5(3):603-613, 1989.

64. Johnson PE: Getting paid by the hour yields more profits. *Proc Am Assoc Bovine Pract Conf*:189-190, 1992.

65. Perry JW: Contract veterinary services are the financial answer. *Proc Am Assoc Bovine Pract*:187-188, 1992.

66. Overby A: Charging by procedure makes our practice profitable. *Proc Am Assoc Bovine Pract*:187-188, 1992.

67. Personal communications: Scott, practice manager, and Lenora Sammons, DVM, owner of Willow Creek Animal Hospital in Reading, PA, June 1998.

68. Sammons ML, Sammons LS: Personnel management in dairy practice: The professional staff. *Vet Clin North Am Food Anim Pract* 5(3): 493-500, 1989.

69. Wutchiette CR, Tumblin DL: Take a look inside the management of today's equine practices. *Vet Econ* (4):80, 1996. (Please note that the graph about the percentages of production paid by practices on p 83 conflicts with the statement on p 82 that 30% of these practices pay 30% of production or more.)

70. Wutchiette CR: Associate pay: Which compensation plan is right for your practice. *Vet Econ* 36(3):48, 1995.

71. Smith BW: Ready, set, coach! *Vet Econ* 38(2):70-75, 1997.

72. Rosenberg R: Production-based compensation doesn't include unpaid charges. *Vet Econ* 38(10):99, 1997.

73. Direct-to-consumer catalogs & pharmacies challenge marketing restrictions. *DVM Mag* 29(6):1, 1998

74. For a more complete explanation of this and other front office procedures, see Drs. Wilson and McConnell's *The Receptionist's Training Manual*, a 195-page "how to" notebook published by Priority Press, Ltd. in 1996, and marketed by AAHA's publications division, 800-252-AAHA, IDEXX Veterinary Information Systems publications division, 800-637-9312, or Priority Press, Ltd., 215-321-9488.

75. *Financial and Productivity Pulsepoints: A Comprehensive Survey and Analysis of Performance Benchmarks*. Lakewood, CO, AAHA Press, p 42, 1998 and p 5, 2002.

76. Garcia E: Employee compensation. *Seminars Vet Med Surg (Sm Anim)* 11(1):41-43, 1996.

77. Pinkleton R: Staff leveraging - Use your staff to build your practice. *Vet Forum* (6):32-34, 1995.

78. Opperman M: Staff members tell all: Where practices excel and where they fall short. *Vet Econ* 35(12):42-47, 1994.

79. Martin P: What can your staff do for you? *Vet Forum* (6):39, 1995.

80. Wutchiette CR, Tumblin DL: Take a look inside the management of today's equine practices. *Vet Econ* 37(4):82, 1996.

81. Jack CJ, Mathew B: Personnel points. *Can Vet J* 36:318, 1995.

82. Opperman M: Evaluating associates: Going beyond the form. *Vet Econ* 37(2):62-65, 1996.

83. Opperman M: How to evaluate your associates effectively. *Vet Econ* 34(10):53-55, 1993.

84. Wilson JF: *The Receptionist's Training Manual*. Eau Claire, WI, IDEXX, 1996. Available in hard copy and on diskette from AAHA, 800-252-AAHA and IDEXX, 800-224-4408.

85. Becker M: Leave burnout behind: Tips from the superstars. *Vet Econ* 34(10):48-52, 1993.

86. Wilson JF: *Law and Ethics of the Veterinary Profession*. Yardley, PA, Priority Press, 1993, p 319.

87. Covey SR: *The 7 Habits of Highly Effective People*, New York, Simon & Schuster, 1989.

88. Lynch TA: *Veterinary Compensation in New England: A Descriptive Study*. North Andover, MA, p 14, 1998.

89. Ideas developed by Drs. Richard Blose and Nick Holland of Shore Veterinarians whose principal practice is located in Ocean View, NJ and who established the performance appraisal ideas contained herein through consultations with the author.

90. Cloud D, Stehr J: Personal communications, Rock Road Animal Hospital, Inc, St. Louis, MO. *Rock Road Animal Hospital Compensation Plan for Veterinarians*. Copyright St. Louis Veterinary Consultants, 1998.

Chapter 4

Basic Employment Benefits

By Jeffrey D. Nemoy, DVM, JD and James F. Wilson, DVM, JD

Veterinary practice owners who employ veterinarians and para-professionals know that quality employees are one of their most valuable business assets. They also know that because of the tax-free status of many employee benefits, well-conceived packages are instrumental in attracting the best applicants and retaining existing employees. Comprehensive benefit packages help enable employees to balance personal and family needs with workplace demands, and thereby create more stable and economically secure family units. This directly affects employees' loyalty, integrity, and productivity which, in turn, affect the profitability of the business.

Although many veterinary practices view themselves as one big happy family, the equitable provision of employee benefits often presents a dilemma. Though most employers usually want to be generous, they also know they cannot provide all the benefits their employees desire. Still, as employers they cannot afford *not* to offer benefits because they help prevent turnover. In fact, a head of a small business management consulting firm based in San Francisco says, "Recruiting, interviewing, and training someone new can cost you more than providing benefits."[1]

Although offering benefits is universal among veterinary employers, the types and value of these perks vary considerably among practices and even within different regions of the country. Depending on lifestyles, family status, and profitability of the practices, certain benefits suit the desires of some employers but not others, while some are in high demand by employees and others are less attractive. Unmarried veterinary associates and support staff in their middle twenties often view higher salaries, flexible or fewer hours, limited volumes of emergency or weekend work, and bonuses as preferable benefits. Less important are life and disability insurance policies, pension plans, or contributions to 401(k) plans. Married employees, in contrast, may view health plans, child care, part-time employment, and flexible time off as their highest priorities. Employees in their late thirties and older tend to be more concerned with job security; health, life, and disability insurance; and profit-sharing or pension plans.[2]

In addition to understanding employees' benefit preferences, employers need to determine (1) which benefits packages are most beneficial and financially feasible for their businesses, (2) which plans are routinely offered in the profession, and (3) whether offering specific benefits to some employees and not others poses a legal challenge. Possible benefits include basic employment benefits (this chapter), health and disability insurance benefits (Chapter 5), life insurance benefits (Chapter 6), ancillary employment benefits (Chapter 7), and retirement benefits (Chapter 8).

RETROSPECTIVE STUDIES AND GOALS

This chapter covers the pros and cons of basic benefits, the value of and frequency with which these benefits are offered to veterinarians, a progressive benefits package based on job performance and seniority, and contract clauses for each of these topics for inclusion in employment agreements.

The contract clauses provided herein were created after analyzing hundreds of veterinary employment contracts from across the United States, the oldest of which was signed in 1987 and the newest in 1999. To assure compliance with local laws, employers are advised to have local legal counsel review the contract clauses before including them in their veterinary employment agreements.

Tables 4.1 and 4.2 analyze the types of basic benefits offered by small, large, equine, and mixed animal practices to male and female associates.

Each year the AVMA publishes data about salaries and benefits for recent veterinary graduates. Table 4.3 provides the data on fringe benefits received by new graduates, as cumulated by the AVMA's Center for Information Management.[3]

LOCATING CONTEMPORARY INFORMATION

The most accurate source of information for local area norms are colleagues in a practice's geographic area. Since discussions of employment benefits tend to be uncommon, though, employers are advised to consult with accountants, lawyers, and practice management consultants. Also, review the norms set forth in this book and check the materials published annually in various veterinary journals and newsletters. These include the annual December, January, or February issues of the *Journal of the American Veterinary Medical Association*, the American Animal Hospital Association's *Compensation and Benefits: An In-Depth Look*,[4] *Veterinary Compensation in New England*[5] and, from time to time, *Veterinary Economics* and the *Veterinary Hospital Management Association Newsletter*.[6]

The *JAVMA* information is cumulated immediately after the graduation of each veterinary class. Because the value of the new graduates' benefits is fairly easily quan-

Table 4.1. Authors' Retrospective Study of 225 Employment Contracts: Percentage of Veterinarians Offered Basic Benefits

	All (N*=225)	Male** (N=83)	Female** (N=130)	Small Animal (N=164)	Equine (N=12)	Large Animal (N=13)	Mixed (N=25)
Vacation Leave	91.1	94	90.8	91.5	75	100	92
Continuing Education	64.9	62.7	65.4	68.3	58.3	53.9	56
Sick Leave	40.6	36.1	42.3	40.5	41.7	38.5	44
Personal Leave	11.2	8.4	11.5	11.7	8.3	7.7	16

* N=number of contracts

** Because some contracts were not identifiable by gender, the number of female and male contracts may not add up to 225.

**Table 4.2. Authors' Retrospective Study of 225 Employment Contracts:
Average Basic Benefits Offered to Veterinarians**

Benefits	All		Male**		Female**	
	Paid days/yr	N*	Paid days/yr	N	Paid days/yr	N
Vacation Leave (paid days/yr)	9.3	197**	9.6	74**	9.3	115**
Continuing Education (paid days/yr)	4.0	113	4.2	37	3.9	69
Continuing Education (financial budget/yr)	$587	109	$612	45	$576	62
Sick Leave (paid days/yr)	4.3	83	4.6	27	4.2	51
Personal Leave (paid days/yr)	2.9	23	2.9	7	3.1	13

Benefits	Small Animal		Equine		Large Animal		Mixed	
	Paid days/yr	N	Paid days/yr	N	Paid days/yr	N	Paid days/yr	N
Vacation Leave (paid days/yr)	9.7	147	8.3	9	7.9	1	8.5	20
Continuing Education (paid days/yr)	4.1	90	3.8	4	3.7	7	3.1	6
Continuing Education (financial budget/yr)	$616	80	$400	4	$450	5	$487	15
Sick Leave (paid days/yr)	4.4	58	4.0	5	3.6	5	3.8	11
Personal Leave (paid days/yr)	2.8	17	2.0	1	5.0	1	3.3	4

*N=number of contracts
**Since some contracts were not identifiable by gender, the numbers for males and females may not add up to the total number of contracts in each category.

tified, this annual study contains accurate and useful data pertaining to the provision of benefits. With respect to salaries, however, it focuses on information available only at the inception of new graduates' employment. This often is misleading because no data are available at the end of the first year of employment to show the impact of production-based compensation for those associates who earn incentive bonuses.

The authors are aware of many new graduates in small animal practice who pro-duced over $300,000 of income for their employers in their first year after graduation. Some new graduates in busy practices with five support staff per doctor produced over $500,000 of income.[7] In cases like these, the base salaries of these graduates were similar to or 25% higher than the means published in *JAVMA*, but their actual compensation for the first year exceeded their base by as much as 40%. No current studies of salaries in veterinary medicine capture this type of discrepancy in reporting the "norms."

Table 4.3. Fringe Benefits Provided by Employers for 1998 and 2001
Veterinary Medical College Graduates

Benefits	Female		Male	
	2001 (%)	1998 (%)	2001 (%)	1998 (%)
Life Insurance	26.1	27.1	31.1	27.4
Medical/Hospital Plan	71.0	64.2	67.2	66.7
Dental Plan	22.2	16.9	21.1	17.7
Cafeteria Plan	2.8	2.8	2.2	4.2
Pension Plan	25.0	17.5	22.9	20.0
Profit Sharing	14.4	12.2	13.8	12.1
Disability Insurance	32.7	32.0	40.1	33.5
Liability Insurance	69.6	69.2	71.1	67.0
Association Dues	60.4	58.7	59.0	54.9
Continuing Education Expense	76.8	73.8	74.1	72.8
Continuing Education Leave	63.1	60.5	62.9	60.5
Paid Legal Holidays	42.3	37.7	40.8	36.3
Sick Leave	51.5	46.1	53.7	50.5
Annual Vacation Leave	75.8	74.9	71.4	73.3
Other	13.2	10.8	9.5	9.8

Costs and varying business philosophies most likely will limit employers from offering their employees every benefit described herein. However, visionary employers who seek the best candidates and desire to retain employees long term are advised to evaluate each benefit, balancing the ability of each to attract and retain personnel with the financial costs for providing such benefits. They can then select the benefits that best fit their own and employees' needs and include those in job offers and employment contracts.

BUDGETARY LIMITATIONS

Employers sometimes must adjust salaries downward to accommodate the increased benefits desired by associates and still keep employee-related costs at acceptable levels. In other cases, employers seeking to hire the best candidates may need to sweeten the benefit pot to offset the lower-than-expected salaries offered. Both parties must recognize that even though employee benefits generally constitute tax-deductible business expenses for employers, what is economically beneficial for employees usually is economically costly to employers.

Veterinary employers cannot afford to allocate more than 23% to 27% of the revenue generated and collected by individual small animal practice associates to payroll expenses for associate veterinarian salaries, benefits, and employer payroll taxes without seriously reducing the business's reasonable and acceptable profit margins. Because of lower fixed cost overhead, these percentages are in the 28% to 32% range for large animal associates. Put another way, associates must recognize that employers can only pay salaries of 17% to 22% of revenue generated by individual small animal associates, or 22% to 27% for large animal clinicians, before adding the costs of benefits and payroll taxes without seriously impairing the business's return on investment and profitability (see Chapter 3 for a comprehensive explanation of this standard).

EMPLOYEE LONGEVITY CONSIDERATIONS

Minimizing employee turnover saves employers costs incurred hiring and training new employees and improves the continuity of care for practices' clients and patients. Conversely, modest levels of employee turnover help reduce the calendar-type increases in wages and benefits expected by long-term employees who are not as productive as they once were or who have reached a production limit in a certain job category.

In some cases, employee turnover is essential to prevent aging employees from receiving salaries and benefits far in excess of their value to the practice. These individuals develop a false sense of importance and value, creating disharmony among more junior employees. Often they feel entitled to their salaries because of longevity, completely disregarding their productivity, attitudes, and negative impact on others at the practice. Further problems are created when practices are sold, because buyers cannot afford nor wish to retain these excessively compensated employees. Therefore, employers must carefully maintain the balance of salary and benefits that rewards and motivates employees equitably without adversely affecting the profitability of the business.

NEGOTIATIONS

To develop trusting and respectful relationships, employers and employees must treat the formulation of the employment contract as a negotiation process and not a dictatorial take-it-or-leave-it endpoint. If pleasant dialogue with good listening and appropriate communication skills cannot be established during discussions of employment contracts, the parties may be served best by going their separate ways. Experience has shown that when employers and employees fail to explain or fully discuss the practice's benefit packages before arriving at oral employment agreements or before signing written contracts, employer-employee relationships are unlikely to survive the contract term. Chances for a successful relationship are even less when considerable disagreement occurs at the negotiation stage and nothing is written down to show what the parties feel they have agreed upon.

There is no doubt that well-conceived benefits packages allow practice owners and managers a competitive edge in attracting candidates while offering nontaxable income to employees. However, all too often employers immersed in the negotiation process fail to effectively explain the employer costs or employee value of the benefits package to job applicants or employees anticipating renewals of their contracts. Additionally, they tend to offer the same packages year after year instead of planning a progressive system of rewards.

To help employees understand the value of packages offered, employers are urged to calculate and provide a written synopsis of the dollar value of individual benefits and the total value of the package. Concerns about money that are discussed but not set forth in writing usually leave both parties wondering what they actually agreed upon. Memories fade rapidly when no written notes or memoranda have been preserved. Even more important, issues involving money that are presented in writing open the door for hypothetical examples, improved dialogue and, hence, a better understanding and appreciation of the value of the benefits offered. Finally, it is hard to argue that a benefit was excluded or different than recalled months after it was discussed when it is recorded in a written agreement.

ANNUAL SALARY AND BENEFITS STATEMENTS

During contract renegotiations, employers are advised to present salary-and-benefits statements to employees using templates similar to the one in Figure 4.1. This enables employees and employers to comprehend the types of employment costs incurred for salaries and benefits each year. As such, it serves as a useful educational tool for employers and a valuable basis for negotiations between the parties.

Employers are encouraged to review the employee salary and benefits statement with employees during contract renegotiations and ask employees if they think they are receiving desirable benefits. Although the answer may be no, the ensuing discussion could lead to further negotiations and perhaps the offering of new or different benefits better suited to both parties. Employees must realize, however, that every increased or additional benefit requested of employers costs money, which, in the absence of increases in fees and/or staff productivity, may be impossible for them to provide, regardless of how attractive and desirable the benefit is to employees.

VACATION LEAVE

A concept often overlooked by employers is the importance of allowing or encouraging employees to use some vacation time during every six-month period and, at the minimum, earn 10 days of vacation time per year. Although employers often view employee vacation time as a hindrance to their veterinary practices, the fact is that such time usually improves the employee's and practice's productivity. Employees and owners working 45, 50, and 60 hours per week for entire years without vacations eventually suffer from fatigue, irritability, and decreased productivity. Ultimately, then, forgoing vacation is detrimental to the practice.

Compared to other countries in the world, the United States offers meager vacation time for employees. It is a well known fact that employers in Europe and Asia have traditionally offered four weeks of vacation time in the first year of employment, a benefit that is unheard for new hires in the United States. In the authors' study, in which approximately 75% of the contracts were for new associates, 8.9% of the employers offered no paid vacation and 17.3% offered only 5 days. This contributes to stress, increased turnover, feelings of exploitation, and decreased productivity of veterinary associates in their first year of employment.

To avoid such employment problems, employers could offer four weeks of vacation time, as do European and Asian employers; however, this is neither economically feasible nor competitive. Instead, considering more reasonable and contemporary options is essential to retaining quality employees and creating successful employment contracts.

Options and issues focusing on vacation time and other benefits have been gleaned from the review of hundreds of employment contracts and are presented herein. By reviewing these options and brainstorming other alternatives, employers and employees can begin to create more harmonious, fair, and enduring employee:employer relationships, benefitting all.

Vacation issues that should be addressed in employment contracts are (1) length, (2) time allotments, (3) calculations for daily vacation pay, (4) eligibility, (5) accruement, (6) scheduling approval, (7) vacation taken in conjunction with paid holidays, and (8) employee terminations and resignations and their impact on the payment of unused vacation leave.

VACATION LENGTH

Assuming competent and well-liked relief veterinarians are available, it makes sense to encourage employees to use their

Employee Salary and Benefits Statement

Employee or Employer's Name _____

Salary   See Chapter 3

Salary (regular and overtime w/o vacation, sick, or CE days) $ _____

Estimated Annual Emergency Compensation @ _____ rate   p. 115 $ _____

Estimated Annual Bonuses or production reconciliation   p. 137 $ _____

            Salary Subtotal $ _____

Salary Payroll Taxes

Federal unemployment taxes paid by employer $ _____

State unemployment taxes paid by employer $ _____

FICA paid by employer (6.2% of salary) $ _____

Medicare paid by employer (1.45% of salary) $ _____

Worker's compensation paid by employer __% of salary varies by state $ _____

         Salary Payroll Taxes Subtotal $ _____

Benefits

Health insurance paid by employer   p. 156 $ _____

Paid/unpaid (circle one) vaca days or hrs _____ at $ _____/day p. 161 $ _____

Paid/unpaid (circle one) sick days _____ at $ _____/day   p. 176 $ _____

Paid/unpaid personal days _____ at $ _____/day   p. 176 $ _____

Continuing education days _____ at $ _____/day   p. 171 $ _____

Continuing education costs for registration, lodging, travel, etc.   p. 173 $ _____

Uniform allowance   p. 267 $ _____

Automobile allowance   p. 268 $ _____

Professional association dues   p. 246 $ _____

Veterinary licenses and/or DEA registration dues   p. 252 $ _____

Value of veterinary professional services for employee's pets   p. 256 $ _____

Miscellaneous (*items that are difficult to track, e.g., animal grooming, bathing, boarding, office birthday parties, meals at staff meetings, holiday parties, discounted vet care and products & other items*) $ _____

         Benefits Subtotal $ _____

VALUE OF TOTAL COMPENSATION PACKAGE $ _____

ESTIMATED TOTAL WORK HOURS SCHEDULED PER YEAR   divided by Hrs/yr

VALUE OF TOTAL PACKAGE PER HOUR WORKED $ _____

Figure 4.1. A sample salary and benefits statement

vacation time in increments of one week or longer. This is because it usually is easier for relief veterinarians to become productive during one- to two-week increments than it is in one or two days at a time. By working five or more consecutive days, staff can get to know relief veterinarians. Additionally, the relief veterinarians can provide better continuity of care for their clients and patients, enhance their acceptance by clients, and increase their productivity.

Although it is ideal for employees to use vacation time for full weeks at a time, vacation time in shorter increments can be equally important and, in many cases, less financially detrimental and stressful to a practice. With this in mind, it is recommended that several days of each year's vacation leave be available for use as single days off to allow employees to accommodate the demands of health-care visits for their children and/or other family members, attend weddings and funerals, accommodate parental commitments at schools or parent teacher organizations, attend to other unexpected demands, or merely "recharge their batteries."

Permitting associates to use vacation time in one- to two-day increments linked to weekends or holidays also allows them to take mini vacations of three to five days, thus getting more distance out of their limited time off. For many, three- to five-day absences are as rejuvenating as a full week's vacation.

There is no doubt that accommodating these types of short-term and often short-notice requests can wreak havoc with scheduling, lead to abuses, and/or precipitate claims of discrimination among employees. Nonetheless, limiting time off to week-long increments or requiring 30 or more days notice can depreciate the value of such vacation time to employees. Thus, employees should be allowed to use at least some of each year's total vacation allowance in short segments, and with minimal notice, to allow them to handle personal or family emergencies.

VACATION TIME ALLOTMENTS

From the author's study, 8.9% of the contracts offered no paid vacation the first year, 17.3% offered only 5 days, and 64% offered 10 days. The authors' experience has shown that the most common vacation allotment to veterinary associates is 10 days per year for the first 5 to 10 years of employment, followed by 5-day increases in vacation time every 5 years thereafter, to a maximum of 15 days.

Employers awarding five-day increases every five years face markedly higher labor costs in the year when longer-term associates earn a full-week increment of additional vacation pay. An alternative to this system is to establish progressive vacation schedules based on yearly increases of one to two days, instead of major five-day increases. This allows employers to spread the additional expense for vacation time more uniformly over each of several years while creating attractive yearly incentives that discourage employees from leaving.

Table 4.4 shows the creativity of seven alternative vacation progressions. For example, in Option 4, 10 vacation days are offered for the first 5 years. During the sixth, seventh, and eighth year, vacation time is increased by 2 days to a total of 12 days per year. This is followed by 1-day increases every 3 years. Thus, the ninth, tenth, and eleventh years will include 13 vacation days per year; while the twelfth, thirteenth, and fourteenth years allow 14 days per year. The fifteenth, sixteenth, and seventeenth years offer 15 vacation days per year, and so on, to a maximum of 20 days per year. Option 5, on the other hand, forces employees to wait a little longer for additional vacation but then offers 15 days immediately. Option 6, seen only occasionally in the profession, is the most generous progression.

Veterinarians opening new practices face numerous start-up expenses. These practice owners could consider offering employees only five vacation days in the

Table 4.4. Options for Vacation Allotments

Year Employed	1	2	3	4	5	6	7	8	9	10
Number of Vacation Days										
Option										
Option 1	10	10	10	10	10	10.5	11	11.5	12	12.5
Option 2	10	10	10	10	10	11	11	12	12	13
Option 3	10	10	10	10	10	12	12	12.5	12.5	13
Option 4	10	10	10	10	10	12	12	12	13	13
Option 5	10	10	10	10	10	10	10	10	10	10
Option 6	10	12	15	15	15	15	15	15	15	15
Option 7	5	8	10	11	11	12	12	12	13	13
Year Employed	**11**	**12**	**13**	**14**	**15**	**16**	**17**	**18**	**19**	**20**
Number of Vacation Days										
Option										
Option 1	13	13.5	14	14.5	15	15.5	16	17.5	18	18.5
Option 2	13	14	14	15	15	16	16	17	17	18
Option 3	13	13.5	13.5	14	14	14.5	14.5	15	15.5	16
Option 4	13	14	14	14	15	15	15	16	16	16
Option 5	15	15	15	15	15	15	15	15	15	15
Option 6	20	20	20	20	20	20	20	20	20	20
Option 7	13	14	14	14	15	15	15	16	16	16

first year to limit costs. Then, to make up for the short vacation time offered initially, in years 2, 3, 4, and 5 they could provide 8, 10, and 11 vacation days, respectively as illustrated in Option 7. Years 6 and on would continue as described in Option 4.

This plan enables new, cost-conscious practice owners to limit costs for vacation in the early years, while allowing employees to receive extra days in their fourth and fifth years. In turn, it rewards productive and long-term employees and reduces employers' costs for employees who do not stay long enough to become eligible for the increased time off.

FIGURING THE DAILY VACATION PAY RATE

Whether associates are paid on fixed monthly or annual salaries, or as a percentage of income generated, when employers provide vacation pay as a benefit, they must determine how much to compensate for each vacation day used. To determine the daily rate of pay for each vacation, sick leave, continuing education, or any other day not worked but for which employees are entitled to compensation, employers must first determine how many days employees are likely to work in a given contract year.

This can be done according to the example set forth in Table 4.5, wherein an associate works 6 days per week but only half days on Wednesday and Saturday. Using this template, adjustments can be made to reflect the actual number of days worked by associates in any practice.

Calculations for Employees on Base Salary

To determine daily vacation pay rates for employees paid flat salaries, divide the yearly salary by the number of full days worked, or scheduled to be worked, in a given year; this is usually around 240. Then multiply that figure by the number of vacation days taken at any one time. For example, Dr. Full-Time is scheduled to earn an annual base salary of $48,000, work 240 days during the full year, and receive 10 vacation days for the year. As part of his annual $48,000 salary, he will receive time off for vacation, for which $2,000 ($200/day) of his annual salary will be paid as vacation pay.

Base Salary Example for Full-Time Employees

$48,000 annual base salary
÷ 240 work days = $200/day

If Dr. Part-Timer is a permanent part-time employee, eligible for vacation time and working 8-hour shifts on Mondays, 12-hour shifts on Thursdays (including evening hours), and a half-day shift on Saturdays, one would need to prorate the yearly salary, converting the number of hours

Table 4.5. Calculations of Work Days Per Year

Days per Year		365
Days off: Sundays	-52	
Half-day: Wednesdays afternoons	-26	
Half-day Saturdays	-26	
Subtotal	**261**	
Holidays (New Year's - 1.5,		
Memorial Day - 1, Independence Day - 1,		
Labor Day - 1, Thanksgiving - 1,		
Christmas - 1.5	-7	
Subtotal	**254**	
Continuing Education (depends on		
factors such as location and income		
available to attend meetings long distances		
from home)	-3	
Subtotal	**251**	
Vacation	-10	
Sick leave (veterinarians never get sick!)	-1	
TOTAL	**240** Work days per year	

worked per year to days. For example, 22.5 hours/week = 2.8 days/week) ÷ 5 days per week = 56% of full time. Now, multiply the number of vacation days earned by the daily pay rate. For example, if Dr. Part-Timer was paid $52,000/year, i.e., $1,000 per week for 56% of full time (2.8 days per week), she would receive 56% of 10 days of vacation time per year, i.e., 5.6 days. If she planned to take one work week's vacation (2.8 days for one of her work weeks), she would receive one week's pay as vacation pay, i.e., $1,000.

Base Salary Example for Permanent Part-Time Employees

Monday = 8 hours, Thursday = 10 hours, and Saturday = 4.5 hours = 22.5 hours/week

22.5 hours/week ÷ 40 hours/week = 56% of full time

$52,000 annual base salary ÷ 52 = $1,000/week for 1 week's vacation pay of 2.8 days

A CONTRACT CLAUSE FOR VACATION PAY WITH A BASE SALARY

A contract clause for vacation pay for those on a base salary might read as follows:

Compensation for each day of an Employee's vacation, sick, and continuing education leave will be paid based upon the average daily salary paid during the contract year.

Calculations for Associates Earning Percentage-Based Compensation

When calculating associates' daily vacation pay, employers should first determine which of the following three percentage-based compensation plans apply.

Plan 1: Percentage-Based Income Without Benefits

These associates generally are paid a specified percentage (24% to 25%) of the gross income produced by their efforts and paid by the clients. Because they receive a significantly higher percentage than the

18% to 22% earned by associates receiving benefits, these veterinary employees do not receive any compensation for vacation pay, sick leave, or continuing education. Instead, money for vacation leave comes from their total annual salaries, and employers do not need to calculate daily vacation pay.

Unfortunately, these employees tend to become accustomed to the higher salaries produced by this compensation arrangement, and many do not budget for time off. The result is that they become reluctant to take vacations or leave because they earn no income when they are gone. In fact, some resent this compensation method, forgetting that the money for their time off must come from their own earnings as a more highly compensated associate rather than as a benefit offered by their employers.

Plan 2: Percentage-Based Income with Benefits but No Base

Under these plans, associates are paid straight percentage commissions (18% to 22%) of the gross income produced by their efforts and paid by clients, without any base salary. Since these associates are paid a lower percentage than those in Plan 1, they receive benefits such as vacation pay in addition to salary.

Because their pay scale is based only on a percentage of income generated, their daily vacation pay rate will fluctuate from week to week and month to month as influenced by their production. To be fair to employers and employees, it is recommended that commission-based employees' daily compensation for vacation time be based upon their average daily salaries during the three months immediately preceding the leave.

Plan 2 Example

Dr. Commission receives 20% of the income generated by her efforts. She has no base salary, but receives a benefits package that includes 10 vacation days. During the 3 months preceding Dr. Commission's vacation week, she worked a total of 60 days and generated $100,000. Her work schedule was such that she worked 5 days per week for a total of 42 hours weekly. Her vacation pay, then, is granted at an average daily pay rate of $333.33/day.

$100,000	income production
x 20%	of income produced
$20,000	in salary
÷ 60	days worked during preceding three months
$333.33	daily

Plan 3: Base Salaries with Benefits or Percentage-Based Income with Benefits, Whichever Is Higher

These associates are paid base salaries plus benefits. They are eligible for additional salary in the form of production-reconciliation compensation at the end of each month or quarter linked to a percentage of the income they generate. Their base salaries routinely are lower than the anticipated earning potential established as a percentage of their gross income. Though both employers and employees expect total compensation to exceed the established base salaries, that is not always the case. Thus, if compensation determined as a percentage of income produced is less than the monthly base salary, these associates still have the safety net of receiving their base salaries plus benefits.

In the event that the percentage-based salaries generated by these associates exceed their base rate of pay, should employers calculate their vacation, sick leave, and continuing education time using their daily income generated salaries or their daily base salaries? To save money, employers prefer to pay these benefits as established by their associates' base salaries.

This is not, however, what the contract stipulates. Furthermore, applying such an interpretation penalizes associate veterinarians who have low base salaries but are excellent income producers. These associates, rightly, expect to receive vacation pay based on their average daily salary as established by their productivity, not their bases.

These different interpretations can create conflict between employers and employees unless agreed upon at the inception of the employment relationship.

Common sense indicates that if associates are highly productive employees, they should be compensated for time off at the higher of these two pay scales. Anything less would be a disincentive. Additionally, the contract language states that these associates will be paid either a base or a percentage, whichever is higher. It says nothing about paying for their time off at the base salary, regardless of how much they are earning on a daily basis.

Thus, when computing the daily rate of pay for highly productive percentage-based associates with this clause in their contracts, employers need to calculate employees' pay based on the average daily salaries they have earned during the three months immediately preceding their time off, or the base salary rate, whichever is higher.

Plan 3 Example

Dr. Fast-Track has negotiated a salary of $80,000/year or 20% of income generated, whichever is greater. If she is working a 240-day work year, her daily base pay would average $333.33/day ($80,000 ÷ 240 = $333.33).

Dr. FT decides to take three days of vacation in October. In looking at the preceding three months of employment, i.e., July through September, she generated $100,000 for the practice, or $12,500 above her base level for that quarter. This is calculated as follows:

$80,000	is the yearly base salary
÷ 20%	of income generated is her rate of compensation
$400,000	of income production needed/year to achieve base salary
÷	
4	quarters in a year
$100,000	income generation/quarter to achieve base pay

$112,500 actual income production
for previous quarter

$100,000 needed to achieve base
for quarter

$12,500 of income production above
base level

Because Dr. Fast Track produced $112,500 of income during the previous three months, she was entitled to a quarterly salary of $22,500. If she worked 60 days during the quarter, this translates into $375/day. This is calculated as follows:

$112,500 quarterly production

× 20% of income generated

$22,500 for this three months

- $20,000 base salary already paid

$2,500 in production reconciliation
compensation for the quarter

$22,500 compensation for the quarter

÷ 60 days worked in the quarter

$375 salary per day

If an employer divided Dr. Fast Track's base salary of $80,000/year by the 240 days she was scheduled to work that year, she would be paid $333.33/day. Because of Dr. Fast Track's excellent productivity, though, she earned $22,500 in the quarter immediately preceding her vacation. If she worked 60 days during the quarter, that translates into $375/day. It is logical, then, that she be paid $375/day for every day of vacation, sick leave, or continuing education used during this time period, rather than that calculated at the lower base salary rate of $333.33/day.

Conflicts may arise when associates' percentage-based income for a given three-month period is less than their base salary. Even though employers would prefer to pay for vacation time for these associates based upon the lower-income-generated figures rather than the base salaries, the contracts for these individuals stipulate that

employees are to receive a base salary or percentage, whichever is greater. That means employers are required to pay for vacation time at the higher base rate, too, instead of the lower income production rate.

A CONTRACT CLAUSE FOR VACATION PAY WITH PERCENTAGE-BASED COMPENSATION

The following clause which deals with vacation pay could be used in employment contracts:

Once Employee has earned percent-based compensation in excess of Employee's base salary, compensation for Employee's vacation, continuing education, and sick leave shall be paid based upon the average daily compensation amount paid to the Employee during the three months preceding the use of such leave, rather than at the base rate for the contract year. If Employee fails to earn percentage-based compensation equal to or in excess of Employee's base salary during the three months preceding the taking of any time off, then Employee's vacation, continuing education, and sick leave will be paid based upon Employee's base salary during the three months immediately preceding such time off.

Employee Eligibility

Ideally, upon completion of the requisite probation or introductory period, employees should be eligible to take half of their vacation time after the first six months, and the other half after or in close proximity to the completion of the first year of employment. In the ensuing years, employee eligibility for vacation time can be as it accrues, although to assure completion of each contract year, some employers prefer to limit eligibility until after completion of each full year of employment. This may appear unfair and impractical to employees. For employers, however, it encourages associates to stay the full length of each contract term rather than resign early.

A CONTRACT CLAUSE FOR EMPLOYEE ELIGIBILITY THAT ENCOURAGES COMPLETION OF THE CONTRACTUAL TERM

The following contract clause could be included to encourage completion of each year of an employment contract:

Employee will be eligible to take vacation time after (six) months of employment. Should the Employee voluntarily resign prior to the completion of the contract year, no vacation, continuing education, or sick leave shall be due or payable, and any prior payments for vacation, continuing education, or sick leave will be deducted from Employee's final paycheck.

ACCRUING VACATION LEAVE

In general, employers should require that employees use vacation leave in the year they earn it rather than saving it from year to year. This diminishes the adverse effects of paying for the vacation time earned during two or more years all in one year. It also minimizes the awkwardness of having employees out of the workplace for lengthy time periods, and encourages compulsive workers to use vacation leave and recharge their batteries more regularly rather than lose it.

The problem with mandatory vacation leave, however, is that it pressures employees to use their vacation leave at inopportune times rather than saving it for special circumstances, such as weddings and honeymoons, long-planned family gatherings, or continuing education seminars at remote locations.

In instances like these, allowing vacation to accumulate helps and motivates employees. Thus, employers are encouraged to be flexible in allowing some vacation time to accrue, rather than forcing employees to use it all or lose it. Contract language that allows for some vacation time to accrue from year to year, with the written consent of employers, helps provide for a modicum

of flexibility while encouraging employees to use their vacation as it is being earned.

A CONTRACT CLAUSE FOR VACATION ACCRUEMENT

The following contract clause addresses vacation accruement:

Employee will earn vacation time at the rate of (5⅓, 8⅓, 10⅓) workdays per full year of employment (or alternatively, at the rate of [0.5⅓, 0.75⅓] workdays per full month of employment). Vacation leave must be used in the year it is earned, and may not be accumulated and carried over from year to year without the written consent of the Employer.

SCHEDULING APPROVAL

Requests for vacation time should be made a specified number of days prior to the scheduled time of absence. Except for family emergencies, associates should be required to give 30 to 60 days' notice prior to taking desired time off and whenever possible be willing, or required, to assist employers in finding acceptable replacements. The specified number of days notice may depend on the season of the year, availability of relief veterinarians or other veterinary coverage, and the nature of the request. If timing conflicts exist with other employees, it seems logical to base decisions on seniority, on a first-come first-serve basis or, perhaps, decide the issue with the flip of a coin.

A CONTRACT CLAUSE FOR SCHEDULING APPROVAL

The following contract clause covers scheduling approvals:

Scheduling of vacation time for periods in excess of 2 days must be presented to the Employer at least (30 to 60) days prior to the start of the desired time off. Scheduling of vacation time for 1 to 2 days off must be made a minimum of (15 to 30) days prior. Employee will assist Employer with locating a replacement veterinarian or risk foregoing the requested time off.

VACATION LEAVE IN CONJUNCTION WITH PAID HOLIDAYS

If the benefits package for employees includes holidays, and the vacation leave is concurrent with a holiday, employees' vacation accounts should be charged only for the workdays taken in conjunction with the holiday. Daily compensation for this time off should be calculated as presented previously, and employees should be paid for the holiday and vacation time separately.

Abuses can occur if associates routinely use vacation time in conjunction with holiday time, leaving the remaining staff or practice owners with the burden of covering busy days adjacent to the holidays. Therefore, some employers have found it wise not to allow associates to use vacation time in conjunction with holidays more than once a year.

A CONTRACT CLAUSE FOR VACATION LEAVE IN CONJUNCTION WITH PAID HOLIDAYS

The following contract clause addresses this concern:

Upon the provision of notice of 60 or more days, Employee may take vacation time in conjunction with holidays (1?, 2?) times per year. Employee must receive written approval by Employer to take vacation time in conjunction with holidays more than the allotted number of times per year.

EMPLOYEE TERMINATION AND UNUSED VACATION LEAVE

To be fair to employees, if employers terminate associates' employment after completion of the requisite orientation and training period but before fulfillment of the specified term, employers should prorate employees' vacation time based on the percentage of the full year actually worked. On the other hand, as discussed previously, employers who wish to encourage employ-

ees to honor the entire terms of their contracts can penalize employees who voluntarily resign prior to the completion of their contracts by withholding all vacation time. Since vacation pay is not required by law, agreements between employers and employees need to be negotiated and stated fully.

A CONTRACT CLAUSE FOR UNUSED VACATION LEAVE AT EMPLOYEE TERMINATION

The following contract clause relating to employee termination and vacation pay could be used in employment contracts:

Should the Employee's employment be terminated by Employer prior to the completion of the requisite orientation and training period, Employee will earn no vacation pay. Should employment be terminated by Employer after requisite orientation and training period but before the fulfillment of the contract term, the Employee's vacation leave will be prorated based upon the percentage of the full year worked for the Employer. In the event the Employee voluntarily resigns at any time prior to the completion of the contract term, no vacation time shall be due or payable, and money paid for vacation time taken prior to such resignation shall be deducted from employee's final paycheck.

EXCEPTIONS TO THE VACATION PLAN

Employers and employees must recognize that at some points during a professional's career, vacation time might be less important than other factors. For instance, associates may need to concentrate on saving money for the purchase of a car, a down payment on a home, or the arrival of a baby. In these situations, employees may seek compensation for vacation time in the form of extra pay rather than as forced vacation.

Alternatively, additional time off at the time of a move or the birth of a baby may be just what the doctor ordered. Thus, flexibility and good communication between both parties are essential.

NATIONAL STANDARDS FOR VACATION LEAVE

As reported in Table 4.3, 76% of female and 71% of male 2001 graduates received annual vacation leave.[8] That study, however, did not indicate how much time off was provided. Based on the authors' three-year study of veterinary employment contracts, 91% of associates received vacation leave. The authors' experience has shown that the most common vacation schedule is 10 days per year for the first 5 to 10 years of employment, and 5-day increases in vacation time every 5 years thereafter.

CONTINUING EDUCATION

The authors' experience has shown that employers providing the most generous continuing education (CE) benefits for their veterinary associates and support staff tend to be the best overall employers. Employers who value CE understand the importance of staying abreast of current professional information and trends and expect staff members to do likewise. They also realize that through their financial commitments to fund the CE costs for associates and willingness to provide time off with pay, they are investing in the future of their manpower resources, hoping to create more loyal, appreciative, productive, and profitable employees in the process.

Time and money are factors in the CE plans of many veterinary practices. With advances in communication technology, CE can be achieved through the use of computers and videos from one's home or at the veterinary practice with minimal expenses and time investments. The following CE suggestions enable veterinarians to further their professional growth without exorbitant registration fees, travel expenses, and extended time commitments:

- attending general and specialty rounds at veterinary schools

- attending seminars provided by various student-organized feline, avian, exotic animal, and equine clubs at veterinary schools

- subscribing to journals that provide articles and supplemental questions for CE credit (e.g., *The Compendium for Continuing Education*)

- utilizing videotapes with supplemental questions for CE credit (e.g., Waltham)

- accessing the AVMA's Network of Animal Health (NOAH) and the Veterinary Information Network (VIN), both of which are less expensive if computer, modem, and Internet access are available for the associate

- frequenting seminars held by local veterinary associations

- helping organize and participating in free or in-hospital seminars offered by pet food and pharmaceutical companies

Financial investments and time commitments for CE cannot always be avoided. In the case of species-based specialties like avian, equine, bovine, feline, or small ruminant medicine, or system-based specialties such as surgery, oncology, dermatology, and internal medicine, there may be only one terrific meeting in the United States each year. For some associates the opportunity for socialization and after-class learning make attendance at formal CE meetings the most valuable medium in which to continue professional growth. Yet, those who have exceptional self-discipline and are great self-starters may be able to stay abreast while studying at home.

State, regional, and national seminars often necessitate traveling to distant locations for several days of educational seminars. Therefore, if employers wish to achieve maximal success from their CE investments, the CE sections of employment contracts should address the following issues: (1) the annual number of days available to employees and whether such time off will be with or without pay, (2) time-in-service requirements for eligibility, (3) scheduling approval, (4) accruement of CE days, (5) which, if any, expenses will be covered by employers, and (6) obligations to present in-hospital seminars about pertinent information gleaned from attendance at such meetings.

CE ELIGIBILITY, SCHEDULING APPROVAL, AND ACCRUEMENT

Ideally, first-year veterinary associates should be eligible for CE benefits after the completion of at least six months of employment, and they should receive a minimum of two to three paid CE days annually. Support staff should be eligible for one to two days of CE and an equivalent or increased amount of education annually thereafter. To discourage early resignations by employees in either category, the allotment of a full CE benefit during the initial and subsequent years should be contingent on completing each year of employment.

Problems arise when new employees are not eligible to attend CE until after the completion of the entire term of their contracts. If they are terminated early or their contracts are not renewed, they become the losers, unable to acquire the desired education or take advantage of this important benefit. Conversely, if they are compensated for their expenses and attendance at seminars but resign prior to completing their contract terms, their employers, who have incurred the cost but lost the value of their CE investment, are the losers.

To resolve this dilemma, employers who have paid for CE only to see employees resign prior to the end of their contract terms should expect to be reimbursed for the CE expenses they have incurred. Conversely, employers who fire staff members after they have completed nine or more months of the agreed-upon term, but prior to the end of the contract term, should not expect to be reimbursed for CE expenditures they have made on behalf of their employees.

In a perfect environment, associates who receive two to three days of paid CE time in the first year of their contracts should be eligible for at least three days in their second and third years, four days in their fourth year and, ideally, five days in their fifth or more years of employment. Reasons for providing such generous CE benefits are (1) to establish incentives that encourage associates to remain with their employers for longer time periods and (2) because it fulfills the need for maturing practitioners to acquire increasing amounts of CE.

To best serve their practices, employers should play a role in deciding the CE topics for their employees. Only if they help employees design their yearly CE attendance can employers enhance the types of services offered by their practices and fill the gaps in each person's education. Requests for attendance at CE meetings should be received by employers a specified number of days prior to the scheduled event. When conflicts exist between two or more associates, decisions can be based on seniority, a coin flip, or the importance of specific CE material to the practice or the employees. In general, employers should require that CE benefits be used in the year in which they are earned, and not allow them to be carried over from year to year without the employers' written consent.

A CONTRACT CLAUSE FOR CE

A contract clause addressing continuing education can read:

Upon completion of (6?, 8?, 9?) months employment, Employee is entitled to (2?, 3?, 4?, 5?) days off with pay to attend continuing education seminars prior to completion of the contract term. Should Employee voluntarily resign prior to the end of the contract term, Employee must reimburse Employer for the expenditures Employer has made on behalf of Employee's continuing educa-

tion. If Employer terminates Employee's employment after (8½, 9½, 10½) months of the contract year but prior to completion of the contract term, then Employee shall not be required to reimburse Employer for continuing education expenditures. If Employee earns CE days and a specified amount of money for CE expenses but has not used the benefit prior to voluntary resignation or Employer termination, no compensation shall be due. Employee must make requests to attend continuing education seminars to the Employer or designated supervisor (15½, 30½) days prior to the scheduled seminar. Employee must use the paid continuing education days during the contract term in which they are earned and cannot accrue this benefit from year to year without the written consent of the Employer.

CE TUITION AND TRAVEL EXPENSES INCURRED

Costs for CE can be very limited (reading journals already received by the practice) or very expensive (flying to a Carribean island for a week of sun and fun plus some education thrown in to qualify the excursion as a business expense). Studies have shown that most practices spend 1% to 2% of gross income to repair and maintain the functionality of the physical plant and equipment in which they practice.[9] Unfortunately, most employers spend less than 0.7% of their gross income maintaining the functionality of the brainpower of their staff.[9] If more practice owners hit a benchmark of 0.8% to 1% for CE expenditures and spread this important benefit out among the entire staff, employee attrition would be reduced, morale would improve, and the profession's clients and patients would be better served. Practice owners and managers who are progressive enough to budget for the continuing education of their employees need to decide which of the following CE expenses will be covered for their employees:

• registration fees

• travel (air, train, auto, taxis, shuttles, and parking)

• housing

• meals ($35/day generally covers reasonable costs)

• wet lab expenses

• entertainment (generally reserved for practice owners)

Costs for registration and banquets or special events can be paid by employers directly or by employees. Within a specified time after returning from CE meetings, e.g., two weeks, employees should have submitted receipts of CE expenses incurred and evidence of completion of courses to their employers. For tax and accounting purposes, records of these transactions should be kept in the employee's file.

It is not uncommon for veterinary employers to dawdle when reimbursing employees for out-of-pocket CE expenses. This tardiness may be due to cash flow shortages, forgetfulness, disorganized bookkeeping and accounts payable systems, retribution for discord in the employer:employee relationship, or procrastination. Thus, it is in the employee's best interest to have clauses included in the contract delineating time periods within which reimbursements should be made. Although employers often omit this issue in their employment contracts, establishing and complying with clear expectations for reimbursement of expenses eradicates staff distrust and confusion about employers' motives and improves staff morale.

A CONTRACT CLAUSE FOR CE EXPENSES INCURRED

A contract clause regarding CE expenses incurred can read:

Employee will receive time off with pay to attend (2½, 3½, 5½) days of veterinary continuing education during the term of each contract year. Additional time off without compensation may be provided upon the mutual consent of the parties.

Costs to cover registration, travel, lodging, (meals?, other incidental expenses?) associated with attendance at professional continuing education meetings required and/or approved by Employer shall not exceed ($350?, $500?, $1,250?) per year. Employee agrees to submit such documentation necessary for Employer to substantiate any reimbursable expenses incurred by Employee within two weeks of attending such meetings. Employer agrees to reimburse Employee only for Employee's accurately documented expenses and will do so within (10?, 15?) work days of receipt of such expense report.

Employees Presenting In-Hospital Seminars

Associates returning from CE nearly always have an enhanced enthusiasm for the practice of veterinary medicine. This stems from learning new material, visits with exhibitors, reviews of autotutorial programs, and from inspiring conversations with classmates and/or colleagues over drinks or dinner. Still, for employers to receive their money's worth from this CE expenditure, newly learned materials should be shared with the practice's veterinarians, support staff, and clientele. Within a specified period of time after returning from a meeting, e.g., two weeks, employers should require that employees present discussions of predetermined topics from the newly learned information by one or more of the following methods:

- preparing a client brochure using layperson terminology

- writing an article for the practice's newsletter

- creating an outline or algorithm of new information for colleagues and support staff

- presenting a 20- to 40-minute seminar to the veterinarians and/or support staff

- drafting outlines for the adoption of new medical, anesthetic, or surgical protocols

A Contract Clause Addressing Employee CE Responsibilities

The following is a contract clause for veterinary employment contracts incorporating a service requirement regarding CE:

In recognition of Employer's investment in furthering Employee's veterinary education, within two weeks of Employee's return from any employer-subsidized continuing education program(s), Employee shall evaluate the new materials that were learned and complete one or more of the following: (1) draft language for a client handout, (2) write an article for the client newsletter, (3) create an algorithm for colleagues and support staff, (4) provide Employer's veterinary and/or support staff with an organized presentation of pertinent information acquired at such continuing education meeting, and/or (5) submit a statement recommending new medical, anesthetic, or surgical protocols.

State Requirements for CE

There is tremendous variation among state laws regarding mandatory CE for veterinarians. For example, some states have no mandatory CE requirements, while others require 20 hours annually. According to one report, 29 of 50 states mandated CE for licensed veterinarians in 1990, and 38 states required it by 1996.[10] With the addition of California in 1998 as another, veterinary CE now is mandated in nearly 80% of the states.

Appendix II lists CE requirements by state, province, or territory, the year the CE requirement was implemented, the mandatory CE hours required per renewal period, and special comments for each jurisdiction.[10]

The special comments reveal specific CE restrictions. For example, some states accept only medical and scientific CE, while other states accept a limited number of hours of nonmedical subjects like practice management in addition to medical/scientific material. Some states accept a certain number of CE hours by online computer or audiovisual materials. Further information can be obtained from the pertinent state board of veterinary examiners.

NATIONAL STANDARDS FOR CE

The authors' study indicates that 65% of employment contracts offered employees CE annually (Table 4.1). The number of paid days and average dollar amounts allocated for employees' expenses were 4 days and $587, respectively (Table 4.2).

HOLIDAY LEAVE

National holidays include New Year's Day, Martin Luther King Day, President's Day, Memorial Day, Independence Day, Labor Day, Veteran's Day, Thanksgiving Day, and Christmas Day. Although employers legally are not required to offer paid holidays, the vast majority provide all of these except President's Day, Martin Luther King Day, and Veteran's Day.[11]

To be complete, employment contracts should address the following holiday issues: (1) employee eligibility, (2) allotments for emergency care and hospitalized patient coverage, and (3) payment options.

EMPLOYEE ELIGIBILITY AND HOLIDAY ALLOTMENTS

Upon completion of the requisite orientation and training period, employees typically receive full pay for the big six holidays, consisting of New Year's Day, Memorial Day, Fourth of July, Labor Day, Thanksgiving, and Christmas. Depending on the availability of staff doctors and local emergency clinics, employees may or may not be required to take emergency calls and/or attend hospitalized cases on one or more of these days. While some practice owners may not plan their holidays with long lead times, new graduates accustomed to school holidays and religious considerations truly expect and need these breaks. To allow for adequate planning, associates

should be apprised of their holiday schedules at least three months in advance.

An interesting alternative in practice many places is to divide holidays into major ones— New Year's Day, Thanksgiving, Christmas—and minor ones—Memorial Day, July 4th, and Labor Day. This allows employees to divide on-call duty, thus capping the number of emergency call days at no more than, e.g., two major holidays and two minor ones per year (the exact number to be determined by employers).

A CONTRACT CLAUSE FOR HOLIDAY LEAVE

Contract language for holiday leave could read:

Upon completion of the (60-day) orientation and training period, paid holidays will include New Year's Day, Memorial Day, Fourth of July, Labor Day, Thanksgiving, and Christmas. The Employee will be required to take emergency calls and/or attend hospitalized cases on (¼?, ⅓?, ½?) of these specified holidays. Should any of these holidays fall on a weekend, resulting in the practice being closed on a weekday in conjunction with such holiday, the Employee will take emergencies and attend hospitalized cases on both the holiday and the day the practice is closed in celebration of the holiday.

Alternatively, the clause could read:

Paid holidays will include full pay for New Year's Day, Thanksgiving, and Christmas (hereinafter called "major holidays") and Memorial Day, July 4th, and Labor Day (hereinafter "minor holidays"). Employee shall not be required to work and/or be on emergency call more than (one?, two?) major holiday(s) and/or (one?, two?) minor holiday(s) per year.

HOLIDAY PAYMENT OPTIONS

Calculations for determining holiday pay for associates are the same as those used for vacation pay. Are employees receiving hourly wages, base salaries, or percentage-based compensation? If they are on hourly wages, they are typically paid for an eight-hour day. When paid yearly base salaries, prorated to monthly or weekly wages, employee paychecks are unaffected by the occurrence of a holiday during a pay period. If employee compensation is production based, readers are referred back to the sections of this chapter calculating daily vacation pay for such employees.

RELIGIOUS HOLIDAYS

Employers should be mindful of religious holidays. For Jewish employees, Rosh Hashanah and Yom Kippur might be offered as paid or unpaid holidays or as paid holidays in lieu of Christmas. The difficulty with this policy is that, unless a countervailing adjustment is made to the person's vacation pay or sick leave, Jewish employees receive one more holiday per year than their Christian counterparts.

For Christian employees, practices that are open on Sundays might consider Easter Sunday as a paid or unpaid holiday. For multi-doctor practices, a blend of Jewish, Christian, agnostic, or atheist doctors works well to accommodate broader work coverage of these diverse religious holidays. Obviously, adjustments to overall vacation, sick leave, and holiday time must be made depending on which religious holidays are celebrated by various employees and owners and how the holidays fall with respect to weekends in each calendar year.

NATIONAL STANDARDS FOR HOLIDAY LEAVE

The AVMA study of employment contracts referenced earlier in Table 4.3 shows that 37% of the agreements provided to new graduates included paid legal holidays. Since most of the contracts reviewed by the authors were silent on this issue, it was not included in their analysis of employee benefits.

SICK AND/OR PERSONAL LEAVE

Paid sick leave is intended to protect staff members against financial losses in the event of short-term illnesses or accidents. Most employers provide some type of sick leave coverage for their employees; however, there are major inconsistencies in the granting and amount of such time off within the profession.

Although sick leave is earned personally by employees, most employers allow employees to use this paid time off to cover medical care for themselves and to attend to the health care needs of their immediate families. A minority of employers compensate their employees for unused sick time.

Compensation for remaining well seems equitable; otherwise, the only employees who profit from this benefit are those who get sick. Though most illnesses are legitimate, employee absences disrupt work schedules, unfairly distribute work loads, reduce the practice's income and, if misused, negatively impact staff morale. Thus, considerable thought should go into the allocation of and methods by which sick leave is granted to employees. Among the myriad issues to be addressed are the following:

- whether sick leave and personal leave should be granted and tracked in the same category or treated as separate benefits;
- whether earned but unused sick leave should be forfeited annually or allowed to accumulate;
- whether sick leave taken prior to or in excess of that which has been earned should be deducted from the employee's final paycheck;
- whether employees who are allowed to cumulate their sick leave from year to year should be compensated for unused leave if they (a) voluntarily resign or (b) are terminated by employers; and

- when employees are allowed to cumulate sick leave and be compensated for days in excess of a specified number, whether the timing of this "well leave" compensation should be on an annual anniversary date, at the employer's discretion, or upon the employee's request.

Differentiating Sick Leave from Personal Leave

While sick leave generally is reserved for personal or family health needs, personal leave constitutes paid time off to attend to personal matters other than health, such as attending school appointments or meetings for the purchase or sale of a home. Time spent and tasks performed during peoples' personal days often are not consistent with vacation time, since employees usually are not on vacation. The use of this time, however, is not and should not be intended to cover personal illnesses. Thus, for clarity and because of the banking options to be discussed herein, employers who wish to provide associates with personal days are encouraged to provide such leave as time off other than vacation or sick leave, and not lump it in with sick leave. "Family" usually is defined as immediate family, or an alternative definition is written in the practice's personnel policy manual.

No norms exist for the provision of personal time. A minority of employers provide such time either (1) on an ad hoc basis as a means of rewarding loyal and long-term employees for exceptional efforts or (2) because they never have thought through these types of issues. Employers are advised to review the variety of other important benefits and read and understand all the issues presented in this chapter before providing employees with annual allocations of personal time. Perhaps, allocating two of each year's vacation days as personal days, to be taken in increments of 2 to 8 hours for family or personal matters is an option.

Sick Leave Allotments

Because of the hassles involved in rescheduling entire days of appointments, veterinary associates rarely call in sick. Instead, they tend to tough it out and hide their illnesses much like members of the feline and avian species. Nonetheless, employment contracts routinely offer associates three to six paid sick days per year, which means such days accrue at the rate of one-quarter to one-half day per month, depending on the employer's generosity and policy.

Employee Eligibility

Employees should be eligible to use paid sick leave for legitimate illnesses after the completion of a standard two- or three-month orientation and training period. Time off for illnesses, accidents, doctor's appointments, or child care responsibilities prior to the completion of the orientation and training period should be treated as leaves of absence without pay.

Sick and Personal Leave Accruement

Most contracts do not allow sick leave to accrue from year to year and, thus, the time not used at the end of each contract year is lost. These "use it or lose it" policies encourage healthy employees to take sick leave despite the havoc it creates in the workplace. Other contracts allow accrued sick leave to be used in future years. This "save it for a rainy day" philosophy encourages employees to retain sick and personal leave time as a short-term disability insurance policy or receive it as a well-leave bonus. The longer employees remain employed, the more value they can create in this benefit and, thus, the stronger the incentive is to remain well and employed at the practice.

An idea utilized by some practice owners is to allow employees to accrue 10 days of sick leave in a "bank account" and, when the minimum balance has been met, compensate these healthy people for unused time in excess of the minimum balance by paying well leave bonuses. The rationale for such a policy includes the following:

- It rewards the healthy without penalizing the sick, because both parties receive compensation for this employee benefit.

- It serves as a strong incentive for employees not to disrupt schedules by calling in sick.

- It encourages employees to remain employed and healthy long enough to take advantage of the excess sick leave bonus policy.

- It serves as an employer-financed short-term disability insurance policy, with no premium costs to employers or employees.

Employees may request payment of their excess sick leave whenever they feel they have enough time off in the bank for their personal comfort. In some cases, this may be as soon as they have more than the minimum 10 days. In other cases, they may decide to wait until they have 20 days in the bank before requesting the excess. For employers who worry about reserves to cover large volumes of banked sick leave, 20- or 25-day caps can be included in contracts.

To avoid being required to compensate employees for unused sick leave at times when the practice's cash flow is low, employers who establish sick leave savings bank plans are urged to reserve the right to time the payments of these well-leave bonuses at their discretion.

A CONTRACT CLAUSE FOR SICK LEAVE ACCRUEMENT

A contract clause for sick leave accruement with no savings bank is as follows:

Employee shall be eligible for sick leave to be used for personal or family ill-nesses after completion of a (two?, three?) month orientation and training period. For Employees who continue employment beyond the established orientation and training period, sick leave shall accrue at the rate of (one-quarter?, one-half?) day per month, commencing with the date of the signing of this Agreement. Sick leave will not be allowed to accumulate from year to year, and any sick leave not used at the end of each contract year will be lost.

Alternative language allowing for sick leave to accumulate in a savings bank would read as follows:

Employee shall be eligible for sick leave to be used for personal or family ill-nesses after completion of a (two?, three?) month orientation and training period. For Employees who continue employment beyond the orientation and training period, such leave shall accrue at the rate of (one-quarter?, one-half?) day per month, commencing with the date of the signing of this Agreement. Employees are allowed to accumulate this leave from year to year, commencing with the original date of employment, to a maximum of (10?, 20?, 25?) days. At the request of Employee, days in excess of 10 held in Employee's "sick leave bank account" will be paid as a bonus as "well leave;" however, the timing of payments will be at the discretion and convenience of the Employer. Sick leave will not be earned during any leaves of absence.

NOTIFICATION REQUIREMENTS

Employers should require associates and support staff to inform their supervisors of their intent to use sick leave no less than one hour before the shift occurs. Twenty-four hour notice is recommended whenever possible. A contract clause covering notice to be provided to employers prior to the utilization of sick leave can be included in the employment contract or, more often, in the practice's personnel policy manual.

Compensation for Sick Leave

Since sick leave, like vacation and CE time, is paid in daily increments, monthly salaries or percentage-based compensation must be broken down into daily segments to calculate compensation. The same methods and examples used to determine daily vacation pay can be applied to sick leave.

Contract clauses covering rates of pay for sick leave of employees paid base salaries or percentage-based compensation are included in the previous sections of this chapter dealing with compensation for vacation pay.

Sick and Personal Leave at Employee Termination

Employers must have compensation policies in place in advance of terminating employees. There are two components of the issues to consider: first, have employees resigned prior to the end of their contract terms or have employers fired them before their contracts expire and; second, how will compensation for unused sick time be handled?

With respect to unused sick time, there are three basic policy options:

1. no year-to-year accrual, i.e., not compensating employees for any of their accrued sick leave;

2. a very generous policy which compensates employees for all sick leave accumulated, including the 10-day minimum balance stored in the bank plus all time in excess of that balance; or

3. a middle-of-the-road approach paying employees only for the value of the sick leave in excess of the minimum 10-day balance.

Beyond choosing a general policy, it should be considered whether sick leave payment will differ depending on whether employees resign or are terminated prior to the end of any contract term. In general, since most employers prohibit employees from cumulating sick leave, it seems reason-able to pay employees who are leaving only for sick leave accrued in excess of the minimum balance required for the bank. This provides an incentive for associates not to use such time off but limits employers' costs when people leave. While providing compensation for all cumulated sick leave is a recommended and admirable position, this may not be financially feasible for some employers. On the other hand, providing no compensation for unused sick leave seems to be a self-defeating policy that encourages employees to use it or lose it, instead of cumulating their own short-term disability protection. Employers are encouraged to consider all the options before applying the one that best fits their management philosophy and financial situation.

As with vacation leave, if employees are terminated by employers prior to fulfillment of the specified term, fair and progressive employers will prorate sick leave based on the percentage of the full year worked. Conversely, it seems fair that employees who inconvenience their employers by resigning prior to completion of the contract term forfeit all sick time not taken.

A CONTRACT CLAUSE FOR EMPLOYEE TERMINATION

A contract clause for employee termination is as follows:

Should the Employee's employment be terminated by the Employer after (6½, 9½) months, payment for the Employee's accrued sick leave in excess of the 10-day minimum balance to be retained for short-term disabilities will be paid by Employer within 10 working days of such termination. Should the Employee voluntarily resign prior to the completion of any contract term, no accrued sick time shall be due or payable.

Another issue surfaces if employers have compensated employees for sick leave and then employees resign prior to the end of the contract term. In most cases, employers simply forego any efforts to recoup their costs. But employment contracts could include a clause allowing employers to withhold prior payments for sick time from the employee's final paycheck. If that is the intent of the employer, the final sentence of the above paragraph would read as follows:

Should the Employee voluntarily resign prior to the completion of the contract year, no accrued vacation or sick time shall be due or payable, and any prior payment for such time will be withheld from the Employee's final paycheck.

NATIONAL STANDARDS FOR SICK AND PERSONAL LEAVE

In the authors' study, the data show that 41% of employees received sick pay (Table 4.1). No analysis was completed of the contracts silent on this issue to determine the frequency with which employers failed to include sick and personal leave in the contract but paid for it anyway.

LEAVES OF ABSENCE

Leaves of absence enable employees to balance family needs with workplace demands, creating stability and economic security for families. Employers offering leaves of absence to promote, maintain, and strengthen the stability of their employees' lives can directly affect the productivity and loyalty of those employees.

With increasing longevity among Americans, our society is facing a larger percentage of elderly people. The consequences will be increasing demands for employees to care for these elderly family members, often in addition to caring for their own children. While leave of absence benefits enable American workers to better handle family responsibilities, the use or misuse of them can be devastating to small business owners.

With the increase in women entering the veterinary workforce, leaves of absence for pregnancy have become commonplace.

In 1980, 9.5% of veterinarians were female. In 1994, 28.7% of veterinarians were female. If the trend continues as projected, by the year 2004, the number of female veterinarians in the United States will equal the number of male veterinarians.

This demographic change also is occurring in other professions. From 1980 to 1994, the percentage of female lawyers increased from 12.8% to 24.8%, the percentage of female physicians increased from 13.4% to 22.3%, and the percentage of female dentists increased from 4.3% to 13.3%.[12]

Even though employees' needs for leaves of absence have grown, employers are not legally mandated and cannot financially afford to provide every type of leave of absence. Beneficial but not legally required leaves of absence include weddings and funerals. Legally mandated leaves of absence include (1) serious health conditions of self, children, spouses, or parents (which, depending on the size of the business, may be governed by the Family and Medical Leave Act); (2) pregnancy leave; (3) medical leave for occupational disability; (4) jury or witness duty, and (5) military leave.[11]

THE FAMILY AND MEDICAL LEAVE ACT

The purpose of the Family and Medical Leave Act of 1993 (FMLA) is to preserve family integrity. This act aims to benefit employees without adversely affecting employers. Eligibility requirements include that the individual

- has been employed by the employer for at least 12 months,

- has been employed for at least 1,250 hours of service during the 12-month period immediately preceding the commencement of the leave, and

- is employed at a worksite where 50 or more employees are employed by the employer within 75 miles of that worksite.[13]

Employers covered by FMLA are required to grant leave to eligible employees for the following circumstances:

- the birth of a son or daughter, and to care for the newborn child;

- the placement of a child with the employee for adoption or foster care;

- to care for the employee's spouse, son, daughter, or parent with a serious health condition; and

- serious health conditions that prevent employees from performing the functions of their jobs.[14]

For the most part, FMLA leave is unpaid. Employees have the right to substitute other types of paid leave such as vacation, sick, or personal leave for FMLA leave. Eligible employees are entitled to a total of 12 work weeks off during any 12-month period for any one or more of the four previously described circumstances.

Employees must provide employers with 30 days written notice prior to taking family and medical leaves of absence.[15] It should state the reason for the leave of absence, the duration of leave, when the leave will begin, and when it will end. If an unforeseeable medical emergency occurs, employees must give notice as soon as possible. Employers can deny FMLA leave if previously specified requirements are not met.

Employers can require seriously ill employees or employees with seriously ill spouses, children, or parents to produce documents from their health care providers substantiating the need for a medical leave. The Department of Labor has developed a form that employees or their family members can use when obtaining medical certification. This form, WH-380, entitled *Certification of Health Care Provider*, meets the FMLA's certification requirements (Figure 4.2).[16] Alternatively, employers can create their own forms as long as they meet the Department of Labor requirements.

A form for employers to use in responding to employees' requests for FMLA leave is presented in Figure 4.3.[16]

During an FMLA leave, employees are entitled to the same group health insurance benefits they were receiving prior to the leave. For example, if employers and employees were both contributing to health insurance premiums, then both continue to contribute at the same level. If the employers were paying the premiums, they are required to continue the payments during the leave of absence.

During leaves of absence, employees are required to report to employers periodically about their health status or that of the family member and their plans to return to work. Upon return from leaves of absence, employees have the right to be placed in the original or a similar job position and receive the same pay, benefits, and working conditions.

In addition to the federally mandated FMLAs, some states have their own family and medical leaves of absence laws. State or local laws that are more stringent than federal laws take precedent. The FMLA of 1993, §825.701, which supports this fact, reads as follows:

(a) Nothing in the FMLA supersedes any provision of State or local law that provides greater family or medical leave rights than those provided by FMLA. The Department of Labor will not, however, enforce State family or medical leave laws, and States will not enforce the FMLA. Employees are not required to designate whether the leave they are taking is FMLA leave or leave under State law, and an employer must comply with the appropriate (applicable) provisions of both. An employer covered by one law and not the other has to comply with the law under which it is covered. Similarly, an employee eligible under only one law must receive benefits in accordance with that law. If leave qualifies for FMLA leave and leave under State law, the leave used counts against the employee's entitlement under both laws.[17]

Certification of Health Care Provider (Family and Medical Leave Act of 1993)	**U.S. Department of Labor** Employment Standards Administration Wage and Hour Division
	OMB No.: 1215-0181 Expires: 08-31-99
1. Employee's Name	2. Patient's Name (if different from employee)

3. The attached sheet describes what is meant by a **"serious health condition"** under the Family and Medical Leave Act. Does the patient's condition[1] qualify under any of the categories described? If so, please check the applicable category.

       (1) _____ (2) _____ (3) _____ (4) _____ (5) _____ (6) _____ , or None of the above _____

4. Describe the **medical facts** which support your certification, including a brief statement as to how the medical facts meet the criteria of one of these categories:

5.a. State the approximate **date** the condition commenced, and the probable **duration of** the condition (and also the probable duration of the patient's present incapacity[2] if different):

b. Will it be **necessary** for the employee to take work only **intermittently or to work on a less then full schedule** as a result of the condition (including for treatment described in Item 6 below)?____

If yes, give the probable duration:

c. If the condition is a **chronic condition** (condition #4) or **pregnancy**, state whether the patient is presently incapacitated[2] and the likely duration and frequency of **episodes of incapacity**[2]:

6.a. If additional **treatments** will be required for the condition, provide an estimate of the probable number of such treatments:

If the patient will be absent from work or other daily activities because of **treatment** on an **intermittent** or part-time basis, also provide an estimate of the probable number of and interval between such treatments, actual or estimated dates of treatment if known, and period required for recovery if any:

b. If any of these treatments will be provided by **another provider of health services** (e.g., physical therapist), please state the nature of treatments:

---

1.   Here and elsewhere on this form, the information sought relates only to the condition for which the employee is taking FMLA leave.
2.   "Incapacity," for purposes of FMLA, is defined to mean inability to work, attend school or perform other regular daily activities due to the serious health condition, treatment therefor, or recovery therefrom.

Figure 4.2. Certification of physician or practitioner (Form WH-380)

c. **If a regimen of continuing treatment** by the patient is required under your supervision, provide a general description of such regimen (e.g., prescription drugs, physical therapy requiring special equipment):

7. a. If medical leave is required for the employee's **absence from work** because of the **employee's own condition** (including absences due to pregnancy or a chronic condition), is the employee **unable to perform work** of any kind?____

b. If able to perform some work, is the employee **unable to perform any one or more of the essential functions of the employee's job** (the employee or the employer should supply you with information about the essential job functions)? If yes, please list the essential functions the employee is unable to perform:

c. If neither a. nor b. applies, is it necessary for the employee to be **absent from work for treatment?**____

8. a. If leave is required to **care for a family member** of the employee with a serious health condition, **does the patient require assistance** for basic medical or personal needs or safety, or for transportation?____

b. If no, would the employee's presence to provide **psychological comfort** be beneficial to the patient or assist in the patient's recovery?____

c. If the patient will need care only intermittently or on a part-time basis, please indicate the probable **duration** of this need:

_____   _____
(Signature of Health Care Provider)   (Type of Practice)

_____   _____
(Address)   (Telephone number)

To be completed by the employee needing family leave to care for a family member:

State the care you will provide and an estimate of the period during which care will be provided, including a schedule if leave is to be taken intermittently or if it will be necessary for you to work less than a full schedule:

_____   _____
(Employee signature)   (Date)

Figure 4.2. Certification of physician or practitioner (Form WH-380) (cont.)

A **"Serious Health Condition"** means an illness, injury impairment, or physical or mental condition that involves one of the following:

1. Hospital Care

Inpatient care (i.e., an overnight stay) in a hospital, hospice, or residential medical care facility, including any period of incapacity[2] or subsequent treatment in connection with or consequent to such inpatient care.

2. Absence Plus Treatment

(a) A period of incapacity[2] of **more than three consecutive calendar days** (including any subsequent treatment or period of incapacity[2] relating to the same condition), that also involves:

(1) **Treatment[3] two or more times** by a health care provider, by a nurse or physician's assistant under direct supervision of a health care provider, or by a provider of health care services (e.g., physical therapist) under orders of, or on referral by, a health care provider; *or*

(2) **Treatment** by a health care provider on **at least one occasion** which results in **a regimen of continuing treatment**[4] under the supervision of the health care provider.

3. Pregnancy

Any period of incapacity due to **pregnancy**, or for **prenatal care.**

4. Chronic Conditions Requiring Treatments

A **chronic condition** which:

(1) Requires **periodic visits** for treatment by a health care provider, or by a nurse or physician's assistant under direct supervision of a health care provider;

(2) Continues over an **extended period of time** (including recurring episodes of a single underlying condition); and

(3) May cause **episodic** rather than a continuing period of incapacity[2] (e.g., asthma, diabetes, epilepsy, etc.).

5. Permanent/Long-term Condition Requiring Supervision

A period of **incapacity**[2] which is **permanent or long-term** due to a condition for which treatment may not be effective. The employee or family member must be **under the continuing supervision of, but need not be receiving active treatment** by a health care provider. Examples include Alzheimer's, a severe stroke, or the terminal stages of a disease.

---

3.   Treatment includes examinations to determine if a serious health condition exists and evaluations of the condition. Treatment does not include routine physical examinations, eye examinations, or dental examinations.

4.   A regimen of continuing treatment includes, for example, a course of prescription medication (e.g., an antibiotic) or therapy requiring special equipment to resolve or alleviate the health condition. A regimen of treatment does not include the taking of over-the-counter medications such as aspirin, antihistamines, or salves; or bed-rest, drinking fluids, exercise, and other similar activities that can be initiated without a visit to a health care provider.

Figure 4.2. Certification of physician or practitioner (Form WH-380) (cont.)

6. Multiple Treatments (Non-Chronic Conditions)

Any period of absence to receive **multiple treatments** (including any period of recovery therefrom) by a health care provider or by a provider of health care services under orders of, or on referral by, a health care provider, either for **restorative surgery** after an accident or other injury, or for a condition that **would likely result in a period of incapacity**[2] **of more than three consecutive calendar days in the absence of medical intervention of treatment**, such as cancer (chemotherapy, radiation, etc.), severe arthritis (physical therapy), and kidney disease (dialysis).

This optional form may be used by employees to satisfy a mandatory requirement to furnish a medical certification (when requested) from a health care provider, including second or third opinions and recertifications. (29 CFR 825.306)

Note: Persons are not required to respond to this collection of information unless it displays a currently valid OMB control number.

Public Burden Statement

We estimate that it will take an average of 10 minutes to complete this collection of information, including the time for reviewing instructions, searching existing data sources, gathering and maintaining the data needed, and completing and reviewing the collection of information. If you have any comments regarding this burden estimate or any other aspect of this collection of information, including suggestions for reducing this burden, send them to the Administrator, Wage and Hour Division, Department of Labor, Room S-3502, 200 Constitution Avenue, N.W., Washington, D.C. 20210.

DO NOT SEND THE COMPLETED FORM TO THIS OFFICE.

Figure 4.2. Certification of physician or practitioner (Form WH-380) (cont.)

Employer Response to Employee Request for Family or Medical Leave (Optional Use Form—See 29 CFR § 825.301) **(Family and Medical Leave Act of 1993)**	**U.S. Department of Labor** Employment Standards Administration Wage and Hour Division

To:_____
(Employee's Name)

From:_____
(Name of Appropriate Employer Representative)

Subject: REQUEST FOR FAMILY/MEDICAL LEAVE

On_____, you notified us of your need to take family/medical leave due to:
(Date)

❑ The birth of a child, or the placement of a child with you for adoption or foster care; or

❑ A serious health condition that makes you unable to perform the essential functions for your job; or

❑ A serious health condition affecting your ❑ spouse, ❑ child, ❑ parent, for which you are needed to provide care.

You notified us that you need this leave beginning on_____ and that you expect leave to
(Date)

continue until on or about_____.
(Date)

Except as explained below, you have a right under the FMLA for up to 12 weeks of unpaid leave in a 12-month period for the reasons listed above. Also, your health benefits must be maintained during any period of unpaid leave under the same conditions as if you continued to work, and you must be reinstated to the same or an equivalent job with the same pay, benefits, and terms and conditions of employment on your return from leave. If you do not return to work following FMLA leave for a reason other than: (1) the continuation, recurrence, or onset of a serious health condition which would entitle you to FMLA leave; or (2) other circumstances beyond your control, you may be required to reimburse us for our share of health insurance premiums paid on your behalf during your FMLA leave.

This is to inform you that: *(Check appropriate boxes; explain where indicated)*

1. You are ❑ eligible ❑ not eligible for leave under the FMLA.

2. The requested leave ❑ will ❑ will not be counted against your annual FMLA entitlement.

3. You ❑ will ❑ will not be required to furnish medical certification of a serious health condition. If required, you must furnish certification by_____*(insert date)* (must be at least 15 days after you are notified of this requirement), or we may delay the commencement of your leave until the certification is submitted.

4. You may elect to substitute accrued paid leave for unpaid FMLA leave. We ❑ will ❑ will not require that you substitute accrued paid leave for unpaid FMLA leave. If paid leave will be used, the following conditions will apply: *(Explain)*

**Figure 4.3. Prototype notice: Employer response to employee request
for family and mediical leave (Form WH-381)**

5. (a). If you normally pay a portion of the premiums for your health insurance, these payments will continue during the period of FMLA leave. Arrangements for payment have been discussed with you, and it is agreed that you will make premium payments as follows: *(Set forth dates, e.g., the 10th of each month, or pay periods, etc. that specifically cover the agreement with the employee).*

(b). You have a minimum 30-day *(or, indicate longer period, if applicable)* grace period in which to make premium payments. If payment is not made timely, your group health insurance may be cancelled, provided we notify you in writing at least 15 days before the date that your health coverage will lapse, or, at our option, we may pay your share of the premiums during FMLA leave, and recover these payments from you upon your return to work. We ❏ will ❏ will not pay your share of health insurance premiums while you are on leave.

(c). We ❏ will ❏ will not do the same with other benefits (e.g., life insurance, disability insurance, etc.) while you are on FMLA leave. If we do pay your premiums for other benefits, when you return from leave you ❏ will ❏ will not be expected to reimburse us for the payments made on your behalf.

6. You ❏ will ❏ will not be required to present a fitness-for-duty certificate prior to being restored to employment. If such certification is required but not received, your return to work may be delayed until certification is provided.

7. (a). You ❏ are ❏ are not a "key employee" as described in §825.217 of the FMLA regulations. If you are a "key employee," restoration to employment may be denied following FMLA leave on the grounds that such restoration will cause substantial and grievous economic injury to us as discussed in §825.218.

(b). We ❏ have ❏ have not determined that restoring you to employment at the conclusion of FMLA leave will cause substantial and grievous economic harm to us. *(Explain (a) and/or (b) below. See §825.219 of the FMLA regulations.)*

8. While on leave, you ❏ will ❏ will not be required to furnish us with periodic reports every_____ _____ *(indicate interval of periodic reports, as appropriate for the particular leave situation)* of your status and intent to return to work (see §825.309 of the FMLA regulations). If the circumstances of your leave change and you are able to return to work earlier than the date indicated on the reverse side of this form, you ❏ will ❏ will not be required to notify us at least two days prior to the date you intend to report to work.

9. You ❏ will ❏ will not be required to furnish recertification relating to a serious health condition. *(Explain below, if necessary, including the interval between certifications as prescribed in §825.308 of the FMLA regulations.)*

The optional use form may be used to satisfy mandatory employer requirements to provide employees taking FMLA leave with written notice detailing specific expectations and obligations of the employee and explaining any consequences of a failure to meet these obligations. (29 CFR 825.301 (b).)

Note: Persons are not required to respond to this collection of information unless it displays a currently valid OMB control number.

Public Burden Statement

We estimate that it will take an average of 5 minutes to complete this collection of information, including the time for reviewing instructions, searching existing data sources, gathering and maintaining the data needed, and completing and reviewing the collection of information. If you have any comments regarding this burden estimate or any other aspect of this collection of information, including suggestions for reducing this burden, send them to the Administrator, Wage and Hour Division, Department of Labor, Room S-3502, 200 Constitution Avenue, N.W., Washington, D.C. 20210.

DO NOT SEND THE COMPLETED FORM TO THIS OFFICE.   Form WH-381

**Figure 4.3. Prototype notice: Employer response to employee request
for family and mediical leave (Form WH-381) (cont.)**

The following is an example of the inter-action between FMLA and state laws:

> If State law provides half pay for employ-ees temporarily disabled because of preg-nancy for six weeks, the employee would be entitled to an additional six weeks of unpaid FMLA leave (or accrued paid leave).[18]

For additional information about the FMLA, practice owners or managers can con-tact the nearest office of the Wage and Hour Division, listed in most telephone directories under U.S. Government, Department of Labor. Alternatively, information can be acquired by writing to the U.S. Department of Labor, Employment Standards Adminis-tration, Wage and Hour Division, Washing-ton, DC 20210. For information about state laws, contact the appropriate State Labor Commissioner's office.

PREGNANCY AND MATERNITY LEAVE

Though the veterinary medical profes-sion is still a male-dominant profession, 67% of veterinary medical students nation-wide are female. As this trend suggests, the number of female veterinarians in the pro-fession will equal the number of male veter-inarians by 2004. With this change in the veterinary profession come additional employment concerns, such as pregnancy-and maternity-related issues.

A major issue is employment discrimi-nation. Federal laws prohibit discrimina-tion based on pregnancy, childbirth, or related medical conditions. These laws require that women be treated the same as other employees with temporary disabilities for all employment-related purposes, includ-ing receipt of benefits.[19] The Equal Pay Act is an excellent example of a federal regula-tory process designed to prevent employ-ment discrimination.

MATERNITY BENEFITS AND THE EQUAL PAY ACT

The Equal Employment Opportunity Commission (EEOC), which authorizes enforcement of the Equal Pay Act, amended that fringe benefits, including maternity benefits, be considered wages. The extant meaning of wages, then, is as follows:

Under the EPA, the term *wages* gener-ally includes all payments made to (or on behalf of) an employee as remuneration for employment. The term includes all forms of compensation irrespective of the time of payment, whether paid periodically or deferred until a later date, and whether called *wages, salary, profit sharing, expense account, monthly minimum, bonus, uni-form cleaning allowance, hotel accommo-dations, use of company car, gasoline allowance*, or some other name. Fringe ben-efits are deemed to be remuneration for employment.[20]

The EEOC uses the following two exam-ples to support that (1) maternity benefits are considered remuneration for employ-ment and that (2) men and women must receive equal remuneration for equal work:

Example 1: An employer provides full temporary disability coverage to its male employees, but it excludes pregnancy and maternity benefits from the coverage it offers to female employees. A female employee alleges that she is being paid an unequal wage because the male employees performing the same job receive full cover-age, while she and other female employees do not. The Commission, in these circum-stances, would find that the employer has violated the Equal Pay Act.[21]

Example 2: An employer provides full temporary disability coverage to all its employees and their spouses, except that it excludes pregnancy and maternity benefits from the coverage it provides to the spouses of male employees. A male employee alleges that he is being paid an unequal wage because female employees performing the same job receive full coverage for their husbands, while he and other male employees do not receive full coverage for their wives. The Commission, in these circumstances, would find that the employer has violated the Equal Pay Act.[21]

It is advisable that employers provide to employees the Employee Salary and Benefits Statement (Figure 4.1) to illustrate the concept that benefits are considered wages. Additionally, employers should be aware that offering temporary disability coverage to some employees but not others usually is unlawful.

LENGTH OF TIME FOR PREGNANCY LEAVE OF ABSENCE

Some states require that employers provide specific periods of time for pregnancy leave of absence. For example, California state law grants a leave of six weeks.[11] Additionally, some states provide for extensions of time in the event of medical complications related to the pregnancy. For example, if a physician required that a mother be bedridden for four months prior to delivery to provide for the safety of the mother and baby, California state law would grant an extension for up to four months.[11]

State Labor Commissions should be contacted to determine the most recent regulations regarding lengths of pregnancy leave requirements.

PREGNANT EMPLOYEES EXPOSED TO HAZARDOUS SUBSTANCES

It is well known that some substances or procedures in veterinary hospitals are dangerous to the fetuses of pregnant employees. Employers must be concerned with the health of the unborn children to avoid lawsuits. However, employers cannot prohibit pregnant associates from working once they are apprised of the risks. The parents rather than the employers must decide what is best for their children.[22]

It is unlawful for employers to exclude employees from working based on reproductive or fetal hazards unless supported by objective scientific evidence.[23] It is recommended, however, that employers have pregnant employees who insist on working in potentially hazardous environments sign statements releasing the employers from liability in the event of a teratogenic defect. Figure 4.4 is an example document that releases employers from liability.[24]

In some situations, it is lawful and financially advantageous to require maternity leave. Examples of legitimate, nondiscriminatory circumstances include incapability of performing job tasks or continual absenteeism, even if it is due to the pregnancy. However, employers are advised to consult with their attorneys before insisting that employees take maternity leave.

PATERNITY LEAVE

Employers covered by the FMLA are required to grant leave to eligible male employees for the birth of a child, care of a newborn, or the placement of an adopted or foster child in their homes. Refer to the section entitled "Family and Medical Leave Act" for more information or resources to contact regarding the FMLA, or contact your state labor commissioner for current state paternity labor laws.

WORKER'S COMPENSATION DURING LEAVES OF ABSENCE

Employees are entitled to worker's compensation benefits for medical leaves of absences resulting from occupational disabilities due to work-related illnesses, injuries, or disabilities. The following are key points that employees should consider regarding medical leave for occupational disabilities:

- Notify employers immediately and fill out accident reports.

- Submit written requests 30 days prior to the leave of absence or as soon as

Date:

Dear _____ :

It is our understanding that you are pregnant and wish to continue working in your capacity as a _____ . You should be aware that scientific evidence indicates that a pregnant woman's exposure to radiation, as well as other types of health hazards, e.g., chemical or toxic hazards and strenuous physical requirements, may pose a significant risk to the fetus. There is a strong likelihood that you and your fetus will be exposed to at least some of these hazards during your pregnancy if you continue to work in your present capacity.

Due to the office's limited staff, you are often the only employee on duty who is qualified or available to perform tasks that could pose a health hazard. While we will attempt to limit your exposure, there inevitably will be times when you must perform the duties assigned to your job.

You may request a transfer to another job assignment and, if a position is available and you are qualified, we will try to accommodate you.

If you decide to continue working for us as a _____ , we will certainly allow you to do so, provided you and your physician deem it safe and you are willing to assume the risks associated with the possible health hazards. If you are willing to take full responsibility for any possible consequences in assuming such risk, please indicate with your signature below. You may request a maternity-related disability leave of absence if you or your physician feel that continued performance of your responsibilities may present a hazard to you or your child.

Please feel free to consult with your physician and attorney before you sign this letter. Please return this letter within ten days of the above date.

If you have any questions, I sincerely request that you contact me.

_____

Employer's signature   Date

_____

Employee's name (please print)

_____

Employee's signature   Date

Figure 4.4. Health hazards during pregnancy release letter

possible; include reasons, date of commencement, duration, and return dates.

- Submit written statements from health care providers verifying the disability and the reasons for the leave.
- Inform employers periodically of your disability status and plans to return to work.[11]

Employers should consider the following regarding medical leave for occupational disabilities:

- Employers must file the incident report with their insurance carriers for workers' compensation purposes.
- Report the injury to the Division of Labor Statistics and Research Department.[11]

For information regarding various mandated lengths of leave, contact the State Labor Commissioner's office in your state.

Funeral Leave

Funeral leave for employees can be in the form of paid or unpaid leaves of absence. For the death of immediate family members, leaves of absence can include days of death, days of mourning, and funeral days. Immediate family members usually include father, mother, sister, brother, spouse, son, daughter, father-in-law, and mother-in-law.

For the death of relatives such as grandparents, uncles, aunts, cousins, or in-laws, employers usually offer unpaid leaves of absence for days on which employees attend funerals. Employees should seek approval for the time off and extra time needed for out-of-town travel.

Professional Liability Insurance

Not to be forgotten among the benefits provided to associates is professional liability insurance. Because of variations in policies designed by different insurance carriers, employers and employees must proceed with caution when addressing this topic in their contracts. Veterinarians or practice owners who have purchased professional liability insurance are termed *certificate holders* in the eyes of their insurance companies.

In general, policies purchased by employers cover themselves, their employees and their volunteers engaged in the provision of veterinary medical services for alleged mishaps which occurred *in the course of employment* during the time a certificate of insurance was in force. Course of employment includes tasks such as taking histories; performing physical examinations; pursuing diagnostic procedures; providing prognoses, phone consultations or advice; rendering treatments; restraining animals for exams and treatments; and prescribing, administering or dispensing drugs and biologicals while generating business for a certificate holder. To determine which activities are covered and which are not, insured parties must read the coverage and exclusion sections of their professional liability insurance polices. For a more comprehensive list of materials on this subject, including a fax-on-demand index, readers are referred to the library of information available from the AVMA PLIT.[25]

Among the important issues to consider involving professional liability insurance are the following:

- purchasing liability insurance that covers legal fees, court costs, and damages related to civil suits for personal injuries suffered by clients or bystanders or for the death or injury of animals or animal tissues belonging to clients;
- determining whether the employee or employer will pay the premium for such coverage;
- knowing whether the insurance carrier's policy allows it to settle a claim on its own initiative or only with the consent of the certificate holder, as does an AVMA policy;

- understanding that professional liability insurance does *not* cover:
  - › costs to defend administrative law complaints for fraud, negligence or incompetence brought by state boards of veterinary examiners;
  - › settlements involving claims by clients where no evidence of negligence exists, i.e., for the public relations value of "having the irate client go away satisfied;"
  - › criminal charges alleging animal cruelty filed by local authorities;
  - › liability arising out of "1-900-pay-per-call" information services;
  - › liability arising out of the intentional performance of a fraudulent or criminal act or omission or an act of actual malice;
  - › liability arising from a veterinary incident caused by a person under the influence of intoxicants, narcotics, or other controlled substances; or
  - › liabilities arising out of agreements wherein the certificate holder guaranteed the results of treatment.
- comprehending that to maintain or support their tax and liability independence, veterinarians who serve as independent contractors should have policies in their own names;
- understanding that associates who provide veterinary advice to friends and relatives during off hours or use their homes as offices to see clients or offer ambulatory veterinary services, and bill clients directly for such efforts instead of through their employers, usually are *not* protected by their employer's policies;
- determining whether an employer's insurance carrier provides protection for employees who are named as separate parties in suits for negligence or whether the company's coverage is extended only to the employer; and
- since coverage can be purchased in increments of $100,000/$300,000, $300,000/$900,000 or $1/$3 million per claim and aggregate, ascertaining whether employers have policies with limits large enough to satisfy the types of claims likely to occur in the course of an associate's employment. When employers have low limits on their policies, it is more important that employees have certificates in their own names in case a verdict involving both parties exceeds the employer's coverage.

Insurance companies selected by the AVMA Professional Liability Insurance Trust (PLIT) have offered outstanding coverage since the inception of the trust in 1962. The PLIT was formed by AVMA as a separate entity for the distinct purpose of establishing malpractice insurance for its members. Nonetheless, other carriers exist through the cooperative efforts and endorsements of state and national veterinary associations. The California VMA[26] and American Animal Hospital Association are examples of two associations that offer plans competing with the AVMA PLIT.

In most cases, employers and employees expect that an employer's professional liability certificate provides coverage to support staff and associates as employees and as individuals. As outlined in the previous bullet list, this may not be the case. This is because not all carriers provide legal protection for employees when they are named separately as defendants in lawsuits. In those cases, employees are stuck relying on the legal counsel and policy limits offered by their employers and hoping they win, rather than relying on legal representation and coverage for damages as named individuals in a lawsuit. Because of this quirk, employers and employees alike should review all of the circumstances cited above at the time they finalize their employment agreements. When an employer's coverage is provided by the PLIT, employees and employers should have separate policies.

In most cases, if employees are required to work exclusively for their employers, the employers pay the costs for both insurance policies. The exception is in instances where employees are engaged in the rendering of veterinary services outside of their employment contracts and, thus, need policies in their own names. In these cases, the employers still may pay full costs or they may split the costs with employees based on their percentage of full-time employment. Sample contract language for payment of professional liability insurance premiums follows:

EMPLOYER shall carry professional liability insurance insuring EMPLOYEE for professional errors, omissions, negligence, incompetence, and malfeasance upon such terms and in such amounts as EMPLOYER shall deem adequate but not less than $1 million per claim/aggregate. **(Lower limit also could be $100,000/$300,000 or $300,000/$900,000 for EMPLOYERS who wish to save money, but these lower amounts are not recommended.)** *Should EMPLOYER's insurance carrier's underwriting policies stipulate that EMPLOYEE needs to have a professional liability insurance policy issued in EMPLOYEE'S name, EMPLOYER will pay for such coverage directly.* **(Alternatively, EMPLOYER will reimburse EMPLOYEE for such expense or EMPLOYEE will pay for such coverage independently.)**

COSTS FOR COVERAGE

Because of the limited value of animal life as a form of property, costs for professional liability insurance in the veterinary profession have been very low and quite stable. Categories are based on the percentage of time spent in small animal, large animal or equine practice, with exclusively equine practitioners paying the highest premiums. AVMA activity classifications are used to determine types of practices. As seen in Figure 4.5, premium costs for coverage move upward based on the volume of services provided for animals with significant market value, i.e., food animals and horses.

In general, AVMA PLIT premiums have gone up by an average of 5% every three to four years.[27]

COVERAGE FOR STUDENTS

Increasing numbers of students from all four years of veterinary school classes are working in veterinary practices as externs, interns, preceptors, or employees. To minimize the risks these future colleagues face from being named as separate parties in suit, the AVMA PLIT has established a policy specifically for students. When students' employers are covered by AVMA insurance, the students working for them can purchase policies naming them as certificate holders for a mere $10 per calendar year. This minimal fee holds true regardless of the number of

Type of Practice	Coverage	Annual Premium
Small animal practitioners	$100,000	$191
Small animal practitioners	$1,000,000	$246
Mixed, predominantly small	$1,000,000	$364
Large animal practitioners	$1,000,000	$1,015
Equine exclusive practitioners	$1,000,000	$2,921

Figure 4.5. Costs for AVMA professional liability insurance coverage.

practices in which the student works in any given calendar year. (800-228-7548)

BAILEE SUPPLEMENTAL INSURANCE COVERAGE

The final concern for employers and employees involves insurance coverage for animals that escape from veterinary practices, are injured while in transit by staff members of veterinary practices, or are attacked by other animals while being hospitalized, groomed, trained, or boarded. Nearly every practice will at one time or another be victimized by one of these risks. Since damages related to these types of circumstances do not involve the provision of medical care, coverage is not routinely available through professional liability policies. Instead, riders or supplemental insurance policies are required to protect employers and employees from this type of liability exposure.

Risks not covered by these types of policies include:

- losses caused by the dishonesty of insured parties or their employees,

- death resulting from natural causes or disease,

- mysterious disappearance,

- losses caused by hostile or warlike actions, and

- losses or loss of use of animal embryos and semen while in storage or transit.

Employers who are unsure of their coverage for these bailment types of risks should check with their insurance agents to assure themselves they are protected. Employees who could be victimized by any of these risks, especially the escape of animals in their care, should ask employers to provide them with verification that bailee supplemental coverage like this in place.

CAFETERIA PLANS

Employers once offered compensation only in the form of salaries or wages, during which time employees were free to use their take-home pay as they wished. Eventually, however, employers began to offer compensation to groups of employees in the form of benefits. Shortly after World War II, government-mandated programs such as Social Security, unemployment compensation insurance, and workers' compensation came into existence. In some cases, employers expanded benefits as a result of union contracts and, eventually, passed these perks on to nonunion employees.

As employers, the government and unions expanded benefits, increases in salaries as a percentage of total take-home pay began to fall. Unfortunately, employees were seldom involved in planning their benefit packages and establishing their financial security; instead, they were forced to accept their employer's or the union's fixed benefits, supplemented by those provided by the government. All too often, employees were unhappy with the benefits offered and, because no one was helping them value those benefits, were unable to appreciate their cost to the employer or net benefit to them as employees.

Some employers began to experiment with benefit plans in order to give their employees choices. Their approach was to direct benefit money into a fund and allow employees to select their choice of benefits by using contributions to the fund. Those *flexible-benefit plans* have evolved into what is known today as *cafeteria plans*. This seldom-used but valuable option for veterinary employees also is known as a *Section 125 plan*.[28]

Employees are individuals with different religious backgrounds, ethnicity, socioeconomic plights, marital and parental status, and physical and mental conditions. Hence, employees have varying needs regarding employment benefits. With this in mind, Congress passed Section 125 of the Internal

Revenue Code of 1954, creating flexible benefits plans called *cafeteria plans*, and thereafter promulgated the rules governing such plans.

Section 125 of the Internal Revenue Code allows employers to create cafeteria plans as devices by which employees choose some of their employment benefits from among an assortment of options. According to the IRS rules,

A 'cafeteria plan' is a separate written benefit plan maintained by an employer for the benefit of its employees, under which all participants are employees and each participant has the opportunity to select the particular benefits that he desires.[29]

The assortment must include a minimum of two benefits, one taxable and one nontaxable. Cafeteria plans must be in writing and cannot discriminate among employees. The written plans must set forth: (1) descriptions of each benefit available under the plan; (2) the plan's eligibility rules governing participation; (3) procedures regarding the election of benefits; (4) the manner in which employers make contributions; (5) the maximum employer contributions available; and (6) the year in which the cafeteria plan operates.[30]

Although Section 125 requires that employers include a minimum of at least two benefits, one taxable and one nontaxable, the section does not set a maximum number of benefits from which employees can choose. Nonetheless, section 125 does limit the kind of benefits available in cafeteria plans.[31]

Nontaxable benefits are those excluded from employees' gross incomes pursuant to the Internal Revenue Code. For cafeteria plan purposes, nontaxable benefits are group-term life insurance up to $50,000 (section 79), health and accident plans (sections 105 and 106), group legal services (section 120), dependent care assistance programs (section 129), and participation in tax-deferred programs such as profit sharing or stock bonus plans (section 401 [k]).[32]

For cafeteria plan purposes, taxable benefits include cash and certain benefits which are typically nontaxable. Certain nontaxable benefits become taxable when included in cafeteria plans: scholarships and fellowships (section 117), van pooling (section 124), educational assistance (section 127), fringe benefits (section 132) such as qualified moving expenses and use of company cars for business purposes, and group-term life insurance exceeding $50,000 (section 79).[31]

Employers establish cafeteria plans in several different ways. *Full flexibility plans* allow employees to convert their benefits packages into either selected benefits or cash or a combination of the two. *Predetermined benefit plans* allow employees to choose prearranged benefits packages. *Core/optional plans* and *flexible spending accounts*, the more common types of plans, are explained in detail below.[33]

Core benefits are the minimum benefits employers provide, typically without any cost to employees. Ideally, core benefits are medical, disability, and life insurance policies which protect employees financially in the event of sickness, injury, and death. No rules exist regarding which core benefits to offer participants; thus, core benefits packages vary among practices offering cafeteria plans.[33]

In addition to core benefits, employees can obtain optional benefits which are paid for by employers' and/or employees' contributions. Optional benefits consist of increasing the quality of one's core benefits or purchasing new ones. For example, employees who receive life insurance policies as core benefits can increase coverage amounts or acquire lower-deductible health insurance policies. Or employees can purchase additional benefits not included in their core policies, such as dental and vision care.[33]

Flexible spending accounts (FSAs) can qualify as cafeteria plans in and of themselves but are often included in more comprehensive plans. FSAs enable employees to purchase additional benefits with pretaxed income.[33] Under an FSA, employees elect to take salary reductions to fund benefits on a before-tax basis.

Employers most commonly establish FSAs for (1) health insurance premiums, (2) reimbursement for out-of-pocket medical expenses not covered by insurance; (3) dependent care expenses; and (4) to enhance benefits lost because participants in the plans contribute less to their social security accounts. Dependent care expense accounts cover costs incurred when caring for children under the age of 13 or persons of any age who are physically or mentally handicapped. Contributions to benefit enhancement accounts often are used to purchase coverage via permanent life insurance policies to compensate for reduced future social security benefits. The need for supplemental life insurance occurs because employees who participate in FSAs have smaller taxable incomes and, thus, their social security payments into the system and benefits received from it are lower.[33]

Participants who elect not to participate in benefit enhancement accounts should sign Release of Liability Documents (Figure 4.6). These documents ensure understanding among employers and employees that participation in flexible spending accounts will reduce future social security benefits.[34]

Release of Liability Form

_____
Participant

_____
Employer

As a participant in the cafeteria plan offered by my employer, I hereby exercise my voluntary right to reject the Social Security Offset Insurance Plan.

I recognize that there may be a reduction of retirement, disability and/or survivor benefits to me and/or my beneficiary as a result of the reduced FICA payments and that the Social Security Offset Insurance Plan was made available to me to replace any future reduction of benefits from the Social Security Administrator.

The rejection of the insurance plan is voluntary on my part and I agree to hold my employer, his employees, the Plan Administrator, and the insurance company harmless from loss due to reduction of any future benefits from the Social Security Administrator.

_____
Date

_____
Participant

_____
Witness

Figure 4.6. Consent forms to release employers from liability

Annual Expense Report

1. Fixed Expenses

    Health Coverage Premiums $_____

    Term Life Insurance Premiums $_____

    Disability Insurance Premiums $_____

    Dental Insurance Premiums $_____

    Indemnity Insurance Premiums $_____

    Other Insurance Premiums $_____

    Total Fixed Expenses Anticipated In The Next 12 Months $_____

2. Variable Expenses

    Out-Of-Pocket Medical/Dental Expenses $_____

    *(Examples include health insurance deductibles,
    uninsured medical costs, check-ups, OBGyn exams,
    travel costs for medical care, medications and
    prescriptions, birth control, dental examinations
    and x-rays, fillings and other routine dental care,
    dentures and bridgework, orthodontia, eye exams
    and treatment, glasses, and contact lenses.)*

    Dependent Care Expenses $_____

    Total Variable Expenses Anticipated In
    The Next 12 Months $_____

    Total Income To Convert Per Year $_____

    Total Income To Convert Per Paycheck $_____

Figure 4.7. Forms to quantify annual expenses

Employees determine their anticipated expenses for the year before utilizing FSAs. Participants can record these expenses in annual expense reports, such as the one presented in Figure 4.7, and submit them to plan administrators. Administrators then deduct the budgeted amounts from employees' pretaxed pay and transfer the money into accounts. To receive reimbursement from accounts for out-of-pocket expenses, participants submit claim vouchers (Figure 4.8) to plan administrators.[34]

ACCOUNT ADMINISTRATION

To help manage their accounts, participants are furnished with monthly reports which include the dollars deposited and spent and the remaining balances. Participants are advised to maintain records of expenses for IRS audits.[33]

Because cafeteria plans are more complex than traditional employee benefits plans, they require effective communications between employers or administrators and employees. Participants must thoroughly understand the plans to take advantage of all the benefits offered. Group and individual meetings between employees and the plan administrator will be required, especially when plans are first installed or new employees brought on board. If claims and selections are handled improperly, errors or overstatements in employees' allocations to an FSA can lead to forfeitures of some of the benefits and disappointed employees.

Claims Voucher

_____
Employer

_____
Employee   SS#

	Declaration Per Pay Period	Incurred Expenses
Insurance Premiums	$_____	$_____
Out-Of-Pocket Medical/Dental Expenses	$_____	$_____
Dependent Care Expenses	$_____	$_____

I acknowledge that I have or will have the necessary documents, such as receipts, vouchers, etc. to support the expenses listed above. The balance unused by the end of the plan year are forfeited.

I certify that the above information is correct and complete:

_____
Employee's Signature   Date

Figure 4.8. Vouchers used to report claims

Once accounts are established, employees are prohibited from making changes during the plan year unless unusual circumstances occur, such as marriage, birth of a child, or termination of employment. Furthermore, the total amount received from the accounts cannot exceed the amount placed in the accounts. Therefore, employees who incur expenses in excess of their account balances must spend taxable income. Moreover, unused balances at the end of the plan year are forfeited to employers. Finally, employees cannot use funds from one account to reimburse costs attributable to another account. For example, employees cannot use funds from their medical expenses reimbursement accounts to pay for child care expenses.[33]

In sum, cafeteria plans offer employers and employees financial and personal advantages. Employers' payroll taxes and employees' income taxes are reduced. Participants are given the opportunity to tailor benefits packages to meet individual needs, reducing dissatisfaction commonly encountered with traditional benefits plans.

The success of cafeteria plans is contingent upon their initial design. Thus, employers are advised to consult with CPAs and insurance agents to determine their plans' objectives, designs, and costs, and to ensure that employers meet all provisions of the Internal Revenue Code, Section 125.

SUMMARY

This concludes the basic employment benefits addressed in most employment contracts. For coverage of a multitude of other benefits, readers are referred to the extensive materials found in Chapter 7, ancillary employment benefits.

REFERENCES

1. Kennedy RR: Creating an attractive employee-benefits package. *Vet Pract Manage* 3(1): 47, 1985-1986.
2. Ibid, p 51.
3. Gehrke BC: *Facts & Figures. Employment of male & female graduates of US veterinary schools, 1998.* *JAVMA* 214(6):789, 1999, Wise JK, *JAVMA* 220(5):600-602, 2002.
4. Collins L, Goebel R, et al: *Compensation and Benefits: An In-Depth Look.* Lakewood, CO, AAHA Press, 1998.
5. Lynch TA: *Veterinary Compensation in New England.* North Andover, MA, 1998.
6. *Veterinary Hospital Managers Association Newsletter.* Albany, NY, July/Aug 1998. (phone 518-433-8911;email VHMA@caphill.com)
7. Genova K: Personal communication, Ann Arbor, MI, March, 1998.
8. Wise JK: The information exchange. Employment of male and female graduates of US veterinary medical colleges, 2001. *JAVMA* 220(5):600, 2001.
9. *Economic Report on Veterinarians & Veterinary Practices.* Schaumberg, IL, Center for Information Management, AVMA, p 163,2001.
10. Moore DA: The state of continuing veterinary medical education. *Calif Vet* 52(4):10-12, 1998.
11. Ericksen BE: *The Staff Personnel Policy Manual.* Los Gatos, CA, Bent Ericksen & Associates, 1998.
12. Gehrke BC: Gender redistribution in the veterinary medical profession. *JAVMA* 208: 1254, 1996.
13. The Family and Medical Leave Act of 1993 §825.110.
14. The Family and Medical Leave Act of 1993 §825.112.
15. The Family and Medical Leave Act of 1993 §825.302.
16. The Family and Medical Leave Act of 1993 Form WH-380 and 381 pp 1007-1008, 1012-1013.
17. The Family and Medical Leave Act of 1993 §825.701 (a).
18. The Family and Medical Leave Act of 1993 §825.701 (a) (2).
19. Title 42 Subchapter VI Equal Employment Opportunities SS 2000e(k).
20. The Equal Pay Act SS 1620.10 Meaning of "Wages."
21. EPA Policy Statement on Maternity Benefits No. 641.
22. *United Auto Workers v Johnson Control*: US SUP. CT., 1991 55 FEP Cases 365.
23. EEOC Guidelines, Pregnancy/Maternity Issues, No. 691, 421:502.
24. Ericksen BE: *Health Hazards During Pregnancy Release Letter.* Los Gatos, CA, Bent Ericksen & Associates, 1995.
25. AVMA Professional Liability Insurance Trust, P.O. Box 1629, Chicago, IL 60690-1629. ph. 1-800-228-7548, fax–on-demand index 1-888-740-7548.
26. Alburger, Bass, DeGrosz insurance brokers, 310 Island Pky, Belmont CA 94002-4110, 1-415-598-0370, web site, http://www.abdi.com.
27. Wilson JF: author's experience.
28. Newkirk R & R: *Introduction to Group Insurance, Fourth Edition.* Dearborn, MI, USA Dearborn Financial Publishing, Inc, 1993, p 79.
29. Internal Revenue Service, 26 CFR Part 1, § 1.125-1 Q-2, May 1984.
30. Ibid, Q-3.
31. Appelman B: Personal communication, Internal Revenue Service, Washington DC, 1997.
32. Internal Revenue Service, CFR 26, s 1.125-2T, Jan 1997.
33. Newkirk R & R: *Introduction to Group Insurance, Fourth Edition.* DearbornUSA Dearborn Financial Publishing, Inc, 1993, pp 79-91.
34. Kendall T: Personal communication, Arden Animal Hospital, Sacramento, CA,1997.

Chapter 5

HEALTH AND DISABILITY INSURANCE

By Alan J. Fishman, CLU, CFP and James F. Wilson, DVM, JD

Mary, age 30, has completed her veterinary education and is interviewing with two veterinary practices in the area. The first offers her a starting salary of $72,000 with no disability insurance coverage. If she is unable to return to work for more than 30 days as a result of an accident or illness, her employment will be terminated and her salary will stop.

The second practice offers a different option. That job has a starting salary of $71,000. In addition, the owner will provide a means by which the practice will continue to pay her salary to age 65 in the event she is unable to return to work after 90 days because of a disability. Which practice should Mary choose?

Most veterinarians would choose the second practice. And herein lies the rationale for disability income coverage. Many professionals would easily spend $800 per year (the cost in this case of disability insurance for Mary) to protect their salaries. Restated, is it logical to spend 2% of one's salary to protect the remaining 98%? We insure our automobiles and homes and, yet, our greatest asset is our ability to earn a living. It is this ability to earn a living that makes all other assets possible.

THE NEED FOR DISABILITY INSURANCE

Mortality risk concerns the probability of death; morbidity the probability of disability. Though many people believe that the chance of long-term disability, defined as a disability lasting more than 90 days, is less than the chance of premature death, consider the following statistics:

- At age 27, the odds of a disability rather than death are 2.7 to 1.

- At age 37, it is 3.3 to 1 greater odds of disability than death.

- At age 42, the odds of disability to death are 3.5 to 1.

- At age 47, there are 2.8 to 1 greater odds of disability than death.

- At age 52, there are 2.2 to 1 greater odds of disability rather than death.

Table 5.1 shows the chance of becoming disabled for more than three months, and the average duration of the disability at the same age.

Only a few options are available when employed veterinarians attempt to replace income lost due to a disability. These

Table 5.1. The Likelihood of Becoming Disabled*

Age	Chance of Becoming Disabled > 3 Months	Average Duration of Disability (years)
25	58%	2.1
30	54%	2.5
35	50%	2.8
40	45%	3.1
45	40%	3.2
50	33%	3.1
55	23%	2.6

* From the 1985 Commissioner's Individual Disability A table and the 1985 Society of Actuaries DTS.[1]

include the use of savings, the sale of liquid or nonliquid assets, loans, family assistance, other sources of household income, and governmental programs such as social security and worker's compensation. It takes most Americans considerable time to build an emergency reserve, and tapping into those savings quickly depletes that reserve if professionals have to rely solely on this source.

Nonliquid assets such as vacation homes, antique cars, stamp collections, and/or family businesses are another possible source of revenue, but they may be difficult to sell quickly. Likewise, fire sales rarely generate a good return on the investment. Increased income from spouses may not be possible or may be inadequate to cover the losses, making it difficult to maintain the family's lifestyle.

Eligibility for social security disability benefits is strict. Disabled parties must be totally disabled and unable to work at any occupation for a year. Moreover, more than half of all claimants are turned down. What about worker's compensation? These benefits are paid only when accidents or injuries are caused in the course of employment, and they are limited by weekly maximums and short benefit periods. Thus, the best choice for replacing lost income is disability income coverage.

DISABILITY INCOME: THE BASICS

Disability income coverage is insurance that protects the earnings of people who are unable to return to work as a result of accidents or illnesses. Professionals can obtain coverage on an individual basis, via group policies, or through veterinary association-sponsored programs.

When a disability occurs, insurance companies generally "issue" (or provide) coverage equal to 55% to 60% of the insured party's monthly income. This percentage drops as monthly income increases beyond $10,000.

Suppose a veterinarian earns $6,000 a month. He or she could purchase approximately $3,900 of coverage, referred to as the *monthly benefit*. Why not 100%? When the premiums are paid personally rather than by the company, the monthly benefits received during periods of disabilities are deemed nontaxable income. Since state and federal income taxes can amount to 40% of wages, disability companies are concerned that people who have coverage in excess of 60% will lack the motivation to return to work.

There is one exception. Since disability insurance companies recognize the earning potential of the young professional, several will offer coverage to senior year students and graduates entering practice without regard to earned income. For example, Provident Life and Accident will provide monthly benefits of $2,000 to senior year students and $3,000 to graduates entering practice.

FEATURES OF THE INDIVIDUAL DISABILITY POLICY

Disability policies include a variety of features, any of which can prove to be vitally important at some point according to life's circumstances (Figure 5.1).

ELIMINATION PERIOD

When disabilities occur, benefits typically are not awarded immediately. The elimination period is the waiting period before the monthly benefits begin. This period is comparable to the deductible in a homeowners or auto policy. The longer the elimination period as cited in one's policy, the lower the premiums. Standard elimination periods include 90 and 180 days.

BENEFIT PERIOD

The benefit period is the time during which monthly benefits are paid. The standard benefit period extends to age 65, at which time benefits from social security and Medicare programs begin for eligible individuals.

NON-CANCELABLE, GUARANTEED RENEWABLE

Non-cancelable, guaranteed renewable policies are policies that cannot be canceled for any reason other than for nonpayment of the premium. Also, the policy's premium cannot be increased for any reason. Policies that are only guaranteed renewable, and not non-cancelable, are slightly less expensive

since companies reserve the right to increase premiums by class of policyholders. A class may be based on, for example, geography, occupational groupings, and/or year of issue.

DEFINITION OF DISABILITY

Insurance companies differentiate disabilities as being conditions preventing insured parties from practicing their own occupations or any occupation. "Own occupation" coverage protects people in their specific occupations, which for veterinarians means they are covered if they cannot return to their jobs as veterinarians. "Any occupation" disability insurance protects people's earnings only if they are unable to return to any occupation. Variations of these standards exist in which policies may combine the own occupation, any occupation definitions, i.e., the first five years will be own occupation and, thereafter, the definition switches to any occupation.

Suppose a veterinarian in private practice earns $80,000, becomes disabled, and is unable to return to the daily grind of running a large practice. Instead, this practitioner decides to become an instructor at a local veterinary technician school, where she earns $55,000. With own occupation coverage, this veterinarian would receive a monthly benefit based on the $80,000 salary. In other words, the earnings from teaching are irrelevant and not considered in the calculations of benefits to be paid.

With any occupation coverage, an individual's monthly benefit is offset by outside earned income. In that case, the monthly benefit would be offset by the $55,000 teaching salary. Candidates for disability insurance are urged to inquire carefully as to the own or any occupation definition in the policies being considered to be sure they are comparing apples with apples when reviewing premium costs for such policies. As might be expected, own occupation policies tend to be considerably more expensive than any occupation policies.

Policy Features - A Comparison			
Policy Features	Company #1	Company #2	Company #3
Non-Cancelable or Guaranteed Renewable?			
Definition of Disability – Own or any occupation? Combination?			
Residual Coverage – Paid only following total disability?			
Automatic Benefit Indexing -If offered, what are the terms?			
Waiver of Premium - How long is the wait before premiums are waived?			
Total Recovery – If offered, for how long?			
Future Insurance Option -What is the maximum amount of additional monthly benefit that can be exercised at one time? How often can this option be exercised?			
Cost of Living Adjustments - Identify the cost of living features, e.g., the percentages offered, & are monthly benefits calculated on a simple or compounded basis?			
Presumptive Loss - This is the loss of sight, speech, hearing, or 2 arms or legs. Will benefits be paid if losses are considered recoverable?			
Survivor Benefits - Are lump-sum benefits offered when the insured dies?			
Capital Sum Benefits - Are these offered in addition to the monthly benefit received via presumptive loss when there is a loss of sight, speech, hearing, or 2 limbs?			
Portability of Discounts - Example: If a discount is awarded to 3 professionals and 1 subsequently leaves the practice, will the remaining 2 lose their discount?			
Exclusions - Are mental/nervous, drugs/alcohol, and/or illnesses for which there is no diagnosis excluded? For how many months will benefits be paid for these conditions?			
Occupational Code - On what occupational code is the premium based, and is it the best class?			
Ratings – An important indication of a company's financial strength. In general, don't consider anything lower than an A-. A.M. Best, S&P, Moody's, and Duff & Phelps rate these companies.			

Figure 5.1. This form can be used to compare features of different disability income policies.

RESIDUAL COVERAGE

Residual coverage is important to professionals who become partially disabled. If they return to work but suffer a loss of income due to loss of time or reduced duties, they receive benefits proportionate to cover the loss. In such cases, residual benefits are based on the percentage of income lost.

AUTOMATIC BENEFIT INDEXING

Many policies include a feature that allows for increases in monthly benefits each year to keep pace with the cost of living. Without this feature, benefits remain as a percentage of a worker's original salary, which eventually would be tremendously inadequate. Automatic benefit indexing increases are offered only during periods of nondisability. Insured parties do not have to accept this increase but may be inclined to do so since no additional medical underwriting is required and the costs for the additional coverage are minimal.

WAIVER OF PREMIUM

Most policies include the waiver of premium feature. With this feature, payment of premiums typically must be continued for the first 90 days of a disability. After that, all premiums are waived.

TOTAL RECOVERY CLAUSE

A total recovery clause is important coverage for self-employed veterinary practice owners and consultants with few or no co-owners whose practices would suffer during prolonged disabilities. Suppose Dr. Joe Practitioner was disabled for three years. During this period, he would lose clients. When he recovered and was able to return to his practice, it would require a period of time to rebuild the client base or referral network. The inclusion of total recovery clauses allows insured individuals like Joe to be reimbursed for their losses until their incomes return to a predetermined percentage of predisability earnings.

FUTURE INSURANCE OPTIONS

Future insurance options riders allow for the purchase of additional increments of insurance as earnings increase without providing further evidence of insurability. Such riders are beneficial for professionals who are concerned that medical problems which surface after their policies have been purchased will make it impossible for them to increase their insurance coverages.

COST OF LIVING OPTION

A cost of living rider allows for increases in monthly benefits during periods of disabilities sufficient to keep pace with the cost of living.

INSURABILITY AND COST

Insurability and the cost of disability income coverage are based on many factors. Except for the common factors of sex, smoker status, medical history, hobbies, and occupational class, industry trends exist that are outside the control of the insured policyholders.

Some companies charge the same rates for both men and women. These are called *unisex rates*. Other companies offer sex-distinct rates for men and women. Because companies have been able to substantiate higher claim rates among women, premiums for this segment of the population are higher.

Medical history is based on height and weight, attending physician statements (or *APSs*), routine blood and urine tests, and medical conditions indicated on the application.

Hobbies also are considered in determining insurability. Recreational activities like car or bike racing, underwater and sky diving, hang gliding, piloting airplanes, and mountain or rock climbing have an impact on the ability or willingness of insurance companies to provide policies.

Insurance companies define the risk in a profession by assigning an "occupational class." The higher the risk associated with an occupation, the higher the premium. Accordingly, for example, the cost of disability income coverage is higher among professional athletes than it is for accountants. The veterinary industry is considered to be relatively low risk. Most insurers place veterinarians in the least risky or next to least risky class. Some insurers go one step further and offer a better occupational class for practitioners who work exclusively with small animals. Practitioners who have large or mixed animal practices usually are placed in slightly higher risk classes than small animal practitioners, presumably because the incidence or severity of claims is higher in equine and large animal practices.

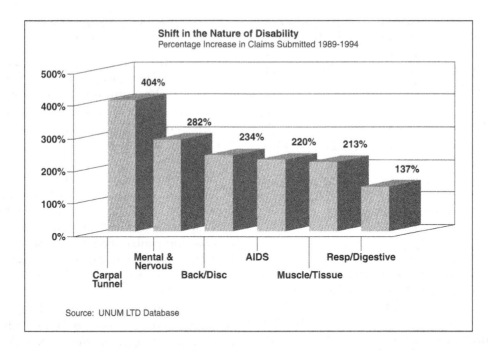

Figure 5.2. This graph shows recent shifts in the frequency of various types of disability claims.

TRENDS IN THE INDUSTRY

Due to the more frequent, costlier claims in the past five years, insurers have had to reevaluate the wording of their contracts and, in some cases, reconsider their presence in the industry. Figure 5.2 illustrates the increasing numbers of claims in various diagnostic codes between 1989 and 1994.

Because of the remarkable increases in the types and numbers of disabilities, considerable changes have been made by many of the top carriers. In the 10 years from 1986 to 1996, 27 out of 64 companies that sold disability insurance exited the market, leaving only 37 companies selling disability insurance. Most of the remaining companies have restricted the definition of disability and/or modified the type of contracts from non-cancellable to guaranteed renewable.

With all the companies departing the industry, many associations and partnerships have formed. Equitable and New England pursued private-label relationships with Paul Revere; National Life of Vermont entered into a private-label arrangement with UNUM (then initiated a co-marketing effort with Paul Revere); New York Life and Penn Mutual presently co-market with Paul Revere; and John Hancock and ILICO co-market with Provident Life and Accident. The bottom line is that there are fewer carriers and more homogenous products. Therefore, disability income contracts which only a few years ago were considered difficult to compare are today becoming difficult to distinguish because of their similarities.

UNISEX RATES

Another trend being seen in the industry is the distinction being made between sexes in determining price. Rates at one time were often the same for males and females, or unisex rates. Today companies usually offer sex-distinct rates. The one exception is association-sponsored plans, many of which still have a unisex rate. Since women are usually charged higher rates than men, association-sponsored plans may prove advantageous to women.

LIFETIME BENEFITS

Lifetime benefits once were common among disability insurance contracts. Now limiting benefits to age 65 is the norm. Thereafter, policyholders must rely on distributions from company pensions, IRAs, personal savings, and governmental programs like social security.

UNDERWRITING

Underwriting in general is becoming more restrictive. At one time, physicians and attorneys were considered great risks in the disability income industry. However, medical doctors now face cost controls and close monitoring from managed care organizations. As incomes have dropped, especially among specialists, some temporarily disabled doctors have found they can earn more from their disability policies than by returning to work. Consider that physicians account for one-third of all premiums but one-half of all claims. In 1994, the peak of the changeover to managed care, claims on physicians with policies over $5,000/month increased 60%; all other claims decreased 7%. Other professions also show increasing numbers of disability claims as well, including attorneys, dentists, and chiropractors.

Certain regions of the country also are seeing the underwriting of disability income policies become more restrictive. Florida and California have higher claims rates than many other states. Because of this, they have been targeted with higher premiums by some insurers.

RESTRICTIONS FOR MENTAL DISORDERS

Until recent years, there were generally no exclusions associated with disability insurance for mental disorders. Policy holders were considered disabled if they were unable to work because of stress, anxiety, addiction to drugs and alcohol, or depression. This proved to be problematic for insurers, though, because mental disabilities are difficult to diagnose and confirm.

Because of this difficulty and the tremendous increase in this type of claim, companies now restrict contract language for mental disabilities. Many carriers today will pay benefits related to disabilities from mental and nervous conditions for only 24 months.

NON-CANCELABLE AND GUARANTEED-RENEWABLE CONTRACTS

Perhaps the strongest provision in most disability income contracts is the non-cancelable feature. The inclusion of this clause means that companies cannot increase premiums on existing policies for any reason. The trend today in regard to this feature is for companies to offer guaranteed renewable contracts, instead, and to permit premium increases for a class of policyholders whose claims experiences warrant price hikes. If the guaranteed renewable contract becomes the industry standard, shopping for the right policy undoubtedly will include a review of previous price increases initiated by the companies under consideration.

OWN OCCUPATION AND ANY OCCUPATION COVERAGE

Payouts and, subsequently, premiums have increased in recent years because of the liberal "own occupation" definition of disability. Because cost is an increasingly important factor in selecting coverage, many of the top carriers have decided to do away with the own occupation type of policy altogether. Thus, the any occupation feature is fast becoming the industry standard.

Group Coverage

Like most insurance, disability insurance can be bought as a group. Group disability coverage is available to companies of varying sizes, including companies with as few as two employees.

There are many similarities between individual and group coverage but just as many differences. Group coverage is a relatively inexpensive way to provide insurance for employees. Its contract provisions are, however, more restrictive than individual coverage.

Noncancelability

In comparing group versus individual policies, it is important to consider the non-cancelable aspect of disability insurance. Whether one has non-cancelable or guaranteed renewable insurance, individual disability income contracts cannot be canceled unless premiums are not paid on a timely basis. Group disability contracts, on the other hand, are priced according to group size, average age of employee population, and industry type, and can be canceled for any reason, including an election by the insurance company not to write coverage.

Level Premiums

Another area where individual coverage proves to be less restrictive than group policies is with premium pricing. Premiums on non-cancelable individual policies cannot be increased for any reason. Premiums on guaranteed renewable individual policies can be increased by class of policyholders only in cases where claims experience warrants such change. In contrast, premiums on group disability contracts can increase from year to year at the insurance company's discretion, usually because of adverse claims experience.

Portability

Individual and group policies also differ in their transferability. Individual policies are portable. Group policies with commercial carriers are not , since insured parties need to be on the payroll to be covered.

For example, a veterinarian works for a large practice and is covered by a group disability contract. If she terminates her employment to begin her own practice, her coverage under the group policy will terminate. Unfortunately, this leaves her with only two options. The first is to secure coverage under another group contract, which will be possible only if she employs at least one other person whom she would like to insure. The second is to qualify for an individual contract, which is a viable option only if she is healthy.

Covered Income

Individual and group contracts differ in regard to what income is covered as well. Individual contracts can provide coverage for base salaries, bonuses, deferred compensation, overtime pay, and retirement plan contributions. Group contracts typically provide coverage for base salaries only.

For example, a veterinary practice pays its partners a low base salary throughout the year and then determines its bonuses at year end as profits permit. If disabled, the professional with a group policy ordinarily would receive a monthly benefit protecting the base salary only. Because many veterinary associates are paid a base salary or percentage of income generated, whichever is greater, disability insurance applicants are urged to determine exactly how "covered income" is defined in the insurance contract.

Riders, Offsets, and Limitations

Riders, as discussed earlier, are prevalent in individual policies. Group policies, on the other hand, offer few.

Individual policies generally cannot be offset by workers compensation or social security payments. Group policies typically allow for these offsets. For example, a veterinarian enduring a disability is entitled to a monthly benefit of $3,000. If this person qualified for disability payments from social security as well, a group contract would reduce the $3,000 monthly amount by the amount received from social security.

Limitations are another area of difference between individual and group policies. Though there are still individual policies that provide coverage for mental, nervous, or alcohol/drug conditions, most group contracts restrict coverage of these disabilities.

REVERSE DISCRIMINATION

While many group long-term disability policies are cost effective in covering the basic disability needs of employees, monthly benefit maximums can leave many professionals with inadequate coverage. The more highly paid the individual, the smaller will be the percentage of income covered by disability income insurance allowed by the insurance provider. This is a condition commonly referred to as *reverse discrimination*. The following example illustrates this concept (Table 5.2):

Peak Veterinary Practice has eight employees, some of whom have worked at the practice more than two years. The owners provide disability income protection as a fringe benefit for employees working greater than 32 hours/week and who have been employed more than 2 years. The practice's existing group disability coverage will protect 60% of an covered employee's salary, to a monthly maximum of $4,000.

While this is adequate coverage for most people in the practice, the two most highly compensated veterinarians will not be sufficiently protected in the event of disability. For example, the owner, whose annual pay is $150,000, would receive the monthly maximum of $4,000 during disability. Compared with a predisability monthly salary of $12,500, the $4,000 benefit is hardly enough coverage because it constitutes only 32% of the owner's salary. Moreover, since the premiums for group coverage generally are paid by the practice, the benefits received during disability are fully taxable to the employee. Assuming the most highly compensated owner is in the 35% combined state and federal tax bracket, the $4,000 monthly benefit is reduced to $2,600, which results in protection for only 21% of this person's salary.

Clearly, group disability coverage can be discriminatory against highly paid practitioners. There are two options to remedy the situation:

- Increase the group's monthly maximum coverage of $4,000 to a level that would protect the higher paid professionals. A problem with this, though, is that it increases employer costs for coverage since some employees will receive higher monthly coverage.

Table 5.2. Levels of Disability Coverage at Peak Veterinary Practice

| Position | Annual Salary | Existing Coverage: 60% of salary, $4,000 monthly maximum | | | |
		Monthly Salary	60% of Coverage	Monthly Maximum	Coverage as % of Salary
Receptionist	$30,000	$2,500	$18,000	$4,000	60%
Vet. Ass't	$20,000	$1,667	$12,000	$4,000	60%
Vet. Tech	$29,000	$2,417	$17,400	$4,000	60%
Vet. Assoc.	$72,000	$6,000	$43,200	$4,000	60%
Vet. Owner	$120,000	$10,000	$72,000	$4,000	40%
Vet. Owner	$150,000	$12,500	$90,000	$4,000	32%

- Obtain supplemental coverage for owners who are adversely affected by the group disability coverage.

The second option is an excellent way to combine the benefits of group and individual disability insurance. Group disability programs are economical for providing needed income protection for most of the employees in the practice. Nonetheless, for individuals whose salaries exceed the minimum coverages provided by group policies and who want the portability, level premium, fewer exclusions, and stronger definition of disability features found in individual insurance contracts, a well-coordinated program offering both group and individual disability coverage makes the most sense. To calculate the amount of supplemental coverage for which a professional is eligible, refer to Figure 5.3.

ASSOCIATION PLANS

Association plans come in many forms. The AVMA has a disability income plan that was initiated in 1957 by veterinarians which is managed under the stewardship of the AVMA Group Health and Life Insurance Trust. This means it is led by veterinarians with legal, actuarial, and sales advisors who market the plan. It is an experience-rated program which allows it to pay dividends, something it has done on occasion.

Association plans generally are one of two types: true association-type plans like the AVMA plan, or discounted individual disability contracts. True association-type plans, like group disability plans, provide basic coverage at affordable costs. Discounted individual disability coverage plans, like those described previously, can be offered when particular insurance companies are endorsed. When a minimum of three members apply for coverage, this frequently allows for a 15% discount in premiums. A 15% discount on a $1,000 annual disability premium will save insured individuals $150, an amount sufficient to satisfy half or more of the cost of the veterinary association's annual dues.

Careful attention should be paid to the any occupation versus own occupation definitions of disabilities with association plans because those with premiums that appear too good to be true often are, and one of the reasons has to do with a more narrow definition of an insured person's disability. Additionally, questions should be asked about the extent of an individual's income that can be insured under the plan. At one time coverage could routinely be obtained for 60% of one's income; with the changes occurring in the industry, some plans now limit coverage to as little as 40% of an insured's income.

The AVMA's excellent insurance program provides disability income coverage with the New York Life Insurance Company. Like most association plans, the coverage is basic and affordable. Determining whether the AVMA coverage is appropriate for veterinary practitioners depends on the individual's particular situation. Like individual disability coverage, AVMA coverage will reimburse veterinarians if they are unable to return to work due to accidents or sicknesses. Moreover, the coverage includes future purchase options, insurance for 60% of an insured's income, cost-of-living adjustments, "own occupation" riders, personalized rehabilitation programs, residual disability benefits, and waiver of premium options.[2] Some of the important features of AVMA coverage are as follows:

- AVMA coverage continues as long as the veterinarian remains a member of the association. If the veterinarian terminates membership, disability income coverage with the AVMA ceases.

- AVMA coverage is not non-cancelable: rates can go up and coverage can be dropped by the existing insurance company. While history has been favorable to those insured through the AVMA trust, it is uncertain how the most recent changes in the disability income

IF A DISABILITY OCCURS, WILL YOUR CURRENT EMPLOYER-SPONSORED GROUP LONG-TERM DISABILITY (LTD) INSURANCE PROVIDE ENOUGH INCOME TO MEET YOUR EXPENSES?

Let's examine YOUR situation: _____

Current Employer Sponsored GROUP LTD Plan Provides _____% of your income
to a MAXIMUM benefit of $ _____ per month.

PROBLEM

YOUR CURRENT MONTHLY INCOME: $_____

NET MONTHLY INCOME (Assuming _____ % Tax Bracket): $_____

YOUR CURRENT GROUP LTD MONTHLY DISABILITY BENEFIT: $_____

NET MONTHLY DISABILITY BENEFIT (Assuming _____ % Tax Bracket): $_____

THE NET MONTHLY DISABILITY BENEFIT OF $ _____
REPRESENTS _____% OF YOUR CURRENT MONTHLY TAKE HOME PAY.

SOLUTION

TOTAL MONTHLY DISABILITY BENEFIT $_____
FOR WHICH PROFESSIONAL IS ELIGIBLE:
Depends on issue limits established by disability company

CURRENT GROUP LTD MONTHLY DISABILITY BENEFIT: -$_____
          $_____   X   80%

Many companies discount group coverage by 20%

DIFFERENCE - AMOUNT ELIGIBLE FOR SUPPLEMENTAL COVERAGE: $_____

RECAP

If the supplemental coverage is purchased with after-tax dollars, the benefit is received tax-free during periods of disability. Total take home pay during disability is as follows:

NET MONTHLY LTD DISABILITY BENEFIT: $_____

SUPPLEMENTAL COVERAGE: +$_____

TOTAL TAKE HOME PAY - DURING DISABILITY:

Represents _____ % of Current Monthly Take Home Pay. $_____

Figure 5.3. Chart used to calculate eligibility for supplementary disability coverage

insurance arena will impact coverages and pricing in the future.

- AVMA coverage for residual disabilities is restrictive: Residual coverage is paid only if a partial disability is preceded by a total disability.

- AVMA coverage does not include automatic benefit indexing.

- AVMA coverage includes a waiver of premium after six months of disability; most commercial policies waive premiums after three months.

If the restrictions in the AVMA or other association-endorsed contracts are of concern, an individual disability income policy may be more suitable. If cost is an issue and the restrictions are of minor importance, the AVMA contract may be appropriate. Which is the best choice? For veterinary practitioners looking for coverage, a combination of group and individual disability income policies may provide the best of both worlds. For independent contractors, consultants, solo practitioners, or professionals who are working in practices with no group disability coverage, the following two options may provide comprehensive coverages at affordable rates.

For those practitioners who are not eligible for any of the valuable AVMA coverage, their best option is to join the AVMA.

OTHER TYPES OF DISABILITY COVERAGE

Three additional types of disability income coverage include overhead expense, buy-sell, and key person.

OVERHEAD EXPENSE INSURANCE

Practice expenses continue during an owner's disability, particularly the fixed expenses for a mortgage or rent, heat, electricity, and employee salaries. Overhead coverage reimburses the practice for these expenses and keeps the doors open until the owner is capable of returning to work. Unlike individual disability coverage, overhead expense policies typically have a short benefit period covering only one to two years. It is within this period of time that veterinarians will be able to judge the possibility of returning to work. If they cannot return and it is likely the practice will need to be sold, the overhead expense coverage helps provide the time needed to effectively market and sell the practice. This coverage is particularly important for solo practitioners who cannot rely on co-owners to pick up the disabled owner's share of the workload.

BUY-SELL INSURANCE

A buy-sell agreement is a legal document between co-owners that identifies the responsibilities each assumes in the event of death, disability, retirement, or termination. Death and disability can be funded with insurance. Though a disability is more common than death at many ages, ironically, many professionals purchase only life insurance to protect against the possibility that a partner will die. The purchase of disability insurance often is the missing page in good planning for succession.

A disability buy-sell policy pays disabled owners for their share of the practice when it becomes apparent their disability will prevent them from returning. Properly drafted buy-sell agreements obligate healthy partners to use these proceeds to buy out the disabled partner's share of the practice. Typically individuals wait one to two years before policy's benefits are paid or the disabled partners become eligible for payment for their ownership interest in the practice. Moreover, practice owners who are the beneficiaries of policies can decide how benefits are to be paid, i.e., as lump sums, in installments, or via combinations of the two.

A disability buy-sell policy is generally a better source of funding than available cash (an unlikely scenario), current income (because this creates a financial drain for the practice), or borrowing (not always a possibility). Premiums for this type of coverage are typically lower than those for individual disability income coverages.

For example, two practitioners are equal partners in a practice worth approximately $500,000. One is age 40, the other 35. Assuming an elimination period of 12 months, a benefit of $250,000 for each policy, and a lump sum payout, the premium for the 35 year old is $1,122.50 per year and the premium for the 40 year old is $1,390. If the payout were changed to monthly installments paid over 60 months instead of a lump sum, the premiums would drop to $741.67 and $978.75, respectively. (Quotes supplied by UNUM Life Insurance Company of America).

KEY PERSON DISABILITY INSURANCE

The loss of a key person such as a veterinarian, assistant, technician, or practice manager to a disability can cause a loss of profits and/or additional expenses incurred in hiring a replacement. Key person disability insurance policies reimburse the practice in the event the key person becomes disabled.

TAXABILITY OF BENEFITS

The taxability of benefits generally depends on who pays the premium. When an individual pays the premium, it is not deductible. Benefits received during periods of disability, though, are tax free. Alternatively, when premiums are paid and deducted by the business, benefits received during disability are taxable to the recipient.

Employers generally are permitted to deduct insurance expenses as a tax benefit only when benefits are provided for all eligible employees. Unlike all other benefits, though, if some important rules are followed, employers can provide disability income coverage for a select few and still receive this deduction. Called a *salary con-*

tinuation plan, this program must meet the following requirements to receive tax-favored treatment:

- The plan must be in writing.

- The plan must be in effect prior to an employee's disability.

- The plan details must be communicated to covered employees.

- The plan can provide for different levels of coverage for different classes of employees or simply provide coverage for a specific class of employee such as veterinarians. Stockholder-employees can be included only if they can be segregated based on length of service, income, or occupational class, i.e., on a basis other than the fact that they are stockholders.

Therefore, practices can provide group coverage for all employees and individual coverage for a few employees and still be permitted tax deductions for both benefits as long as a salary continuation plan is properly designed. One caveat, though, is that deductions are not permitted for sole proprietors, partners, and most owners of S-Corporations, i.e., types of corporations that permit income and expenses to flow through to the shareholders.

An alternative program is the executive bonus. Let's say an employer wants to provide disability income coverage for a selected employee and still receive a deduction. A salary continuation plan will not work if the employer is uninterested in covering other employees in the same class. Instead, the employer can give the selected employee a bonus equal to the premium and the employee can use the bonus to purchase the needed disability income coverage. This bonus generally is tax deductible by the practice, assuming the total compensation for the employee is considered reasonable when compared to the services rendered. The executive bonus program may be advantageous for sole proprietors, partners, and owners of S-Corporations not permitted deductions in salary continuation plans.

Premiums paid for overhead expense coverage are tax-deductible business expenses, but benefits received during a disability are taxable to the business. Since the benefit is merely a reimbursement for paid expenses, the result is a tax wash. Premiums paid for buy-sell and key person coverage are not tax deductible by the practice.

As with all tax matters discussed in this book, consultation with professionals specializing in these matters is essential. Local laws vary, and tax laws change from year to year. Tax attorneys, accountants, and insurance agents all can assist in these matters.

STEP RATE POLICIES

Many disability companies offer step rate policies. These are policies designed for young professionals wherein policy premiums are low for several years, begin to increase some years later, and eventually level off for the balance of the contract (typically to age 65). The advantages include low premiums in the early years and premium increases as earnings increase. The one disadvantage is that the total premium outlay to age 65 is higher.

DISCOUNTED POLICIES

As mentioned earlier, members of associations that endorse particular disability income insurance companies will generally receive multi-life discounts of 15% on the premiums. This discount is also offered by non-association-endorsed disability companies to practices wherein three or more professionals or nonprofessional applicants apply for coverage. A common mistake occurs when professionals purchase disability income coverage on their own. By failing to coordinate their efforts and purchase insurance with others in the practice who also need coverage, they lose the benefit of the multi-life discount.

Two owners of a veterinary practice can purchase coverage from the same carrier, include a third—perhaps a technician, assistant, or receptionist—and each will receive the multi-life discount. If the disability income coverage is paid by the practice as part of a wage continuation plan, the multilife discount typically pays for the coverage of the third person. Consider this example: Two veterinarians purchase disability insurance with combined premiums of $4,000. If they decide to include the receptionist, a 15% discount on their policies, $600, would more than pay for the receptionist's $450 premium.

IMPAIRED RISK

Applicants with no preexisting medical conditions generally can obtain what is called *standard coverage*. When medical conditions exist, disability companies can exclude coverage for disabilities resulting from these conditions (called *exclusions* or *riders*), charge an additional cost (called a *rating*), restrict some of the benefits (i.e., reduce the benefit period), or simply deny coverage. If a rating is applied, one option is to increase the elimination period. Assuming the applicant has adequate cash reserves, an increase in elimination period from 90 to 365 days may reduce the cost of the premium to an affordable level.

If there is some uncertainty about the degree to which a preexisting medical condition will affect the application process and underwriting decision, agents can informally inquire about coverage with several top companies. This saves a great deal of time and identifies which companies may be more flexible in dealing with a particular medical condition. Although it may seem odd, different companies evaluate risks differently.

There are several disability companies that offer unique programs should an applicant be denied coverage. One such company offers what is called a *graded benefit* type of program. This company denies very few applicants and does not exclude preexisting medical conditions. The disadvantages include relatively high premiums, reduced benefit periods (typically two to five years), and graded benefit amounts. Under the latter provision, this company pays only 25% of the monthly benefit if the applicant is disabled in the first year the policy was issued, 50% if disabled in year two, 75% if disabled in year three, and full benefits in years four and after.

SELECTING AN AGENT

Good sources to check with when seeking an agent include fellow professionals and national, state, or local veterinary associations. Agents who specialize in the veterinary profession are more likely to understand the risk management issues confronting veterinarians and, therefore, are better prepared to support their recommendations. Moreover, agents who have cultivated strong relationships with individuals in the profession depend on satisfied clients for referrals and to help them build successful practices.

In selecting the right individual, technical competence, objectivity, and chemistry are important. As for technical competence, a good agent will ask the following questions during the first meeting.

- What is your projected income for the year?

- To what level do you expect your income to increase in years 5, 10, and 25? This is an important question to ask in assessing how much, if any, future insurance options should be purchased.

- What type of liquid emergency reserves do you have? In other words, how long could you live without a paycheck?

- What type of educational debt load are you carrying?

- How long would it take for you to return to your present income level if

you were disabled for two years?, five years?, ten years? Self-employed professionals must consider this when determining whether a total recovery rider is necessary.

Also, good agents will address the following key issues in designing the most comprehensive disability income programs:

- the difference between guaranteed renewable and non-cancelable policies;

- the differences in the definitions of disability, i.e., the inability to return to one's own occupation or any occupation;

- preexisting medical conditions which may adversely impact the underwriting of the case; and

- the economics and policy features of individual, group, and association coverage.

Objectivity is important in determining whose interests are being served. Some agents sell primarily for one company, while others sell for multiple companies. The latter may be more objective in assessing an applicant's needs and recommending the right coverage. Good agents understand the differences among the top companies and are able to discuss policy details, including exclusions. A basis of comparison among companies will either reinforce initial thoughts or identify a better choice.

Selecting an agent ultimately may be decided upon chemistry or comfort level. Some agents may rush the process or appear insensitive to the applicant's particular circumstances. Good agents will listen, answer questions, and understand that service, not product, is the most important factor in building a mutually rewarding relationship.

This section would not be complete without some comments on replacement of disability income policies. A replacement occurs when an agent replaces an older policy, in many cases sold by another agent, with a new disability income policy. As discussed, the industry trend is to restrict policy features and increase premiums. Therefore, older policies have become more valuable and in most cases should not be replaced. Agents who recommend replacing existing policies with ones they are selling should be asked to provide written comparisons of the policies. Only after the benefits and costs are clearly summarized can applicants make correct decisions.

FINAL THOUGHTS

Some companies believe the non-cancelable feature of disability income policies is to blame for the more restricted, costlier insurance we have today; others believe it is the way disability has been defined. Still others believe that exclusions are necessary to better manage claims and redirect focus on catastrophic illnesses. Whatever the cause, the disability income industry is undergoing rapid changes. It is evident that philosophical differences among disability companies have reshaped and will continue to reshape this product and its features.

CASE STUDIES

CASE #1

George Smith, DVM, is a board-certified consultant working at multiple practices specializing in cardiology. He recently purchased an ultrasound machine with a cost in excess of $100,000. The lease payments alone run close to $650 a month. Dr. Smith is particularly concerned about prolonged disability and the impact this would have with his network of referrals cultivated over the years. Recommendation: Secure individual disability coverage and, if possible, be sure total recovery is included. Moreover, overhead expense coverage should be purchased to protect the monthly lease payments.

CASE #2

Nancy Wilcox, VMD, is the majority owner of a large practice in western Pennsylvania. She has 2 partners, an associate veterinarian, and 12 employees, for a total of 15 people working at the practice. Dr. Wilcox is interested in coverage for all employees and is particularly concerned with securing the most comprehensive coverage for the three owners. She decides on a group disability program to provide a base level of protection for all employees, and supplements the group policy with individual disability income coverages for the three owners. By using the same insurance company for the three individual disability policies, she is able to secure a 15% discount for additional policies. In addition, Dr. Wilcox will consider the benefits of disability buy-sell policies for the partners.

CASE #3

Tom Wilson, DVM, is an associate with a mixed practice in Waupaca, Wisconsin. His wife is an attorney with a local firm, and she has disability coverage through an individual policy. While Dr. Wilson recognizes the importance of disability income protection, his family's rather substantial inheritance places them in a comfortable financial position. He decides to obtain coverage for only a portion of his income. He purchases both an individual policy and an AVMA group policy.

CASE #4

Margaret Shevlin, DVM, is an associate with a practice in Texas. Her benefits include a group disability program which protects 60% of her earnings, to a monthly maximum of $3,000. Her annual compensation is above the $60,000 threshold protected by the group policy; moreover, Dr. Shevlin's family lives in Orinda, California and she hopes to return to her hometown within three years to start her own practice.

Dr. Shevlin should supplement the group coverage offered by the practice with an individual policy. This individual policy will bridge the gap in coverage resulting from the reverse discrimination discussed earlier. Also, if she adds the future insurance option rider to this policy, Dr. Shevlin will be able to purchase additional increments of coverage without providing evidence of insurability when she leaves her present employment.

EMPLOYEE HEALTH COVERAGE

One of the most important, yet confusing fringe benefits for employees to consider is health care coverage. The confusion involves three major issues and three minor ones. Among the more easily addressed minor ones are: (1) tax deductions for employers and tax savings for employees; (2) lower premiums for employees whose health care is provided through membership in employers' group plans; and (3) access by employees to better plans than they could purchase independent of their employers. Among the major ones are: (1) understanding the various types of health care coverage available in today's markets; (2) selecting the most desirable one; and (3) keeping abreast of the rapid changes in plans providing and laws regarding health coverage.

THE MINOR ISSUES

Because health coverage is a business tax deduction for employers and is not considered by the IRS to be taxable income for employees, the tax savings on this benefit for employees is remarkable. Since health care coverage generally costs between $1,500 and $3,000 per year per employee, and much more for families, the tax savings for employees can be considerable. Depending on the party's age, health status, and taxable income, tax savings of as much as $450 to $900 per individual are available for employees, most of whom will be taxed at a 30% state and federal combined rate.

Secondly, employers who provide health coverage for their employees allow them access to participation in group plans. In most cases this means that premiums for this coverage cost considerably less than comparable plans purchased by individuals on the open market. Even more important, however, is the fact that employer-paid health care plans force employees who otherwise may not seek out nor budget for the costs of such insurance to obtain coverage.

Lastly, employees with preexisting health problems often can obtain coverage only if they are members of groups. With employment comes a right to enroll in a plan simply because one is employed by the employer, irrespective of former employment or health history. This option may not exist when people apply for health coverage as individuals.

THE MAJOR ISSUES

Health insurance and the shifting laws and insurance company policies that regulate this complex field can be confusing for staff members and small business owners to navigate. It is no surprise, then, that according to a *U.S. News and World Report* article, three fourths of Americans are worried about their health care coverage, one fourth cannot figure out their bills, one fifth can't pay them, and half are upset that doctors' treatments are based on the plan's coverage rather than what is best for the patient.[3] Equally disconcerting is the fact that in 1998, General Motors, the largest private-sector purchaser of health care in the United States, spent a staggering $1,200 per vehicle built just to cover the health care costs of its employees.[3]

For employees and employers to avoid the quagmires involved in choosing a suitable plan, they must have a clear understanding of the types of health coverage options available and some of the common terms encountered.

Types of Health Care Coverage

Health care coverage can be divided into two broad categories: fee-for-service and managed care. Managed care plans differ from traditional fee-for-service, or indemnity, plans in that they are characterized by "the existence of a single entity responsible for integrating and coordinating the financing and delivery of services that were once scattered between providers and payers".[4] Managed care plans encourage patients to use the services of health care providers who belong to their plan. Instead of paying a monthly fee for coverage and seeking care for individual services as they would under a fee-for-service system, patients (or employers) are charged monthly or quarterly premiums in advance and patients pay only a small co-payment for certain services, depending on the specifics of the plan.

FEE-FOR-SERVICE HEALTH CARE

Before the popularity of managed care plans in the 1990s, health insurance coverage consisted almost exclusively of fee-for-service plans. These plans, which still exist in small numbers, allow patients to visit the physicians of their choice, and the physicians are reimbursed for each service performed. Invoices are either billed directly to the insurance companies by the providers or are paid directly by patients, who then request reimbursement from their insurance carriers. Premiums for these plans tend to be considerably higher than those for managed care plans, since patients are not restricted in their choices of doctors or treatments.

During the golden age of medical science following World War II, new drugs, equipment, and medical techniques helped increase the average life span of Americans from 63 years to 76 years by 1996. Under the fee-for-service model, doctors and hospitals had a financial incentive to throw every-

thing they could at every patient's malady. The more procedures, the more income they earned. The third-party payment insurance systems prevalent at the time had the same incentives because they simply raised premiums to match costs. The institution of Medicare in 1965 further institutionalized the blank check mentality, under which the government and private insurance companies were expected to pay virtually all bills submitted.[4]

The long-term result of the fee-for-service system was extraordinary health care inflation. Whereas in 1980 Americans spent $247 billion on health care, or 8.9% of the gross domestic product (GDP), by 1990 that figure had risen to $697 billion, an alarming 12.1% of the GDP. Projections for the early 2000s were for costs to rise to as high as 16% of the GDP, remarkably higher than Japan's 7.2% or Canada's 9.6%. Something had to give, so insurance premiums rose exorbitantly, copayments by insured patients increased, and benefits were reduced.[3]

By 1995 managed care had taken hold and Americans were spending $988 billion on health care, or 13.6% of the GDP. This was still a lot, but much less than the $1.07 trillion, 14.8% of the GDP that the Congressional Budget Office had forecast only three years earlier. The savings were due largely to the rapid exit from fee-for-service health care into managed care.

Generally, fee-for-service insurance policies place broad restrictions on covered medical expenses. These include restricted coverage on health issues such as pregnancies, fertility workups, mental health care, and substance abuse expenses. Thus, it is important for employers who seek coverage for themselves and their staff and employees who wish to evaluate the extent of their coverage to read sample policies carefully before selecting a carrier. Since the details and comparisons of policies are difficult for lay people to assess, consultations with unbiased insurance agents usually are essential to help compare the options.

Also important in the choice is a determination of the co-insurance and deductibles specified in the policy. Deductibles determine how much insured parties are required to pay before their insurance coverage kicks in. Two hundred fifty to five hundred dollar deductible policies are common, with some rising to $5,000 to keep costs competitive with managed care. Co-payment policies requiring that insured parties pay 20% of the first $5,000 by insured parties are common. Thereafter, the policies most often cover 100% of specified expenses up to a maximum of $1 million during the term of the policy.

In addition to co-payments by policyholders, some of these plans now require a utilization review process, i.e., a case-by-case review of medical care to ascertain suitability and essentiality. This process can range from pre-hospital admission screening by carriers to second opinions and hospital discharge decisions. Because of their high cost, traditional fee-for-service plans with no restrictions are rapidly becoming extinct in most areas of the country.

MANAGED CARE

Managed care can be subdivided into three specific types of plans: (1) health maintenance organizations, or HMOs; (2) preferred provider organizations, or PPOs; and (3) hybrids, such as point-of-service (POS) plans.

HMOs

HMOs have been in existence for more than 50 years and are the best known and earliest form of managed care. They are the strictest of the managed plans and provide total care in the form of a combination of insurance companies, physicians, and hospitals. The HMO covers all medical expenses, provided patients use medical professionals and facilities within an approved network.

Members of HMOs or their employers pay monthly premiums and co-payments (usually between $5 and $15) each time they visit a doctor. Patients must select primary care physicians who approve all care, referrals, and hospital admissions. These physicians, also known as *gatekeeper physicians*, must be consulted first each time a health-related problem occurs, and patients usually are not allowed to seek the care of specialists unless the gatekeeper physicians approve. HMOs may deny benefits if members use medical providers outside their plan's network, in which case patients bear full responsibility for the medical expenses incurred.

Some consumers view HMOs as inflexible since noncompliance with plan regulations can result in a reduction or complete denial of benefits. The use of capitation reimbursement policies by some HMOs has also been a point of contention. A capitation basis for physician reimbursement means that the insurance company pays the physician a fee per member, per month, whether the patient visits the physician or not. This means the risks for losses are borne by the physicians in the plan, not the parent insurance companies. This financial arrangement has been criticized as an incentive for physicians to minimize the number of visits, services, referrals, and medical care, contrary to the needs of their patients.

Despite problems inherent in managed care and specific to HMOs, these plans can provide benefits to business owners and employees. According to an American Association of Health report by the Lewin Group, managed care helped Americans save between $116 billion and $181 billion in health care costs from 1990 to 1996. If employers had passed those savings on to workers, the average worker would have gained an extra $228 per year in take-home pay ($408 per couple). In states like California, where 37% of people belong to HMOs, the savings would have amounted to $770 per family.[3]

Many managed care plans have formal systems designed to improve and review the quality of care provided.[5] These systems can eliminate much of the wasteful care and many of the duplicative tests that have plagued traditional fee-for-service plans and caused costs to escalate so remarkably. To benefit patients and keep costs down, managed care also emphasizes preventive care and early detection.

A 12-year study by RAND (an independent research organization) found that patients who belonged to HMOs had 40% fewer hospitalizations and saved 28% in health care costs as compared to patients in traditional indemnity plans, without adversely impacting their quality of care.[5] Other studies have found that mortality rates, treatment results, and the rates of nonelective surgery were the same for private patients and those in HMOs.[5] Some HMOs reward quality care by conducting patient satisfaction surveys. The higher the physician rates in these surveys, the more they will be paid by the HMO. With advantages like those listed above, and 12% lower annual premiums on average as compared to indemnity plans, the appeal of HMOs to many businesses is easily understood. Today, three out of four Americans insured through their employers belong to some type of managed care plan.[3]

Although physicians have complained bitterly about the loss of their independent medical decision-making rights and deteriorating patient care, a September 1997 *Journal of the American Medical Association* article refutes many of those claims. The study reported that older patients suffered through fewer episodes of "potentially ineffective care" (hospital jargon for care that prolongs an inevitable death). Treatment in the last six months of life for those over 65 accounts for 21% of all Medicare spending. Moreover, the care often is futile, painful, degrading, and unwanted. The article showed that HMO patients were 25% less likely to suffer though such undesired care.[3]

According to a study in the *American Journal of Public Health*, managed care also seems to do a better job of finding breast, cervical, colon, and melanoma cancers— sooner than fee-for-service plans. Additionally, the

Health Affairs journal reported that open-heart surgery patients in such plans were more likely to be steered to high-volume facilities that experienced fewer deaths and lower fatalities.[3] William M. Mercer's book *Demanding Medical Excellence: Doctors and Accountability in the Information Age* states it well when it says, "The problem with all these people who are not being killed is that very few people know it. Your doctor doesn't say, "You know, I was going to recommend inappropriate surgery but because of managed care, I won't.'"

PPOs

Preferred provider organizations, or PPOs, are at the opposite end of the managed care spectrum. Their numbers are growing, and they represent a balance between traditional fee-for-service plans and HMOs. They are similar to HMOs in that they offer networks of health care providers with whom they have negotiated discounted billing rates. Members are strongly encouraged to see physicians within the network, and are penalized with lower reimbursement rates if they seek outside treatment. Unlike HMOs, PPOs do not require patients to see primary care physicians first, thus allowing members to consult with specialists without prior approval. Overall, PPOs attempt to balance the competing interests of cost control and patient free choice by combining aspects of traditional health insurance with managed care initiatives.

Point of Service Plans

Point of service plans, sometimes referred to as *open HMOs*, have primary care physicians coordinate all care and make necessary referrals. In theory, patients are encouraged to seek treatment within the network but are allowed to see outside physicians. In practice, out-of-network deductibles, co-payments, and low reimbursement rates usually are so cost prohibitive that many members cannot afford this option.

Employers usually incur lower premiums with POS plans than with fee-for-service options or PPOs since the coordination offered by gatekeeper physicians substantially reduces costs.

SELECTING THE RIGHT HEALTH CARE PLAN

The delicate task for employers is to select plans that balance the quality and extent of services offered with their costs. The task for employees is to understand the nature of the plans offered by their employers and, when choices exist, select the plan that best suits their needs. Careful examination of plans for features such as the geographic location of physicians, labs, and hospitals in the network, the availability of wellness programs, provisions for emergency care, and coverage for chronic diseases is essential.

The National Committee for Quality Assurance (NCQA), a Washington-based nonprofit organization, has been working with HMOs and business organizations to develop a standardized set of criteria by which to judge HMO health plans.[6] They created the HEDIS 3.0 (Health Plan Employer Data and Information Set), with over 60 measurements of plan performance in the areas of quality of care, access to care, and patient satisfaction. The report cards generated by HEDIS rate plans according to specific criteria but do not rank them overall.

The American Accreditation Healthcare Commission is another nonprofit organization that focuses on managed plans in general and PPOs in particular.[7] In many states, information about health care plans is available from that state's Department of Insurance or the Department of Health. Before selecting plans that are right for employees and practice owners, each party should ask to see the most recent report card, inquire as to whether the plan is accredited (and if so, by whom), and check with the state regulatory departments for any additional information available.

HEALTH CARE OPTIONS FOR VETERINARY PRACTICES

Increasing health care costs have forced employers to seek creative solutions when selecting coverage for themselves and their families or offering it to their employees. Veterinarians who are members of the American Veterinary Medical Association (AVMA) are eligible for AVMA health insurance through an indemnity plan underwritten by New York Life. The plan is both national and international in coverage and does not rely on a fixed network. In some areas the AVMA plan offers a preferred provider network option in which participating health care providers offer fixed-fee service for AVMA policyholders.[8]

Of particular importance is the fact that the AVMA health plan is available to new graduates at discounted rates and offers delayed payment options unavailable elsewhere. This plan has the added benefit of portability, which means policy holders can take their coverage with them should they change jobs. Many state VMAs offer health care coverage for employers and employees through agreements with local insurance brokerages in their states. In Pennsylvania, for example, HMOs, PPOs, and indemnity plans that are equal to or better than the AVMA plan are offered through Blue Cross and Blue Shield. Information about such plans can be acquired by contacting the state VMAs in which employers and employees work.

Although it requires payments to two different carriers, veterinary employers can offer health insurance through one company to their technical and support staff while offering a different company's plan, such as that of the AVMA, to their employed veterinarians. In some cases, though, health insurance carriers require that a certain percentage of eligible employees (usually 75%) enroll with their company to assure a large enough size group for eligibility. Employers are urged to check the specific requirements of the employers' primary carrier before purchasing coverage.

In other cases, small employers can offer dual or triple option plans. Dual option plans allow employees to select between indemnity and HMO plans, or a PPO and an HMO plan, from the same carrier. Triple option plans offer all three. In such plans the rates are blended for the programs, usually resulting in lower costs. The advantage of this for employers is that they can pay one bill and limit their administrative costs.

Cafeteria plans, discussed in depth in Chapter 4, are yet another creative option for offering health benefits. Congress first authorized cafeteria plans in 1978 under Section 125 of the Internal Revenue Code. A cafeteria plan, or "Section 125 plan," provides employer and employee tax advantages by allowing participating employees to select benefits from a menu of choices, from which the name *cafeteria plan* is derived. These plans allow health contributions and deposits to flexible spending accounts to be made with pretax dollars.

Employers favor these plans because they help attract and retain quality employees while simultaneously reducing costs through payroll tax savings and efficient use of benefit dollars. Flexible benefit plans are attractive to employees since they are able to pick and choose among various tax-free benefits and levels of coverage, creating custom plans tailored to each individual. By setting up Section 125 plans, employers can also institute flexible spending accounts (FSAs) to allow certain expenses to be paid by the employee with pretax dollars. A "health-FSA" is for health and dental expenses that are not covered by the employer's insurance, including deductibles, co-payments, and noncovered items such as eyeglasses.

Cafeteria plans have limitations that make them less attractive to some businesses. All participants in the plan must be employees, thereby excluding sole proprietors and partners of a partnership from participating. If the business is an S-corporation, employees who are greater than 2% owners are excluded from Section 125 plans. C-corporations that have not elected "S" status with the Internal Revenue Service have no restrictions on eligibility. Other limitations specify that all contributions must be made through salary-reduction agreements, and the plans must meet certain nondiscrimination, election, and enrollment requirements. One of the eligibility test standards specifies that the plan must uniformly benefit all employees in the classes designated as eligible to participate, and it cannot discriminate in favor of highly compensated individuals. Thus, veterinary employers who offer cafeteria plans must be certain they do not discriminate in favor of their employed veterinarians.

Some small businesses have found that purchasing alliances can make health insurance more affordable and accessible. California sponsored the first state purchase alliance for small businesses in 1993, and since then 15 other states have adopted similar plans. Generally these plans target companies that employ 3 to 50 people, and most require that employers pay certain percentages of the premium or a flat fee based on the lowest-cost plan. Alliances also typically mandate participation by 75% of a company's eligible employees. The primary benefit offered by purchasing alliances is lower cost of premiums due to volume purchasing. Other attractive features include guaranteed coverage and renewal, and businesses that employ persons with high-cost medical histories are not charged excessively high premium rates. More information on purchasing alliances can be obtained by contacting the Institute for Health Policy Solutions in Washington, DC.[9]

THE EFFECT OF NEW HEALTH INSURANCE LEGISLATION ON SMALL BUSINESSES

On July 1, 1997, major provisions of the Health Insurance Portability and Accountability Act (HIPAA) of 1996 went into effect. HIPAA guarantees that insurers may impose only one 12-month waiting period for any preexisting condition treated or diagnosed in the previous six months. Any prior health care coverage without a break of 62 days or more will be credited toward the preexisting exclusion period. Pregnancy is not a preexisting condition, and newborns or adopted children enrolled within the first 30 days are not subject to the 12-month waiting period.

Prior to HIPAA, persons with preexisting conditions were limited to HMOs or, rarely, other insurance plans that would accept them for coverage without evidence of insurability during the initial or open enrollment period, which usually occurs once a year. The enactment of HIPAA has been a boon to the mobility of employees with family members who suffer from expensive or chronic diseases. Because of this legislation, they are no longer locked into their existing jobs to maintain their health coverage. HIPAA does not mandate that employees be entitled to the same type of health care coverage; it simply guarantees that employees will be able to obtain coverage if their new employers offer it.

Employees who lose health coverage due to job termination or decreased work hours are eligible to purchase coverage for themselves and their families for limited time periods through COBRA (Consolidated Omnibus Budget Reconciliation Act). Employees have 60 days after termination of employment to accept COBRA coverage, and they are responsible for paying the total cost of their insurance premiums.

Under HIPAA, insurance companies that sell to the small group market cannot turn down any small employer who applies for coverage, so even companies with only two employees will be eligible. In addition, insurance companies must continue insurance coverage for any businesses that request renewal, regardless of the health status of the employees. HIPAA aids the self-employed by increasing the percentage of a premium that can be deducted from income taxes to 60% of the premium in 1999, and more in future years. It also establishes tax incentives for the purchase of long-term care insurance.[10]

While the benefits of HIPAA are numerous, it does not address the quality or comprehensiveness of health care offered by employers, nor does it encourage employers to offer any coverage. The cost savings associated with greater competition among providers could be offset when small businesses hire people with health problems and add them to their plans, thereby increasing costs for all employees. Administrative costs will also rise as small companies attempt to comply with HIPAA provisions. Nonetheless, HIPAA was an important legislative step in filling some gaps in the health insurance industry, even though more work still is needed.

WHAT'S IN STORE FOR THE FUTURE

For all the changes that have occurred in the past decade and cuts in health care costs achieved through managed care, the industry still faces formidable challenges. Like a recurring disease, inflation is continuing and costs are eating away at HMO profits. Though managed care has brought with it considerable cost savings, it is not without its problems. It does nothing for the millions of Americans without insurance. The old fee-for-service insurance system covered poor, uninsured people through overcharges to those with insurance. Because neither doctors, patients, nor insurance companies were insisting that bills reflect actual care given to individual patients, hospitals calculated bills in manners that covered all their costs of operation. Although this was, in essence, a hidden tax on the self-employed who paid their own way and employers who provided insurance for their employees, the system provided a financial safety net to cover health costs for the uninsured.

When managed care hit with a vengeance in the 1990s, insurers began negotiating fees. To control costs, they insisted that their policies would cover only the costs of care actually provided to their insured patients. As their power grew, they also set limits on costs that provided no discernable medical benefits, such as lengthy postdelivery hospital stays for new mothers and brand name drugs where evidence showed no benefit over the use of generics. However, when uninsured Americans kept coming through their doors, and hospitals could not morally or legally turn them away, they began cutting costs by cutting staff. Although hospital administrators insist that the squeeze has not affected the quality of care, some have pointed to reductions in nursing staff and hospital comforts as an undesirable consequence of this trend.

Another concern is that today's managed care companies have a high percentage of young, healthy insured customers. While this currently is an attractive business model, it is at odds with the demographic trends of a country whose average age and, thus, need for medical care is rising rapidly. The result, according to Arthur Caplan, Director of the University of Pennsylvania's Bioethics Center, is that "What we think we're in now with cost containment and rationing (of medical care) is nothing compared to when the (baby) boomers age."[4]

The changeover from the fee-for-service insurance concept of health insurance to managed care has been a historically necessary response to a crisis in the country's health care system. Coping with the next set of challenges will not be as easy and will require improving the managed care system of delivery as well. It also will require that Americans take better care of their own health to reduce costs. If readers think the provision of health care as a tax-free benefit from employers is important today, it will become even more important in the future.

Glossary of Health Care Insurance Terms

Allowed Expenses: The maximum amount a plan pays for a covered service.

Balance Billing: The practice of providers billing patients for all charges not paid for by the insurance companies. Balance billing is prohibited under some managed care plans.

Benefits: Medical services for which insurance plans will pay, in full or in part.

Claims: Notices to insurance companies that insured persons have received care covered by their plans. This is also a request for payment.

Closed Panel: A managed care plan that contracts with physicians on an exclusive basis for services and does not allow those physicians to see patients from another managed care organization.

Co-insurance: A term that describes shared payments between insurance companies and individuals. This figure is usually given in percentages, such as insurance companies paying 80% of covered charges, and members paying the remaining 20%.

Co-payment: The insured member's portion of a cost for a service, usually a flat fee such as $10 for an office visit. Usually a plan will require co-payments without a deductible (HMO, POS), or co-insurance and a deductible (indemnity, PPO plans).

Covered Expenses: The expenses for which health plans will consider paying for services, as defined in the contract.

Deductible: A portion of the covered expenses (usually $100 to $500) that insured individuals must pay before insurance coverage with co-insurance goes into effect. Deductibles are usually based on calendar years.

Formulary: Listings of drugs that physicians may prescribe. Physicians are requested or required to use only formulary drugs unless there are valid medical reasons to use nonformulary drugs.

Maximum Out-of-Pocket: The most money insured patients can expect to pay for covered expenses. This limit varies with each plan, with some companies counting deductibles, co-insurance, and co-payments towards the limit, and others not. Once the limit has been met, the health plans pay 100% of certain covered expenses.

Network: Selected groups of physicians, hospitals, laboratories, and other health care providers who participate in each managed care plan's health delivery program. Providers agree to follow the plan's procedures, permit the monitoring of their practices, and provide certain negotiated discounts in exchange for a guaranteed patient pool.

Preauthorization: An insurance company policy requiring insured parties or their primary care physicians to notify carriers in advance of certain medical procedures in order for those procedures to be covered expenses.

Premiums: Monies paid to health care plans for coverage. Premiums are usually paid monthly and may be paid in part or in total by employers.

Primary Care Physicians (Gatekeeper Physicians): These physicians coordinate and manage the medical care of HMO and POS patients. Primary care physicians usually are family physicians, internal medicine physicians, or pediatricians. These doctors see patients for all medical services, refer them to specialists when necessary, and coordinate all hospital and other medical care.

Providers: Suppliers of health care services. They could be physicians, hospitals, therapists, home nursing care organizations, etc.

Usual, Customary, or Reasonable Charges: The average cost of a specific medical procedure in an insured party's geographic area. This is the maximum amount some insurance companies will pay for certain covered expenses. They also are referred to as *allowed expenses* and reflect providers' retail costs for services.

USEFUL REFERENCES

Caprio K: Small Business Insurance Pools. Biztalk, 1996-1998, http://www.biztalk.com.

Carlson G: Managed Care: Understanding our Changing Health Care System. Community Decisions for Health, Managed Care, http://www.reeusda.gov.

Health Council of South Florida Consumer Guide, The Insurance Maze, http://www.med.miami,edu/HCFS.

Health Insurance Association of America, Guide to Health Insurance, April, 1997, http://www.hiaa.org.

Heller GB:*Penn Bar Assoc Quart* (July):93-116, 1998.

Insurance News Network: GAO Report: HIPAA Isn't Working. 1998.

Martin E: New Health Insurance Provisions Affect Small Business. Small Business Information, 1997, http://sbinformation.tqn.com.

NJ Health Pages:Your Guide to Managed Care, 1996-1997, http://www.nj.com/healthpages.

Palo Alto Medical Foundation: A Simple Guide to Health Insurance, http://204.162.243.22/hplans.

Taft J: Balance Quality, Services When Choosing Benefit Plans. *Austin Bus J* (Sept):1997.

Tie R: Filling the Gaps in Employer-Provided Insurance, Part 2, http://nestegg.iddis.com.

Value Design: Flexible Benefits Plan Design, Interactive Benefits Web, Frequently Asked Questions, 1998.

References

1. Disability Table A, *Transactions*, Society of Actuaries, 1985, Vol 37, p 449.

2. Hoban CM: Disability income insurance: Is your protecton adequate? *JAVMA* 215(2):155, 1999.

3. Brink S: HMOs were the right Rx: Americans got lower medical costs but also more worries. *U.S. World & News Report*, March 9, 1998.

4. Heller GB: *Penn Bar Assoc Quart* (July): *93-116, 1998.*

5. NJ Health Pages, *Your Guide to Managed Care*, http://www.nj.com/healthpages.

6. The National Committee for Quality Assurance can be contacted at (202) 955-3500, 2000 L Street NW, Ste, 500, Washington, DC 20036.

7. The American Accreditation Healthcare Commission can be reached at (202) 216-9010.

8. For information on the AVMA health coverage plans, readers are encouraged to contact (800) 621-6360.

9. Institute for Health Policy Solutions, 1444 I Street NW, Ste 900, Washington, DC, 10005; (202) 857-0810.

10. Martin E: New Health Insurance Provisions Affect Small Business, @Small Business Information, 1997, http://sbinformation.tqn.com

Chapter 6

LIFE INSURANCE

By Alan Fishman, CLU, CFP®

Most veterinary practice owners do not offer life insurance as a fringe benefit for their employees. However, some do and, in the event of their death or that of key employees, the insurance accommodates the orderly transition of practice ownership. Thus, it makes sense to include an analysis of life insurance here to allow for better financial planning for practice owners and employees who may wish to receive life insurance as part of their fringe benefit package.

Life insurance is a product designed more than 150 years ago to spread the financial risk associated with the loss of life among a large group of people. Despite its simple premise, the industry has become very complicated. Product portfolios have expanded to include many variations of the traditional term and permanent life insurance coverage.

Like the disability income industry, societal factors have contributed to these changes. The emergence of the two-wage-earning family and the fact that individuals are living longer into retirement than ever before have expanded the purposes for which today's life insurance products are purchased. A generation ago, people's major financial concern focused on dying too soon; today the concern also is in living too long to be able to support oneself adequately in retirement.

THE PARTIES TO A LIFE INSURANCE CONTRACT

Fundamental to the discussion of life insurance is an understanding of the definition of the parties involved in the contract. They are as follows:

- Applicants (or policy owners) are the individuals or entities applying for coverage.

- Insureds are the individuals being insured.

- Beneficiaries are the individuals or entities who receive the death benefit proceeds of the life insurance policies held on the insureds.

Though technically beneficiaries are not parties to life insurance contracts between insured parties and their insurance companies ("irrevocable" beneficiaries are the exception), declaring who the beneficiary of an insurance policy will be also is an important concept to master. The beneficiary can be an individual related to the insured party, a co-owner of a veterinary practice, the corporation or other entity that owns the practice, or an employee of the business. Two examples will help illustrate the roles above.

- Robert Saslow, DVM, applies for life insurance on his own life to provide needed income for his wife in the event of his death. Dr. Saslow is the owner of the policy and the insured; his wife, Sarah, is the beneficiary.

- Mary O'Donnell, DVM, a veterinary practice owner, applies for life insurance on Seth, the office manager and someone considered to be a key professional. Referred to as *key person coverage*, Dr. O'Donnell needs the coverage to reimburse the practice for lost revenues associated with Seth's management of the practice and the costs associated with locating, hiring, and training his replacement. In this example, the veterinary practice is the owner and the beneficiary; Seth, the office manager, is the insured.

TERM LIFE INSURANCE

All types of insurance coverage fall into one of two types: term life or permanent life. Term life insurance, as the name suggests, provides coverage for finite periods of time, or terms. It provides guaranteed death benefits in return for specified amounts of premiums paid for a stated number of years. In the early stages of most professionals' lives, term is the least expensive type of life insurance to purchase. Similar to auto or homeowners insurance policies, an insured party receives protection against loss for the term of the policy. If there is no claim under the policy, there is no benefit to be paid. At the end of the period for which coverage was provided, there are no refunds or payouts and, instead, all premiums paid will have been lost.

Some term plans renew annually, with premiums increasing each year, while others provide coverage for specified numbers of years, with premiums remaining level for the term of the contract. The different forms of term life insurance policies are annually renewable, decreasing term, and level term.

ANNUALLY RENEWABLE

With annually renewable term policies (also called *guaranteed renewable* and *yearly renewable*, premiums increase each year. In comparison to the other term policies listed below, annually renewable life insurance plans offer lower premiums in the initial years of the policies. This type may be suitable for individuals whose financial resources are limited or whose financial obligations are not permanent.

DECREASING TERM

With decreasing term insurance, premiums are level and coverage decreases with time. This type of insurance is suitable for financial obligations that reduce with time, like home mortgages and payments on the purchase of veterinary practices.

LEVEL TERM

This type of insurance offers level premiums for a stated number of years. Popular coverages include 5-, 10-, 15-, 20-, and 30-year level terms. Though premiums may be scheduled to remain level for a stated time period, they may not be guaranteed for the entire period (for example, a 20-year level policy may be guaranteed for all 20 years, or for only 5 years).

Level term policies are most suitable for situations in which coverage is needed for a predictable period of time. For example, a level term policy would be appropriate for a veterinary practice owner applying for a loan to expand a practice. Banks often will require that they obtain life insurance policies to protect their loans in the event the owners die prior to the time the loans are repaid. Since most practice loans are repaid over 10 years, the most appropriate coverage in this case would be a level term policy for 10 years.

REENTRY

With term insurance, companies often offer level rates for a certain period of time, after which insured parties need to requalify medically to continue their policies. Medical requalification is called *reentry* into the policy.

For example, a company offers level rates for 10 years and then permits insured parties to medically requalify for new rates in Years 11 through 20. By allowing the insured to requalify, or reenter, in Year 11, the insureds can attempt to qualify for lower rates thereafter. If the insured parties decide not to reenter, or they do not medically qualify for the lower rates, the original higher rates will prevail.

CONVERTIBILITY

Convertibility allows for the conversion of term policies into permanent life policies without requiring medical examinations or additional underwriting review by insurance companies. Some companies permit convertibility of level term policies during the level premium period only, i.e., a 15-year level term policy may be convertible for only 15 years. Other companies are more flexible and offer the convertibility feature to age 65 or later. Because convertibility is an important concept and one that is commonly used to differentiate policies, purchasers of life insurance need to understand its advantages when comparing costs and coverages for various policies offered by insurance agents.

PERMANENT LIFE INSURANCE

Permanent life insurance policies are designed to stay in force throughout an insured's entire life. To meet this objective, premiums generally are level throughout the life of the insured and, in the early years, are higher than those charged for term life insurance policies. Why the difference? Permanent life policies include two components: (1) a term cost for the "pure protection" provided by the death benefit and (2) a cash or policy value element. It is this cash value that differentiates the two types of policies. Moreover, it is the buildup of cash value over time that often keeps the coverage in force.

Life insurance has many tax benefits. Permanent life policy values grow tax advantaged and generally can be accessed by selecting several distribution options available to policy owners. If coordinated properly, policy values can be withdrawn with minimal tax consequences, since distributions are taxed on a first-in first out (FIFO) basis. In other words, distributions are treated as a return of capital until policy amounts withdrawn equal amounts of premiums contributed. Accumulated values withdrawn in excess of "basis" generally are treated as taxable income, unless policy owners choose to classify these distributions as loans. Determining the most advantageous way to withdraw policy values can be difficult, though, and should not be made without consulting a life insurance professional.

A description of whole life, universal life, variable universal life, and variable life insurance policies follows. Each enjoys the tax-advantaged features described previously. In reviewing the various forms, particular attention should be paid to the factors on which policy values are calculated and the different degrees of product guarantees.

WHOLE LIFE

Considered the most traditional form of permanent life insurance, whole life policies build cash value by investing portions of premiums collected in conservative vehicles like corporate bonds of intermediate-term maturities. Of all the types of permanent coverage, whole life has the strongest guarantees built into the contract. In return for paying the stated premium for the life of the contract, the policy owner is rewarded with a death benefit that is guaranteed for the life of the contract.

Cash values in a whole life contract include a guaranteed portion and a dividend portion. Though not guaranteed, a company's ability to meet originally projected or illustrated dividends is predicated on the company's management and minimization of mortality costs and operating expenses versus its gains from the performance of its investment portfolio.

One disadvantage of whole life insurance policies is the inflexibility of modifying premiums. Premiums can be "internally funded" only if sufficient cash values exist to do so. When this occurs, the policy's dividends can be applied against premiums due. However, unlike universal and variable universal policies, whole life premiums cannot be reduced during periods of favorable investment performance.

Universal Life

Universal life policies differ from whole life policies in that they separate the three elements common to all permanent policies, these being the pure cost of the protection (or term cost), the expense element (or the administrative costs associated with the policies), and the cash value. Separating these components allows for more flexibility in that policy owners can generally modify the policy face amount or adjust the premium in response to changing needs. Moreover, net premiums collected are invested in interest-sensitive vehicles so that investment returns can be more favorable in high interest rate environments or, conversely, unfavorable in low interest rate environments. There is generally an interest rate minimum or floor below which the contract will not earn a lower rate.

Since the investment risk is shifted in part to the policy's owner, premiums are somewhat lower than those seen with whole life policies. Although premiums can be lower, these policies offer fewer guarantees. A low interest rate environment for an extended period can require an increase in premium costs down the road. This was the case in the mid 1990s with universal life policies sold during the high interest environment of the eighties.

Variable Universal Life

Variable universal life insurance is similar to universal life, with one major exception. Unlike other types of permanent coverage, the policyowners direct where the net premiums are invested. These investments are referred to as *sub-accounts* and are similar to the mutual funds available from mutual fund families. In fact, the investment managers and objectives often are one and the same. The value of the account at death or retirement is based solely on the performance of the underlying investments. Like universal life policies, policyowners can modify the policy face amounts or adjust the premiums in response to changing needs. Unlike the other two types, there are fewer guarantees.

Variable Life

Variable life policies incorporate the strong features found in the whole life and the variable universal life policies summarized above. In return for minimum guaranteed death benefits, premium payments usually are level.

Hybrid Policies

In addition to the term and permanent types of coverage, many policies sold today are a combination of the two. Referred to as *hybrid policies*, these combine the benefits of whole life policies with those of term life policies. Individuals looking for strong guarantees at affordable costs may find these types of policies a better alternative than either whole or term policies.

SECOND-TO-DIE, OR SURVIVORSHIP POLICIES

Life insurance policies can be issued on one life or more. While most policies cover a single life, various forms of policies have been manufactured to meet particular niches and/or special needs. Second-to-die, or survivorship policies cover two lives and pay death benefits only after the second death. Two major advantages of this type of policy include lower premiums compared to two individual policies, and more liberal underwriting. This means that since insurance companies are obligated to pay death benefits only after the death of a second person, coverage usually can be secured in cases where one insured is not particularly healthy. Possible uses include the payment of estate taxes or to provide for key person coverage and practice buyouts.

Though large estates (couples whose net worth is above $1,300,000 in 1999 and $2 million in 2006) can be subject to taxes, the amount due is generally postponed until the death of the surviving spouse. Estate taxes can be as high as 55% of an individual's taxable estate and are due within nine months of death. Since many large estates may not have the necessary liquidity to pay these amounts, survivorship policies are beneficial because the proceeds are paid after the surviving spouse dies.

Survivorship policies also can be used to provide key person coverage. Consider this example:

Susan Thompson, DVM, has two professionals she considers important to the growth of the practice. Though she could absorb the loss of one of these individuals, the practice would suffer if both were to die. In this case, a survivorship policy could be used to reimburse the practice for lost revenue and expenses incurred to hire experienced veterinarians after the death of the second associate.

In addition, survivorship policies can be used to purchase practices, as illustrated in the following example.

Charlie and Sandy Koenig, DVMs, a couple from Louisiana, have owned a successful practice for over 20 years. Not far from retirement and concerned about the continuity of their practices, they have entered into an arrangement with an employee who has demonstrated the desire and talent to manage the practice. In this scenario, the dedicated employee is the owner and beneficiary of a survivorship policy on the lives of the Koenigs. When both owners die, the employee will have the funds necessary to buy the practice.

FIRST-TO-DIE, OR JOINT-LIFE POLICIES

First-to-die, or joint-life policies, cover two or more lives and pay death benefits after the first death. When insurance proceeds are most needed at the first death, premiums can be lower with a joint-life policy than with two individual policies. These policies can be most advantageously used for funding buy-sell arrangements, key person protection, and with working couples in need of insurance protection when the first spouse dies. A joint-life policy can be less expensive than two individual policies.

The joint-life (first-to-die) policy is appropriate in situations where liquidity is needed at the first death. In buy-sell arrangements between two equal partners, cash is needed for the surviving partner to buy out the deceased partner's interest in the practice. For key person protection, consider the following example.

Lloyd Meisels, DVM, employs two valuable associates he hopes will one day purchase his practice. Instead of obtaining policies on each to reimburse the practice for the cost to replace these professionals, he opts to secure one joint-life policy to guarantee that needed funds will be available at the time of either person's death.

Finally, the design of the joint-life policy may be appropriate for working couples who need to insure against the loss of either spouse.

Carol Reed, DVM, and Jim Reed, CPA, a Texan couple, each earn approximately the same salary and have determined their need for life insurance to be about the same. They have two children. They would like their insurance to offset the lost income of a deceased spouse and provide for the educational needs of their children. A joint-life policy may be less expensive than two individual policies, and it would ensure that the necessary money is available when the first spouse dies.

LIFE INSURANCE POLICY RIDERS

Though most life insurance contracts are reasonably similar, policy owners can tailor coverages to meet their needs by selecting from a variety of optional features, called *riders*. The most commonly offered riders are described below.

WAIVER OF PREMIUM

This rider waives premium payments during periods of disability. It is especially important for individuals who have no or inadequate disability income coverage.

ADDITIONAL INSURANCE

This rider permits additional increments of coverage to be purchased at specified times without requiring medical examinations or additional underwriting. It

may be especially important for concerned individuals whose families have a history of medical conditions.

ACCELERATED BENEFITS

A more recent addition to the menu of options, the accelerated benefits rider allows for an advance of a portion of the death benefit when the insured has a terminal illness or is required to stay in a nursing home. Many policies offer this rider without an extra charge.

ACCIDENTAL DEATH BENEFIT

For a nominal cost, the accidental death benefit rider doubles the policy face amount when the insured dies of accidental bodily injury.

POLICY SPLIT OPTION

The policy split option rider is used with survivorship policies. In the event of divorce or a tax law change favoring the need for policy proceeds to be paid at the first death rather than the second, this rider permits the separation of a joint life policy into two individual polices. Generally, the more competitive companies will offer this rider at no charge and require no medical underwriting.

EXCHANGE RIDER

This rider permits an exchange of permanent life insurance policies from one insured to another. It is most applicable with the key person coverages described below and is needed when valuable employees who leave practices are replaced with new valuable employees. This rider averts the need to surrender one policy and secure a second one on a new employee. By maintaining the same policy and changing only the name of the insured, policy values are not reduced a second time by acquisition costs and other expenses associated with the first year of a policy. However, underwriting acceptance of the second key employee is required.

ISSUES OF INSURABILITY

Similar to disability income, the underwriting of life insurance applications is the process of reviewing the appropriateness of particular risks, including but not limited to the following factors:

- Preexisting medical conditions

- Routine blood and urine test results

- Attending physician statements (APSs)

- Smoker status

- Height and weight

- Family medical history

- Occupation

- Hobbies: including racing, underwater and sky diving, hang gliding,

- piloting planes, mountain and rock climbing

- Alcohol or drug use

- Auto vehicle driving records

Unlike disability income coverages, life insurance pricing is more favorable for women than men. Since women live longer than men, the premiums for two identical 35-year-old individuals, one male and one female, would be lower for the female. Risk characterization for both sexes also may be treated differently among disability income and life applications.

With disability income coverages, companies offer standard rates to applicants with no medical conditions or modify the price and/or coverage in some way to accommodate for unfavorable risk. For life insurance, companies also can offer standard rates for applicants with no medical conditions, but for applicants with exceptional health, they may offer what is called *preferred rates*. Applicants considered unhealthy for any reason can be assessed

additional flat charges or rating increases (additional percentage cost increases), or they can be denied coverage. Although companies will offer different rates predicated on one's health, they generally do not modify coverages for life insurance applicants.

INDIVIDUAL APPLICATIONS FOR LIFE INSURANCE

The proceeds of one's life insurance can be used to pay off home mortgages, student loans, or credit card debts; fund college; or provide income for surviving spouses. To determine the amount of life insurance that is needed, agents should ask individuals about their personal and career goals, risk tolerance, and the extent to which liquidity may be needed to meet emergencies, opportunities, and other obligations. Referred to as *risk assessment*, this process incorporates a "needs analysis" type of approach.

The rule of thumb traditionally has been that young people need approximately five times their annual salaries in life insurance coverage. Like any rules of thumb, though, this oversimplified method has many drawbacks. A thorough needs analysis highlights the factors on which a more comprehensive determination is made.

Life insurance generally is purchased to address two needs: cash and income. Cash needs are the expenses associated with or presented upon the death of an individual. To determine the appropriate amount of coverage to satisfy the cash expenses, individuals should address the following issues:

- mortgage or rent - What is the remaining balance to be paid off on the residence? In the event of the death of a spouse, survivors may wish to live debt free in their homes. For renters, perhaps a 5- or 10-year reserve fund would be an appropriate safety net.

- debt liquidation - Though most federally guaranteed educational loans build the cost of life insurance into the loan repayment schedule, there may be other student loans, credit card debt, or other outstanding debts that need to be paid off in the event of a death.

- child and home care fund - If children are present, life insurance should provide funds sufficient for several years of day care and domestic services.

- educational fund - It is highly unlikely that surviving spouses will be able to fund the college education of all children without some type of supplemental income. Thus, when life insurance is being purchased, the number of children likely to attend college must be considered as well as the desires for them to attend community colleges, private or state universities, Ivy League schools, and/or graduate schools. Eligibility for scholarships or grants in aid also should be factored in.

- immediate money reserves - Expenses associated with death include medical, hospital, burial, probate, attorney's, and executor's fees. Depending on the state, inheritance or state death taxes may be due. For larger estates, i.e., those in excess of $650,000 for individuals and $1,300,000 for married couples in 1999 or $1.0 and $2.0 million, respectively, in 2006, federal estate taxes must be considered as well.

- emergency reserves - Surviving spouses may need money to deal with unexpected bills, medical emergencies, auto expenses, or home repairs. To avoid the payment of these costs from the surviving spouse's monthly income or savings, additional money derived from life insurance can help.

After careful consideration of the cash needs above, the next step is to determine the income needs for the surviving spouses. During this process the following questions are addressed:

- What amount of money is needed for the family to maintain its current lifestyle?

- How much of the lost household income will need to be replaced?

- If the surviving spouse did not work outside the home, will he or she wish to or be able to return to the workforce? In what capacity and at what salary?

- If the surviving spouse did work, will that party wish to or be able to continue to work? Because of the ages of the children, would it be better if the surviving spouse did not have to work outside the home?

- To what extent will social security contribute? Generally speaking, children under the age of 18 will receive support from Social Security.

Once again, some examples will help illustrate this planning process.

Rob earns $70,000 as a veterinarian and his wife, Jill, earns $50,000 as a controller for a local hardware store. Together, their annual household income equals $120,000. Assuming Rob were to die, Jill probably would not need the entire $120,000. Instead, based on a study by the Bureau of Labor Statistics, she would need about 70% of their combined incomes, or $84,000. If support from social security for the couple's three- and six-year-old daughters amounted to approximately $12,000 each year, Jill would have an annual shortfall of about $22,000 ($84,000 less her salary of $50,000, assuming she continued to work, and less the social security payments of $12,000).

This annual shortfall, or additional income needed, can be replaced by life insurance. How much should be earmarked for this shortfall? What is a reasonable rate of return? If we assume an 8% annual return, Rob would need approximately $275,000 of life insurance to replace the $22,000

($22,000/.08). This assumes that Rob wants the shortfall to be replaced with earnings only and wishes to leave the principal intact.

The above example illustrates the need to secure $275,000 of life insurance to cover income needs. Let us assume Rob and Jill calculated their cash needs at Rob's death to be as follows:

- retire home mortgage: $150,000
- pay off student loans: $30,000
- provide for child care: $80,000
- initiate an educational fund: $50,000
- establish an immediate money fund: $20,000
- build an emergency fund: $35,000

The cash needs above equal $365,000. Combined with the predetermined income need of $275,000, the total need for life insurance comes to $640,000.

While this method certainly is more comprehensive than the five times salary rule of thumb mentioned earlier, it is not without its drawbacks. Certain components of cash needs and income needs were approximations, e.g., college costs and child care. Furthermore, the current value of money to be used to meet expenses at some future date was not taken into account. Computer calculations are essential for a more comprehensive method of identifying life insurance needs. Competent and contemporary life insurance agents have access to software packages that can be used to customize appropriate amounts of death benefits to the needs and desires of each client.

SPOUSAL INSURANCE AND INHERITANCE EQUALIZATION

Two other individual applications of life insurance include spousal insurance and inheritance equalization. Spousal insurance generally is purchased for spouses who work in the home. A brief description of this concept was addressed previously when cash needs were discussed. In addition to providing child care, spouses who work in the home contribute significantly to the costs of maintaining the home. Wage-earning surviving spouses will need to replace these services and can do so by purchasing sufficient insurance on these spouses to cover expenses associated with child care and household cleaning and cooking services.

Inheritance equalization is an issue in some situations and may be considered in cases like the following:

Richard Drumm, DVM, and his wife, Karen, have a net worth of approximately $900,000. Their estate consists of the following: a home worth $250,000, a veterinary practice worth about $500,000, and investments valued at approximately $150,000. They have two children, Danielle and Lauren. Danielle is studying to be a veterinarian and is in her last year of a residency program. She looks forward to joining dad's practice. Lauren is graduating soon from college and is interested in becoming a teacher.

Richard and Karen have met with an estate attorney and are planning the disposition of their assets when they die. Richard is particularly concerned with future ownership and management of the practice. Cash flow shortcomings may prevent him from paying Danielle the salary she may command with her specialty working in another larger practice. Therefore, he is uncomfortable having her buy the practice when he is ready to retire. Furthermore, she has no interest nor aptitude for management.

Herein lies a bigger problem. Since the veterinary practice represents a large portion of their estate, if Danielle inherited the practice, the balance of the estate would not represent an equal portion for Lauren. The answer to this dilemma? Richard can purchase insurance on himself to cover the shortfall so that Danielle inherits the practice and Lauren receives her equal share of the estate with cash from the life insurance.

Business Applications for Life Insurance

There are many business applications for life insurance. Though the details are not within the scope of this book, insured professionals need to appreciate their importance in the area of benefits. To that end, group insurance coverage, funding for buy sell agreements, deferred compensation plans, key person coverages, and the concepts of split dollar and reverse split dollar are discussed herein.

Group Coverage

Like group disability coverage, group life insurance offers an affordable means of providing coverage for practices of all sizes. For larger practices, particularly those with more than 10 employees, liberal underwriting of applicants often is another benefit. So long as coverages do not exceed certain levels, physical examinations are not needed and requested medical history is minimal.

Group life coverages cannot discriminate in favor of a selected few parties within a business. All eligible employees, generally those who work a minimum of 30 hours/week, must be included. While there is little flexibility as to who must be covered, there is some flexibility in plan design. The following three methods highlight the differences on which coverages can be based:

1. fixed amount: This places all employees, regardless of position, in the same category. A practice that offers $15,000 of coverage for each employee is an example of this method.
2. percentage of compensation: The most common of the three methods, percentage of compensation bases the amount of coverage on a multiple of employee compensation. Since it is tied to salary, it rewards the employees who are more

highly paid and presumably the most responsible for the success of the practice. A practice that offers two times salary would be an example of this method. To limit the exposure of coverages offered and minimize the cost, a maximum may be included, e.g., two times salary to a maximum of $100,000.
3. by position: This method bases its coverage amount on the position of the employee. Practices that offer $50,000 to veterinarians, $25,000 to technicians, and $15,000 for clerical support exemplify this method.

To prevent practices from setting up schedules of coverages by position that discriminate against lower-paid employees, as set forth in the third method above, there are two restrictions. First, the amount of coverage in any one position can be no greater than 2.5 times the amount of coverage in the next lowest position. And second, the amount of coverage for the lowest position can be no less than 10% of the amount of coverage in the top position. There also must be a reasonable expectation that each position will include more than one employee.

Table 6.1 highlights these restrictions. In this table, Plan A is unacceptable for two reasons. First of all, the technicians cannot be provided with coverage 2.5 times less than the amount offered the veterinarians ($40,000 represents the minimum acceptable coverage for the technicians). Secondly, clerical employees cannot be offered coverages lower than 10% of those offered the veterinarians ($10,000 represents the minimum acceptable coverage for the clerical positions). Plan B is acceptable.

Before concluding discussion on group life insurance coverage, some comment on taxation is warranted. Generally speaking, the cost to provide the first $50,000 of coverage is tax deductible to the employer and not taxed to the employee. Assuming the benefit is paid entirely by the employer, the cost of the insurance above this amount becomes taxable income to the employee.

Table 6.1. Amounts of Coverage

Job Position	Plan A	Plan B
Veterinarian	$100,000	$100,000
Veterinary Technician	$ 35,000	$ 40,000
Veterinary Assistant	$ 25,000	$ 25,000
Clerical	$ 5,000	$ 10,000

FUNDING FOR BUY-SELL AGREEMENTS

Veterinary practices generally are considered small, closely held businesses. In most cases, practices contain two assets; the ongoing value of the business, i.e., the practice, and the real estate. The primary asset of the practice is the goodwill attributed to (1) the professional(s) who operate and manage it and (2) the business's name, location, and reputation, also known as the "blue sky" or intangible asset value. The equipment, instruments, furnishings, drug inventory, and other tangible assets constitute a lesser percentage of the practice's value.

Because so much of a practice's value is attributable to its intangible assets, particularly the name, management, and drawing power of the owner, it can be difficult to sell in the event of death. When coowners are involved, the prospect of practice continuation following the death of one party can be planned. Such agreements are legal documents among coowners that identify the responsibilities each assumes in the event of death, disability, retirement, or termination. Here, the concern is with the death of a coowner and the liquidity needed to buy out the deceased owner's share of the practice.

Ray Sprowl, DVM and Jill Smith, VMD are equal partners in a small animal clinic in Santa Monica, CA. The practice has been valued at approximately $1,000,000. They have retained the services of an attorney to draft a buy-sell agreement. The agreement obligates Ray to buy out Jill's husband in the event of Jill's death and obligates Jill to buy out Ray's wife in the event of Ray's death. The buy-sell agreement has provided a market for the deceased partner's share of the practice and, assuming the needed liquidity is available, will assure the continuation of the practice for the surviving partner. To accommodate the needed liquidity, each partner obtains a $500,000 life insurance policy on the life of the other partner.

To illustrate this example, Ray is the owner and beneficiary of a policy on Jill and vice versa. In the event of Jill's death, Ray will receive the $500,000. He is then obligated, pursuant to the buy-sell agreement, to use this money to buy out Jill's share of the practice. Ray is now the 100% owner of the practice and Jill's husband has received the agreed-upon value for her share of the practice.

The policies in the above example were owned by the veterinarians. This type of arrangement is known as *cross-purchase* life insurance. While there are other types of buy-out arrangements, like *entity purchases* or *wait and see*, consultations with accountants and attorneys specializing in these matters can identify which scenario is best. Veterinarians need only understand the importance of coordinating the benefits of well-drafted buy-sell agreements with life insurance, and the dangerous implications of one without the other.

Funding for Nonqualified Deferred Compensation Plans

Retirement plans are one way to defer income. Though employers need to comply with strict Employee Retirement Income Security Act (ERISA) and Internal Revenue Service guidelines, these plans enjoy the benefits of being IRS-qualified programs. By adhering to predetermined eligibility rules, vesting requirements, funding limitations, and periodic filing deadlines, employers receive tax deductions and employees receive tax-deferred growth on the contributions. With continuing tax law changes that limit the extent to which owners can benefit from these qualified plans, successful veterinarians may look for alternatives or supplemental types of plans.

Nonqualified deferred compensation plans permit business owners or key employees to postpone receipt of a portion of income until some later date. In essence, this is an unsecured promise by a practice to pay a benefit to an owner or key employee in the future. Compared to the qualified types of plans, these nonqualified programs are less regulated and permit veterinarian-owners to discriminate in selecting who participates and the extent to which each participant benefits. Nonqualified plans do not impose funding, vesting, or participation requirements.

Unlike qualified plans, the contributions made by employers to deferred compensation programs are not deductible. However, the benefit to the recipients is that the deferred income provided through this vehicle is not taxed until retirement, when presumably they are likely to be in lower marginal tax brackets. In its true form, deferred compensation is an employee-motivated program, i.e., it is the employees who voluntarily decide to defer portions of their salaries they otherwise would receive today so that those earnings are received when they are in lower tax brackets later.

Another form of deferred compensation known as a supplemental executive retirement plan, SERP, is one which is employer motivated. In this case, it is the employer who decides to provide supplemental retirement benefits in addition to salary or an existing pension program.

Although deferred compensation represents an unsecured promise to pay a future benefit, practices generally attempt to fund such programs on an ongoing basis and do not wait until retirement to satisfy the financial obligations from working capital. To ensure sufficient funds are set aside, vehicles such as mutual funds and life insurance can be used. The latter choice is common.

Life insurance is a unique product that offers tax-deferred accumulation of wealth and death benefit protection. When it is offered as a benefit, for example, veterinarian-owners can provide key employees with supplemental income by accessing policy cash values in retirement or by providing an employee's spouse with preretirement death benefits in the event the key employee dies prior to retirement. Additionally, a waiver of premium rider can ensure continued funding in the event employees are unable to return to work because of a disability.

Amounts contributed to deferred compensation programs can be determined in several ways:

- based on a flat amount where the practice contributes $5,000 a year for an employee;

- by basing it on a percentage of salary, i.e., the practice contributes 10% of the employee's salary; or

- by defining the benefit at retirement, i.e., the employee receives $50,000 a year at age 65 for a period of 10 years.

The chosen methodology is generally spelled out in the deferred compensation agreement, a document that includes the employer's promise to pay, the employee's responsibilities, and a vesting schedule that governs what portion of contributed amount vests with the employee and/or the length of employment needed before the employee is entitled to receive the contributions. Veterinary owners can offer deferred compensation programs to two employees and provide for different contribution formulas and vesting schedules.

With many common arrangements, contributed amounts generally are owned by the business and therefore are subject to claims by creditors in bankruptcy or subject to termination by new owners. On the other hand, trusts may be used to segregate and protect assets from attack by new owners. Since the design and funding of deferred compensation programs are extremely complex, professionals are encouraged to seek counsel from attorneys specializing in these matters. An example situation follows.

> Richard Cohen, DVM, has an interest in saving for retirement but understands that he would need to contribute for all other employees if he implemented an IRS-qualified retirement plan. Total salaries for the practice equal $300,000; Dr. Cohen's salary is $100,000. The maximum he can contribute to a traditional profit sharing plan is $45,000. His portion of the contribution, $15,000, represents only 33% of the entire contribution. His true cost to implement this qualified plan is as follows:

Total contributions	$45,000
Less taxes saved (assuming a 31% tax bracket)	$13,950
Net contribution	$31,050
Less Dr. Cohen's contribution	$15,000
Net cost to Dr. Cohen	$16,050

In this example, $16,050 is the cost to implement a qualified plan. An alternative is the nonqualified deferred compensation program. Though there is no deduction for amounts contributed, a $15,000 contribu-

tion to a SERP would be less expensive than the $16,050 cost of the qualified retirement plan. In addition, the nonqualified deferred compensation program requires minimal administrative costs and imposes fewer rules regarding eligibility, vesting, and contribution limits than traditional IRS qualified profit sharing plans.

KEY PERSON INSURANCE

The importance of key person insurance coverage, as described earlier, cannot be understated. Successful veterinary practice owners all hesitate to open their doors without adequate property and casualty insurance covering fire, wind, water, theft, and professional liability insurance. Like many small businesses, the practice's success often can be attributed to one or two key employees.

The effects of the death of a key employee can be devastating. Financial institutions that have provided credit may become concerned, clients may lose confidence, and other employees, perhaps other key employees, may seek employment elsewhere or fear for the future.

Key person coverage cannot replace valuable employees. It can, however, protect against the loss of income and provide the time necessary to find, hire, and train the best candidate. How much coverage is needed? While it is difficult to place a value on a key person, the practice's CPA and insurance agent should address the following issues in determining the most appropriate amount of coverage:

- How much does the key person contribute to the profits of the practice?

- How much would that employee's loss cost the practice?

- How long will it take to find a replacement?

- How much will it cost to train this individual?

Split Dollar Coverage

Split dollar coverage is not a type of life insurance. Rather, it is a technique for sharing the benefits (cash values and death benefits) versus the costs (ownership and premiums) of permanent life insurance policy between two parties. These parties generally include individuals in need of life insurance and individuals or entities with the financial capacity to purchase the coverage. Given as an employee benefit, split dollar coverage can be used to attract and retain young professionals who may not be able to afford the premiums.

In the most common split dollar coverage scenario, employers pay all or a portion of the life insurance premium, and key employees receive the coverage with only minimal expense. Though the premiums paid by the practice can be substantial, employers can be reimbursed in the future for these payments by tapping into the cash value in the policies and/or agreeing on a predetermined split of the death benefit. Ownership agreements include the following:

- collateral assignments: Employees own the policies but "rent" or assign ownership privileges to employers, usually in amounts equal to the outlay of premium payments.

- endorsements: Employers own the policies on the lives of key employees with endorsements added that address the split of ownership. That is, employers "rent" the death benefit component to the employee.

A variation of the split dollar coverage is the reverse split dollar, in which the traditional roles presented above are reversed. With reverse split dollar coverage, it is the practice that wishes to obtain the life insurance coverage on a key employee. When coupled with the provision of a supplemental retirement income for the same employee, reverse split dollar can provide an attractive benefit. The employee controls the cash value, and the employer receives the death benefit.

Recent rulings by the IRS have affected the tax aspects of split dollar, and therefore life insurance professionals and attorneys specializing in these matters should be sought in reviewing the many variations that exist and in determining whether these programs provide the stated benefits.

Choosing the Right Company

A life insurance policy is only as good as the company that issues it. Of the approximately 1,225 life insurance companies in operation today, there have been relatively few financial failures. The fact that these recent failures involved several well-known companies, though, makes the selection process more important. To identify the right company, people seeking insurance need to consider company ratings, company type, licensing issues, investment strength, illustration integrity (whether their financial projections are reasonable), and miscellaneous financial factors including lapse ratios, expense ratios, and 10-year dividend comparisons.

Of the factors listed above, ratings are certainly the easiest to obtain. A.M. Best, a long-time, objective observer of the life insurance industry, rates companies for financial strength by using letter grades. Other rating services, like Standard and Poors, Moody's Investor Services, and Duff and Phelps, provide similar measures of financial strength. And, while company ratings are important, purchasers of life insurance need not become overly concerned with minor differences when comparing companies. Consider these comments from *Best Week 5/94*:

We believe, based on factual analysis, that insurers rated B+ and above maintain secure financial strength and shouldn't be competitively disadvantaged to a point where they are automatically selected against or excluded from consideration.

Rating organizations rate only the financial strength or claims-paying ability of the insurance entity. Though this is important, a top rating does not necessarily mean top policy performance and/or policyholder satisfaction. A few companies have boasted top ratings in the past when they were taken over by state regulators shortly thereafter. A thorough review of company ratings is a good starting point, but it should not be the final determinant.

TYPES OF LIFE INSURANCE COMPANIES

The two main types of life insurance companies are mutual and stock. Stock companies have always outnumbered mutual companies (fewer than 100 of the approximate 1,225 life insurance companies are mutual); but until recently, mutual companies represented the largest percentage of assets. Then, several large well known mutual companies changed to stock ownership and stock companies now account for close to 84% of all assets.

Mutual companies are owned by their policyholders and have a fiduciary responsibility to treat all policyholders fairly. Since policyholders are owners of the company, they share in the profits (by receiving dividends on their policies). Stock companies, in contrast, are owned by their shareholders. Their primary objective is to increase stockholder values.

The percentage of company profits returned and the parties to whom they are returned can represent important differences between company types. Most mutual companies adhere to a concept referred to as the *contribution principle*, which splits profits among policyholders in the same proportion as premiums paid on the policies contributed to that profit. This method of equitable distribution prevents one policyholder or group of policyholders from subsidizing another group.

Many stock companies are owned by parent holding companies. In reviewing the financial strength of stock companies, individuals should analyze the flow of funds between these entities. A recent A.M. Best Report is helpful. It reviews how much money the parent has invested in the stock company, what volumes of dividends have been returned to the parent, and whether stockholder dividends have been paid in excess of company profitability.

Licensing is another important factor governing the activities of insurers. Each state creates its own rules and monitors companies licensed within its boundaries. And, while the National Association of Insurance Commissioners (NAIC) would like to establish minimum standards for all states, some state insurance departments are stronger than others. New York, for example, is considered the most demanding and most aggressive state in which to conduct business. Moreover, some of their regulations are considered extraterritorial, requiring companies that do business in New York to satisfy those particular regulations in every other state in which the company operates. It is because of these burdensome extraterritorial rules that many companies decide to bypass the New York marketplace. In fact, only about 11% of all companies are licensed to do business in the state of New York. Because of the state's regulatory strengths, individuals who seek additional levels of company financial strength and scrutiny may wish to restrict their search to those companies licensed in New York.

In the eighties, some insurance companies were hurt by investing heavily in junk bonds (debt instruments issued by companies of questionable strength that pay relatively high interest). Others were hurt by poor investments in real estate. As a result, financial strength is an important factor to consider when selecting an insurance company. It pays to ask the right questions, such as

- How much of the company's investment assets are in noninvestment grade, or junk bonds?

- What percentage of the investment portfolio is in the stock market?, and

- Are any real estate mortgages in the investment portfolio?

If the answer to any of these questions is yes, what percentages of the investments are delinquent or in default? Other financial measures that need to be addressed include

- lapse ratio: the percentage of total policies that lapse, or cancel. This is considered a measure of policy strength. The lower the better.

- expense ratio: the percentage of company expenses to total revenue. This is considered a measure of profitability. Again, the lower the better.

- 10-year dividend comparisons: a comparison of dividends paid against dividends illustrated (projected) over a 10-year period. Considered a measure of illustration integrity, this reflects company profitability. Here, higher is better.

When selecting a mutual fund or stock in which to invest, investors should review past performance in the form of annual returns for one, three, and five years before investing. With life insurance, the decision is often predicated on future performance. This information is generally found in company illustrations and computer printouts which project how policies may perform given a set of variables, including interest rates and dividends, neither of which are guaranteed. With increased product complexity and performance based more on the financial markets than guarantees, illustrations may be less dependable in predicting future performance. In 1996, the NAIC developed a new model regulation on sales illustrations to address this concern. The purpose was "to provide rules for life insurance policy illustrations that will protect consumers and foster consumer education."

Included in this model is a requirement, for example, that agents' and applicants' signatures accompany each illustration used to sell a policy.

As of 1/1/2002, 37 states have adopted the model regulation in whole or in part, and it is expected that the remaining states will follow suit in the next several years.

Many policies are sold today by spread sheeting the numbers and selecting the lowest premium. In the words of Aristotle, "People prefer an attractive impossibility to a less attractive probability." With new legislation and a better understanding of the factors used to generate illustrations, companies are on a more level playing field and consumers are better equipped to make the right decision.

CHOOSING BETWEEN TERM AND PERMANENT LIFE INSURANCE

Applicants need to consider all parts of their personal equations in choosing between term and permanent life insurance. To start, for example, over what period is the coverage needed? Logically, one would assume that temporary needs in the form of loans, key person coverages, and children's needs might best be protected with term insurance. Meanwhile, permanent needs such as supporting a spouse and/or family, and estate and inheritance taxes might best be protected with permanent insurance. With the assistance of good insurance advisors, applicants must match the products with the needs. Some examples follow.

- Jill has secured a 10-year loan with the local bank to start a veterinary practice. To protect the bank's interest, the loan officer has asked Jill to purchase life insurance. The logical choice? Ten-year level term insurance.

- Bob's wife, Karen, works at home and is busy raising their three children. The youngest child is six. Concerned with the impact his wife's premature death would have on the children, Bob would like to protect the family for a period of about 15 years. It is at the end of this period that the youngest child is likely to graduate from college and no longer be a dependent. Again, the logical choice is term insurance—probably 15-year level term insurance.

In these cases, the period for which the coverage was needed was easy to establish. Unfortunately, the decision can be more difficult than this. Say two people get married and have a child at the age of 35. Assume the husband earns $80,000 and the wife works part time and earns $18,000. The life insurance professional determines the need for coverage on the husband is approximately $400,000. As discussed earlier, there are two needs typically addressed with the purchase of life insurance:

- cash needs: to pay off the mortgage, cover tuition costs for the children, and satisfy other costs, and

- income needs: to replace the higher wage earner's salary and maintain the lifestyle to which the family has grown accustomed.

The cash needs portion generally can be satisfied with term insurance, since these obligations will decrease with time. On the other hand, the income needs portion will generally increase with time because as incomes increase, peoples' lifestyles become more expensive. It is this need that may best be solved with permanent insurance. Determining the proper mix of permanent and term insurance can be addressed only when the objectives and all of the necessary facts are considered.

In addition to solving temporary needs, term insurance is the right choice in situations where cash flow is tight. While the term-versus-permanent decision is important, it must not supersede the more critical issue, i.e., determining the proper amount of coverage. If after determining the proper amount of coverage, individuals cannot afford the premiums for permanent coverage, term insurance is the logical choice. Most term products permit conversion from term to permanent insurance at some future point without the need for medical evaluations of applicants.

A caveat relating to the popularity of 20-year level term insurance needs to be mentioned. As its popularity has grown, so too has its misapplication. Individuals need to be careful when solving permanent needs with this product.

In many cases, the 20-year level term product is purchased only to protect a family's cash needs addressed earlier. Rarely, the objective is to convert it to some form of permanent life insurance. In 20 years an insured's mortgage may be nearly paid off and the children no longer dependent on mom and dad. If only the needs brought about by a death are addressed, the family may be left without life insurance at the wrong time. Because of this, additional questions to be asked include:

- What will the 35-year-old breadwinner be doing 20 years from the inception date of the policy?

- At age 55 will the insured's mortgage payment be high or low?

- Will the family's children have graduated from college?

- Will insurance be needed to provide income for a surviving spouse?

- Will funds be needed for graduate school or weddings?

At best, the 20-year level term product is an inexpensive way to provide coverage for 20 years. However, by underestimating the period over which coverage is needed, policies may be dropped short of their intended purpose. Unless individuals can state with unwavering certainty that their needs for life insurance will end in 20 years, deciding between term and permanent insurance can be a complex decision. Practitioners must understand these concepts and, with the help of insurance professionals, select the coverage or combination of coverages most appropriate for their situations.

LIFE INSURANCE AS AN INVESTMENT

Permanent life insurance offers many benefits. Aside from the permanent coverage it offers, the cash accumulation can be an advantage. As discussed earlier, the cash value receives tax-advantaged status inside a life insurance contract. These tax-advantaged features include tax-deferred growth on the cash buildup and tax-favored treatment on distributions from the policy when the insured party retires.

Recognizing the benefits these contracts offer, there are laws which limit the amounts that can be contributed to policies. If contributed amounts exceed this threshold, policies will be considered investments, and withdrawals no longer will receive tax-advantaged treatment. While many have argued that the 6% to 8% return on investment expected with a traditional whole life policy may not be competitive compared to the recent double-digit returns of the stock market, more risk-tolerant individuals can choose the variable universal life insurance policy. With this product, the cash values can be invested in separate accounts similar to mutual funds, allowing for opportunities to earn more competitive returns. The issue here is not the product, but rather the application of the product which will determine its viability as a competitive investment.

There are many costs included in life insurance policies including the cost of insurance, sales commissions, and other expenses, particularly in the first year. To maximize the cash accumulation component in the policy, individuals should maintain long-term objectives and be willing to own the policies as they would any other investment for retirement. In addition, the following conditions need to be addressed in determining whether life insurance fits a particular situation:

- Individuals should take advantage of all tax-deductible retirement vehicles first.

- They should be in a relatively high tax bracket.

- Participants should have a death benefit need.

- They should be in good health.

Because contributions made to retirement programs such as 401(k)s, IRAs, and pension plans have tax deductions up front, the best place to start when saving for retirement is with these plans. These deductions and the tax-deferred growth these programs offer usually will generate larger balances than life insurance at retirement. Therefore, life insurance should not be used as an investment vehicle unless these tax-deductible programs have been exhausted first. As with any vehicle offering tax-deferred growth, individuals in higher tax brackets will benefit most. Insurance applicants should not consider life insurance as an investment if they are in the lowest tax brackets.

In addressing the benefits of life insurance as an investment, it must be remembered that the cost of insurance included in the premium can be major. Thus, if no death benefit needs exist, applicants may wish to consider other tax-advantaged investment vehicles such as annuities rather than life insurance.

Additionally, veterinary professionals should not consider life insurance for investment purposes if they are in poor health. Unless individuals can qualify for standard or preferred health, the high cost of insurance will allow little growth of the investment component.

SELECTING AN AGENT

As with disability insurance, discussed earlier, technical competence, objectivity, and interpersonal chemistry all are important in selecting an agent. Beyond that, the following points are worth consideration:

Is the agent well versed in the variety and uses of products available in the marketplace today?

- Does the agent keep abreast of current insurance, tax law, estate planning, and business issues?

- Will the agent take a macro or micro look at an individual's financial picture?

Some agents have an expertise in only one area of the financial service profession; others are multidimensional in scope and capable of addressing the client's financial planning objectives as well. Is the agent in the business of selling products or providing solutions to problems? The latter may place a greater emphasis on planning and will be more likely to address an individual's concerns. Professionals looking for competent counsel may restrict their search to agents who are CLUs and/or ChFCs, acronyms for Chartered Life Underwriters and Chartered Financial Consultants. These designations are awarded to agents with a demonstrated expertise in the area of life insurance and financial planning.

As with disability income policies, agents may recommend that existing life insurance policies be replaced. The practice is fairly common with term policies, since competition among insurance companies has brought premiums for this type of coverage down in recent years. With permanent life policies, though, the benefits from replacements are limited. There are new sales loads and expenses with a new policy, much of which has been paid with the existing policy. There also may be surrender costs in transferring cash values from one policy to another. To determine the appropriateness of a replacement, the Society of Financial Service Professionals has developed a policy replacement evaluation form known as the *Replacement Questionnaire* (RQ). If an agent suggests replacing a permanent policy, be sure the insurance professional has completed this form and that its conclusion justifies the recommended action.

FINAL THOUGHTS

Most people understand the benefits of life insurance in their personal lives. Its unique characteristics and many assets also can make it a tremendous benefit to offer in the workplace. Thus, practice owners and associates should appreciate the multidimensional utility and leverage of life insurance in a variety of situations and applications before making investments in life insurance or discarding options for this type of financial planning.

Chapter 7

ANCILLARY EMPLOYMENT BENEFITS

By Jeffrey D. Nemoy, DVM, JD and James F. Wilson, DVM, JD

Ancillary benefits are an integral part of any employment package. While salary is paramount, benefits offered can carry enormous weight in terms of how potential employers are perceived and in terms of whether or not a job is ultimately desirable. Table 7.1 analyzes the frequency with which the various benefits were offered in the authors' study of 225 contracts.

Verbal agreements alone regarding ancillary benefits are subject to misinterpretation, change over time and, ultimately, problems between employers and employees. Employees may not fully realize their responsibilities related to receipt of benefits. Detailed descriptions of all employment benefits therefore should be clearly written into employment contracts. Specific language should be used to avoid any misunderstandings that could lead to problems. To assure compliance with local laws, employers are advised to have local legal counsel review the sample contract clauses herein before including them in their own veterinary agreements.

This chapter describes a wide variety of ancillary benefits, most of which would be offered to associates, but some of which might also be applicable to support staff. Those covered include

- professional association dues
- professional licensing fees
- DEA registration fees
- employee pet care plans
- pet health insurance
- travel and moving allowances
- speaking engagements
- uniform allowances
- use of automobiles
- health club memberships
- child care
- housing allowances
- loans for new employees

PROFESSIONAL ASSOCIATION DUES

Employers need to weigh the value of veterinary association memberships when deciding whether or not to pay associates' dues. Numerous benefits offered by national, state, and local veterinary medical associations are often unrecognized by practice owners and associates. The multitude of benefits offered by the American Veterinary

Table 7.1. Veterinarians Offered Ancillary Benefits in a Study of 225 Employment Contracts*

Benefits	All (%)	Male** (%)		Female** (%)		Sm. Animal (%)		Equine (%)		Lrg. Animal (%)		Mixed (%)	
National association dues	60.6	63.9	53/83	58.5	76/130	65.0	106/164	50.0	6/12	38.5	5/13	45.8	11/24
State association dues	52.0	54.2	45/83	50.0	65/130	59.2	97/164	25.0	3/12	23.0	3/13	37.5	9/24
Local association dues	38.7	38.6	32/83	36.9	48/130	44.5	73/164	8.3	1/12	15.4	2/13	29.2	7/24
Professional license fees	28.1	30.5	25/82	26.9	35/130	25.6	42/164	58.3	7/12	30.8	4/13	17.4	4/23
DEA registration dues	15.1	15.7	13/83	14.6	19/130	16.5	27/164	8.3	1/12	15.4	2/13	16.7	4/24
Employee pet care plans	12.0	8.4	7/83	13.9	18/130	13.4	22/164	0	0	7.7	1/13	16.7	4/24
Moving allowances	4.4	8.4	7/83	2.3	3/130	3.7	6/164	0	0	0	0	8.3	2/24
Uniform allowances	8.0	7.2	6/83	7.7	10/130	9.2	15/164	0	0	7.7	1/13	8.3	2/24
Health club memberships	0	0	0	0	0	0	0	0	0	0	0	0	0
Child care	0.4	0	0	0	0	0	0	0	0	0	0	0	0
Housing allowances	0.9	0	0	1.5	2/130	0.6	1/164	0	0	0	0	4.2	1/24
Loans for new employees	0.4	1.2	1/83	0.8	1/130	1.2	2/164	0	0	0	0	0	0

* This study included 225 employment contracts in the U.S., the oldest of which was signed in 1987, the newest of which was signed in 1998 and most of which were written between 1995 and 1998.[1]

** Since some contracts were not identifiable by gender, the number of male and female contracts does not add up to 225.

Medical Association, the American Animal Hospital Association, and the California Veterinary Medical Association (as representative of a state organization) are described below.

Practice owners and associates should address the following issues to determine which organization(s) provide the most value: (1) the educational needs of the practice owner, associates, and support staff; (2) the career goals and interests of the owners and employees over the next 5 to 10 years; (3) the benefits offered by various associations; (4) the costs incurred for individual and, perhaps, multi-doctor memberships; (5) the importance of the political activism and clout of the association; and (6) whether benefits offered by the association merit the costs of membership.

THE AMERICAN VETERINARY MEDICAL ASSOCIATION

Power in numbers is the force that the members of the American Veterinary Medi-cal Association (AVMA) use to access the corporate rates and services of companies. The many services provided to members lend tremendous value to AVMA membership. These include

- AVMA Membership Directory and Resource Manual
- *The Journal of the American Veterinary Medical Association* or *The Journal of Veterinary Research*
- AVMA group health and life insurance trust
- AVMA professional liability insurance trust
- AVMA worker's compensation insurance
- discount on Sprint long distance rates for business and residential telephones
- AVMA gold Mastercard, which has no annual fee and a fixed rate
- Allied Van Lines, North American Van Lines, and Mayflower Transit discount prices for interstate moves

- Budget and Alamo corporate vehicle rental rates

- a placement service for job seekers and job suppliers

- career counseling

- a relief veterinarian registry

- free and/or reduced dues to new graduates, interns, residents, and graduate students

- discounts to the Network of Animal Health (NOAH)

- access to the AVMA library located at the headquarters in Schaumburg, Illinois

- access to the AVMA Foundation, which supports veterinary medical research and disperses the revolving student loan fund of the Auxiliary to the AVMA and the Disaster Relief Emergency Fund

For the costs of AVMA memberships or more information about the services offered, call AVMA Member Services at 1-800-248-2862 extensions 237 or 238; or write to AVMA Member Services, 1931 N. Meacham Road, Suite 100, Schaumburg, IL 60173. On the Internet, the AVMA web site address is http://www.avma.org.

THE AMERICAN ANIMAL HOSPITAL ASSOCIATION

Since 1933, the American Animal Hospital Association (AAHA) has provided members with resources to ensure continued professional growth. AAHA offers three types of memberships, which include (1) hospital memberships—practices that meet AAHA standards are eligible for membership, and associate veterinarians at these practices can hold individual memberships; (2) affiliate memberships—individual members at noncertified AAHA practices; and (3) management associate memberships—office managers affiliated with certified or noncertified AAHA practices.

Associates with the first or second type of membership are entitled to the following benefits:

- membership directory

- the *Journal of the American Animal Hospital Association*—members receive six scientific publications bimonthly

- *Trends* magazine—members receive six management publications bimonthly

- proceedings of the annual meeting

- discounts on continuing education and access to a vast library of veterinary publications, videotapes, interactive computer programs, and audiotapes

Management associate members are entitled to the following benefits:

- membership directory

- *Trends* magazine

- copies of the spring and fall management conference proceedings

- discounts on continuing education and publications

AAHA offers all members a variety of consulting services for routine questions. Some services or in-depth consulting is provided on a reasonable fee-for-service basis. Contact AAHA at 800-252-AAHA to receive fee information about the following consulting services:

- architectural review service

- practice exit/retirement strategies

- associate buy-in/buy-out issues

- employee contract issues

- valuation/appraisal assistance and referral

- facility and practice expansion

- when to hire an associate or manager

- staff and staffing issues

- partnership issues

- compensation and benefits

- demographics of a practice area
- choosing a banker/lawyer/accountant
- understanding financial statements
- a client-needs survey

In addition to the above benefits and consulting services, AAHA hospitals are privileged to use the AAHA logo for hospital stationery, literature, and yellow page advertisements. They also are permitted to advertise on the AAHA worldwide web site to inform local, traveling, or relocating pet owners of their availability and services. For readers interested in viewing the AAHA worldwide web site, their address is http://www.healthypet.com. Topics available include: about AAHA, hospital locator, pet planet newsletter, pet care tips, and pet care library. The library has information about behavior, common animal health problems, the human/animal bond, nutrition, and preventative care. For more information about the services and costs of AAHA memberships, call 1-800-252-2242 or write to the American Animal Hospital Association, PO Box 150899, Denver, CO 80215-0899.

STATE VETERINARY MEDICAL ASSOCIATIONS

All states have state and local veterinary associations that track legislative activities affecting veterinary medicine, promote the profession on a local level, offer continuing education, and provide opportunities for camaraderie within the profession. The quantity and quality of membership services differ everywhere due to the tremendous variation in populations of veterinarians by state. The California Veterinary Medical Association is the focus of this discussion because of the size and depth of the services it offers.

The California Veterinary Medical Association (CVMA) is an outstanding state veterinary medical association devoted to promoting the veterinary profession. Its goals are to protect the rights of veterinarians, to create a positive public perception of CVMA members, to provide continuing education, and to save members money. These goals are accomplished by offering the following services (some free and others at discount prices) to CVMA members:

- membership directory
- *California Veterinarian*, a scientific journal
- *Update*, a timely newsletter covering issues that are hot off the press
- continuing education programs
- no membership charge to UC Davis veterinary students/residents nor for first-year graduates of all veterinary schools; and discounted dues for veterinarians in their second, third, and fourth years after graduation
- group insurance such as veterinary professional liability insurance, workers' compensation, and business automobile insurance
- OSHA consultations, workshops, and compliance kits and updates
- CA veterinary regulatory manual
- doctor and staff personnel manuals
- regulatory survival seminars
- complaint mediation (between consumers and veterinarians)
- credit union memberships
- no-annual-fee gold Mastercard
- privilege of using the CVMA Logo on stationery and in yellow page advertisements
- pet emergency posters for clients
- amusement park discounts
- car rental discounts
- materials for schools and community group presentations
- resource libraries on-line

Addresses and phone numbers for all state and local veterinary associations can be found in the *AVMA Membership Directory and Resource Manual* under the section entitled *State and Local Veterinary Medical Associations of the United States.*

Who Should Pay Professional Association Dues?

The majority of employers reimburse employees or pay professional membership fees for the AVMA and state veterinary medical associations (VMAs) directly. The authors' study of 225 employment contracts showed that it is less common for employers to pay membership fees for local VMAs; 60.6% and 52% of employers paid national and state professional association dues respectively, while 38.7% paid local dues.[1]

It is vital to the veterinary profession that local, state, and national veterinary and veterinary technician associations promote their professions and safeguard their political and legislative interests. Often the activities of committees for public relations, legislation, scientific convention, practice act revisions, and political action go unnoticed by members but produce huge benefits for the organization and the profession.

Because of these more subtle benefits as well as the obvious ones enumerated herein, employers are urged to pay membership dues for associates and technicians in full or at least in part. A $400- to $600-per-person annual dues expenditure for national, state, and local organizations will seem expensive for employers of multiple veterinary associates. But individual payments of that amount may be impossible for veterinary technicians whose salaries are often very low or for recent veterinary graduates, whose average individual educational debt in 1998 was nearly $60,000.

If costs seem excessive in multi-doctor practices, payment of 50% of dues in year one of employment, 75% in year two, and

100% for years three and after could be offered. New graduates generally are offered free or discounted memberships for their first few years after graduation anyway, so dues may be nonexistent or low at first.

Since this is a generous employee benefit, some employers elect to reward employees who stay at the practices for the duration of their employment terms and penalize those who do not. They accomplish this by covering the costs of employees' dues only during their terms of employment and requiring that their employees reimburse them for the costs of these and other benefits if they resign early. Applicable language on this issue is either placed in Employers' personnel policy manuals or added to their employment contracts.

This proration of benefits based on a continued employment policy also can be applied to other types of benefits that lend themselves to proration. In addition to association dues, this includes DEA registration fees, costs for veterinary or veterinary technician licenses, continuing education allowances, and, in some cases, vacation leave. Contract language for reimbursement of benefits can be drafted in two ways: (1) providing each particular benefit independent of the others or (2) included as a general policy covering reimbursement of all such benefits via a separate clause dealing with this issue generically.

A CONTRACT CLAUSE FOR PROFESSIONAL ASSOCIATION DUES

In most cases it is easier and more cost effective for employers to pay association dues and receive the tax benefit of this business expense than it is for employees to pay such dues and pursue a tax deduction for the expense. If employers do not pay the dues, employees must pay them themselves and file Schedule A, itemized tax returns, or Schedule C, independent trade or business tax returns to receive any tax deduction for the expense. Thus, the following clause is recommended in employment contracts:

Employer will pay Employee's dues for membership in the AVMA, State VMA, and AAHA (or AAEP, AABP, AAFP, etc.), and Local VMA. Employee accepts that if Employee resigns before the end of the term of this agreement, Employer may at Employer's option, bill Employee for or withhold from Employee's final paycheck, a prorata share of association dues paid by Employer for that portion of the year after which Employee no longer is employed by Employer.

SAMPLE CONTRACT LANGUAGE REQUIRING REIMBURSEMENT FOR ALL BENEFITS

To limit employee benefits to time periods prior to employee resignations, clauses similar to the following can be added:

Employee accepts that if Employee resigns before the end of the term of this agreement, Employer may at Employer's option, bill Employee for or withhold from Employee's final paycheck, a prorata share of all benefits that have been prepaid by Employer for the portion of the year after which Employee no longer is employed by Employer.

PROFESSIONAL LICENSING FEES

Veterinary medical license fees vary from state to state, ranging from biennial fees of $200 to annual fees of $450.[2] Since fees are considerable, contracts should address whether employers or employees incur the costs. For current information regarding state fees for veterinary licenses, readers can review the "Digest of Veterinary Practice Acts" section of the *AVMA Membership Directory and Resource Manual.*

WHO SHOULD PAY PROFESSIONAL LICENSING FEES?

Employers or employees should analyze the "exclusive service" sections of their vet-erinary employment agreements when deciding who will pay professional licensing fees. While most contracts require that employees work exclusively for their employers, some fail to address this issue, and others allow ancillary employment with the employer' approval.

The exclusive service sections of veterinary employment contracts usually are written in one of three ways: in an employer-slanted manner, in a neutral style, or in an employee-friendly way. Employer-slanted exclusive service sections typically prohibit employees from working for any other veterinary employers. Under such circumstances, it seems only equitable that these employers pay their employees' licensing fees.

Neutral-style agreements allow employees to engage in ancillary veterinary employment as long as employers approve in advance a written request for a waiver of the exclusive service requirement. In these situations, if employers deny extracurricular employment, employees are required by contract to practice veterinary medicine only for their employers. Given that employers in this situation retain a modicum of control over employees' professional time, employers should pay a percentage of the licensing fees equal to the employee's percentage of full-time employment.

Employee-friendly exclusive service contract sections generally state that employees must devote only the majority of their time to the practice of veterinary medicine for their employers. In this type of situation, employees may engage in other employment provided that their employers are apprised of such activity and it does not interfere with employees' performance or productivity. These types of exclusive service sections enable employees to have more control and flexibility over the use of their licenses and, therefore, it seems appropriate that employees pay the licensing fees. Equally logical, however, would be a policy stipulating that employers pay a percentage of the license fees equal to the employee's percentage of full-time employment.

In the authors' study of veterinary employment contracts from 1987 through 1998, 80% of the agreements had exclusive service sections. Of these, 53%, 24.4%, and 2.7% were employer friendly, neutral, and employee friendly, respectively. Employers paid professional license fees 28.1% of the time.

A CONTRACT CLAUSE FOR LICENSING FEE PAYMENTS

In employer-friendly contracts, where employees are employed exclusively by their employers and "are expected to devote such time and attention as necessary to perform adequately the duties enumerated in their contracts," the following language can be used:

Employee's professional licensing fee for (name of state) shall be paid by Employer.

In a more neutral style contract, employees are employed exclusively by the employer and are "expected to devote such time and attention as necessary to perform adequately the duties enumerated in the contract, unless provided with a written waiver of this requirement signed by Employer." In such situations a licensing fee clause might read as follows:

Employer will pay a percentage of Employee's professional licensing fee for (name of state) equal to the Employee's percentage of full-time employment.

In those cases where employee-friendly exclusive service sections are used, stipulating that employees are "expected to devote the majority of their time, attention and energies to the practice of veterinary medicine with the Employer but may engage in other employment so long as Employer is apprised of such employment before Employee agrees to perform such services and provided such ancillary employment does not materially interfere with Employee's performance or productivity

while employed by Employer," the following clause is appropriate:

Employee's professional licensing fee for (name of state) shall be paid by Employee or alternatively,

Employer agrees to pay a percentage of Employee's professional licensing fee for (name of state) equal to the Employee's percentage of full-time employment for Employer.

DRUG ENFORCEMENT AGENCY REGISTRATION

DEA REGISTRANTS AND AGENTS

As with many issues in law, the legal quagmires surrounding the ordering, prescribing, dispensing, and administering of controlled drugs can be complex and the penalties for transgressions severe. Employers and associate veterinarians, thus, are urged to study the subsequent section carefully when discussing this employment topic and formulating a plan for their practices.

Veterinarians who register with the Drug Enforcement Agency (DEA) using the address of their employment site, i.e., registrants, can order, administer, dispense, and prescribe controlled substances. Veterinarians who do not have DEA registrations but who are employed at practices where practice owners and/or supervisors have registrations can administer and dispense controlled substances as agents or employees of those registrants. They cannot, however, order or prescribe controlled drugs. The following statements in the Code of Federal Regulations (CFR) are the foundation for the above explanations about registrants, employees, and agents:

(a) The requirement of registration is waived for any agent or employee of a person who is registered to engage in any group or independent activities, if such agent or employee is acting in the usual course of his business or employment.

(b) An individual practitioner, as defined in §1304.02 of this chapter, who is an agent or employee of another individual practitioner (other than a mid-level practitioner) registered to dispense controlled substances may, when acting in the normal course of business or employment, administer or dispense (other than by issuance of prescription) controlled substances if and to the extent that such individual practitioner is authorized or permitted to do so by the jurisdiction in which he or she practices, under the registration of the employer or principal practitioner in lieu of being registered him/herself.[3]

During contract negotiations, employers and employees should discuss whether associates should be registrants or agents and, for associates who become registrants, which party will pay the registration fee. The following categories of veterinary associates are those who need to concern themselves with these issues:

- veterinarians who work at multi-doctor practices

- associates employed at more than one practice

- relief veterinarians who serve as independent contractors

PRACTICES EMPLOYING MULTIPLE DOCTORS

Owners of multi-doctor practices should consider whether their new associates need to register with the DEA. Although CFR § 1301.24 enables veterinarians to administer and dispense controlled substances as agents or employees of registrants, they cannot order or prescribe these drugs. Therefore, if the work schedules of registrants and agents do not overlap, there may not be anyone in the office to sign prescription pads or call pharmacies with prescriptions when they

are needed. To resolve this problem, employers have the following options:

1. Register only enough associates so that one of them is available at all times during the work schedule. The benefits of this solution are (a) fewer $210 DEA registrations, (b) reduced management time locating and/or filling out application renewals and drug order forms, and (c) fewer registrants per practice and, thus, decreased risks of abuse. The pitfalls of this option are that (a) employers may find it difficult to ensure that at least one registrant is on the premises at all times and (b) the practice's registrants will be held accountable for errors and/or abuses of all other associates at the practice who do not have their own registrations but, instead, serve as agents of the registrants.

2. Require that all associates have their own DEA registrations. This option enables all associates to order, administer, dispense, and prescribe controlled substances with ease. The detriments to this plan include (a) increased costs, (b) increased time and confusion filing the paperwork and maintaining drug inventories and records for multiple registrants, and (c) with the proliferation of DEA registrations, increased volumes of drugs and order forms on hand and, thus, increased opportunities for staff abuse.

In summary, because 10% to 20% of all veterinarians will abuse alcohol or other drugs during their lives to the extent that it affects their work,[4] employers and employees are advised to have candid discussions of how DEA registrations will be handled before employment relationships and contracts are finalized.

ASSOCIATES EMPLOYED AT MULTIPLE PRACTICES

Associates working for several practices need to evaluate their DEA status at each practice and decide whether they want or need to have DEA registrations at all of them. As discussed previously, CFR § 1301.24 enables veterinarians to administer or dispense controlled substances as agents or employees of registrants. This eliminates the costs of multiple registrations as well as the difficulties encountered maintaining individual inventories of controlled drugs at each site but does not allow unregistered associates to prescribe such drugs. Additionally, for this policy to work, employers of associates working at multiple practices must be willing to trust their part-time employees to dispense and/or administer drugs from their inventory with accuracy, honesty, and integrity, and to maintain good records.

INDEPENDENT CONTRACTOR VETERINARIANS

Relief veterinarians who function as independent contractors must review two distinct issues when dealing with DEA registration decisions: whether they are independent contractors according to IRS guidelines and whether they can serve as agents under CFR § 1301.24.

The IRS requires veterinarians who seek independent contractor status to establish independence from the practitioners for whom they work. The IRS guidelines, discussed in detail in Chapter 10, distinguish employees from independent contractors by focusing on three general areas: behavioral control, financial control, and relationships between employers and workers. In general, if businesses have the right to direct and control their workers, the workers are employees; if not, the workers more likely are considered to be independent contractors.

Under this theory, the IRS could contend that veterinarians who act as agents or employees for purposes of DEA registration may be relinquishing control of their independence to the practice owners upon whose DEA registration they are relying. In doing so, they may have weakened their independent contractor status under the IRS guidelines.

On the other hand, independent contractors could argue that since CFR § 1301.24 provides that veterinarians dispensing or administering controlled substances as agents are exempt from registering with the DEA, their independent contractor status is not altered. The rationale for this position is that they are serving merely as agents of the registrants for whom they work and not as employees. To further this position, they could argue that to minimize duplicative DEA registrations and maintenance of duplicative controlled drug inventories, they have chosen to administer and/or dispense controlled drugs as agents of the veterinary practice owners for whom they work while "acting in their normal course of business" as independent contractors.

The glitch with all of this is that to be truly independent of the control of the practices for which they work, independent contractors also must be able to prescribe controlled substances. Therefore, in the end, it appears that the only safe course of action independent contractors can take is to obtain their own DEA registrations.

This can be done by using one's home address as the place of business instead of registering at each practice at which one works. Independent contractors must realize, however, that any controlled substances they order then will be delivered only to the address at which they are registered, i.e., the home address. Although this approach may satisfy IRS requirements and allow veterinary associates to prescribe controlled substances, it is a major inconvenience that all controlled substances must be delivered to their home, where often no one is there to accept deliveries.

WHO SHOULD PAY THE FEES?

A contract consideration often overlooked by employers and employees involves which party should pay the three-year $210 DEA registration fee.

Employers are advised to pay associates' DEA registration fees when

- employers of multi-doctor practices require that their employees have DEA registrations in their own names.

- employers include exclusivity clauses in employment contracts which preclude associates from working for any other veterinary employers.

Since employees in these situations are limited to using their DEA registrations only for their employers, clients and patients, it seems logical that the employers pay the fees.

In either of these cases, employers can consider the following payment options:

- paying the full $210, three-year fee on behalf of employees at the time employees start working for employers.

- requiring that employees pay the fee but reimbursing them $70/year at the beginning of each employment term.

- requiring that employees pay the fee but reimbursing them $70/year at the end of the employment term, thereby providing some motivation to stay the entire year.

- paying the entire $210 in year one, but withholding a pro rata share of this amount from the final paycheck in the event that employees stay fewer than three years.

Associates should consider or be expected to pay their own DEA registration fees in the following situations:

- when they are employed at multiple practices and use their DEA registrations for clients and patients of all the practices.

- when they are relief veterinarians hired as independent contractors.

CONTRACT CLAUSES FOR DEA REGISTRATION

Four sample contract clauses regarding DEA registration follow:

1. *At the beginning of the contract term, Employer will pay Employee's full three-year DEA registration fee or, if Employee already has paid such fee, Employer will reimburse Employee for the pro rata share of such registration that is covered by the term of this Agreement. Upon termination of employment, Employee will notify the DEA of Employee's change of employment location.*

2. *At the beginning of each year of the contract term, Employer will reimburse Employee for the pro rata share of Employee's three-year DEA registration fee covered by the term of this Agreement (i.e., $70 for a one-year term, $140 for a two-year term, and $210 for a person completing a three-year term). Upon termination of employment, Employee will notify the DEA of Employee's change of employment location.*

3. *At the end of each year of employment, Employer will reimburse Employee for one-third of Employee's three-year DEA registration fee. Upon termination of employment, Employee will notify the DEA of Employee's change of employment location.*

4. *At the beginning of the contract term, Employer will pay Employee's full three-year DEA registration fee. However, Employer reserves the right to seek reimbursement or to withhold funds from Employee's final paycheck sufficient to cover that portion of the three-year DEA registration period during which Employee fails to work for Employer. Upon termination of employment, Employee will notify the DEA of Employee's change of employment location.*

RESOURCES FOR ADDITIONAL DEA INFORMATION

The DEA's publications entitled *The Physician's Manual* and *A Pharmacist's Manual* provide basic information on the Controlled Substances Act of 1970, which is the most pertinent to physicians and pharmacists. These booklets can be obtained from the United States Department of Justice, DEA, Office of Diversion Control, Liaison and Policy Section, 600-700 Army Navy Drive, Arlington, VA 22202; phone 202-307-7297.

Additional information can be acquired by accessing the DEA web site, located at http://www.usdoj.gov/dea/deahome.htm. An on-line database of current DEA statutes is available at the Government Printing Office's web site, located at http://www.access.gpo.gov. Individuals without a legal background, though, will discover that statutory language is burdensome and difficult to understand.

The most practical reference focusing on DEA rules and regulations for veterinary medicine and containing samples of most DEA forms is located in the Controlled Substances chapter of the *Law and Ethics of the Veterinary Profession* textbook, published by Priority Press, Ltd., P.O. Box 306, Yardley, PA 19067, phone 215-321-9488. DEA issues covered in that publication include

- classifications of controlled substances

- applications, registration renewals, terminations, and address changes

- obtaining and completing controlled substances order forms

- using powers of attorney documents to order controlled drugs

- rules for record keeping

- inventory protocols and requirements

- lending controlled drugs to others

- administration of controlled drugs by nonveterinary staff members

- DEA registrations for animal shelters

- security of stored controlled substances

- dealing with thefts or losses

- programs for chemically impaired veterinarians

If further help is needed, the appropriate DEA Divisional Office, Appendix L of the *Law and Ethics of the Veterinary Profession* textbook, veterinary board, or state controlled substance agencies can provide it.

In summary, reviewing many resources is critical to gaining a complete understanding of the issues associated with the use of controlled drugs. A failure to do so may expose practice owners, employed associates, and relief veterinarians to devastating criminal and/or financial consequences.

EMPLOYEE PET CARE PLANS

Whereas most veterinary students of the 1950s and 1960s did not have personal pets while in school, the majority of today's students and new graduates have multiple pets. Additionally, support staff usually have numerous pets. Thus, employee pet care costs can be burdensome for practice owners who do not address this issue in their employment contracts or personnel policy manuals. Employers are urged to establish well-conceived plans that achieve the following objectives:

1. Discourage hospital theft:

   Employers who have plans in place may be able to reduce product theft. Typical reasons for product theft can be one or more of the following: (a) employees become aware of the difference between employer and client costs and are resentful when asked to pay the markup fees, (b) employees have numerous pets and become overwhelmed with the financial responsibilities of ownership, (c) employees have unsupervised access to the practice's products, and (d) hospitals have inaccurate or no inventory controls in place. In addition to brainstorming different strategies that can be used to prevent product theft, employers are advised to consider employee pet care plans as a solution. These plans enable employees to obtain veterinary products and services for personal pets and be charged the employer's costs plus a specified percentage. Such plans reduce employee resentment related to standard markups and ease the financial burdens for the many kind-hearted veterinary employees who own numerous pets.

2. Encourage employee familiarity with products and professional services:

Employees who have first-hand experience with product effectiveness, techniques for administering these products, side effects, and post-treatment responsibilities can help employers in several ways. They can give feedback to practice owners regarding product efficacy, side effects, and ease of administration; they can provide clients with informative and credible explanations of the practice's products and professional services; the practices will likely sell more products and professional services because employees are familiar with and endorse them; and clients will perceive knowledgeable veterinary associates and support staff as a positive reflection of the practice.

3. Attract new staff and maintain existing employees:

Since many of today's veterinary employees have multiple pets, offering pet care plans is a valuable benefit that gives employers a competitive edge in attracting quality employees.

NUMBERS OF PETS COVERED BY THE PLAN

The number of pets owned by employees varies greatly. Some employees will own 1 to 2 pets; some are good-hearted "collectors" owning as many as 5 to 10; and others are breeders or show circuit participants. Animosities may develop among employees if they perceive that some fellow workers receive thousands of dollars of discounted pet care each year while others receive only limited benefits.

Employers of large numbers of employees most likely will find it necessary to limit the numbers of animals that qualify for pet care discounts. To minimize costs and dis-

parities among employees, the University of Pennsylvania teaching hospital caps discounts at four animals, identified at the beginning of each year. Practice owners are urged to limit the numbers of animals that qualify for their employee pet care discounts to prevent abuse by some staff members and subsequent ill will among the others.

EXAMPLES OF EMPLOYEE PET CARE PLANS

Three examples of employee pet care plans follow. Variations of these plans depend on profitability of the practice and the generosity of the owners. Regardless of the plan implemented, employers are advised to establish the following procedures with employees:

- Maintain individual medical records on each employee's pets.

- Record sales of veterinary products or professional services in each pet's medical record contemporaneously with the provision of care.

- Require employees to pay charges within 15 to 30 days of the time products are dispensed or services rendered.

Example 1. Subsidized Plans allow employees to obtain products such as flea sprays, pet foods, medications, vaccines, and laboratory samples sent to outside laboratories at cost for their personal pets. No charges are assessed for veterinary services such as surgery, in-house diagnostic laboratory work, and hospitalization for employees' personal pets. Such plans are extremely generous for employees, but there is one caveat with them. Doctors may be inclined to spend insufficient time, performing only cursory physical exams and diagnostic work-ups, be reluctant to send lab samples to outside laboratories, and prescribe the least expensive medications. This, in turn, creates awkward relationships with staff members, who would prefer full access to their doctor's best efforts and the highest quality medications.

Example 2. Partially Subsidized Plans allow employees to obtain products for personal pets, i.e., flea sprays, pet foods, medications, and vaccines, and to send samples to outside laboratories and be charged for these items at the employer's cost plus 10%. This percentage covers costs incurred by employers to order and stock products and pay the fees billed by the outside laboratories. Fees for in-house veterinary services such as surgery, dentistry, diagnostic laboratory work, and hospitalization performed for employees' personal pets (during employees' time off) on employers' premises are charged at 25% to 50% of the employer's standard fees for such services. If doctors or employees enlist the assistance of other staff members to provide veterinary services during working hours, employees are charged at 50% to 60% of standard fees.

The 25% to 50% of employers' standard fees covers the expenses incurred by employers for hospital supplies used while performing professional services; ordering and stocking those supplies; and maintaining and cleaning the facilities, instruments, and/or equipment used. The 50% to 60% of employers' fees covers all the previous expenses plus something for the time paid for the additional staff members.

Example 3. Minimally Subsidized/No Profit Plans allow employees to obtain products for personal pets, i.e., flea sprays, pet foods, medications, and vaccines, and send samples to outside labs, and be charged for these items at the employer's cost plus 20%. Fees for veterinary services such as surgery, diagnostic laboratory work, and hospitalization performed on employees' personal pets during their scheduled workday are charged at 70% to 80% of the employer's standard fee for such services. This covers the employer's cost for the veterinary services but disallows any employer profit.

A CONTRACT CLAUSE FOR EMPLOYEE PET CARE PLANS

1. The following sample contract language is for a subsidized plan:

Employee is entitled to obtain from Employer products such as flea sprays, pet foods, kitty litter, leashes, bandage materials, medications, and vaccines, for Employee's personal pets and have diagnostic samples sent to outside laboratories and be charged for these items at Employer's cost. No fees will be charged for veterinary services such as surgery, anesthesia, in-house diagnostic laboratory work, dentistry, radiographs, hospitalization, fluid therapy, catheterizations, ear irrigations, splints, bandages, and casts performed on a limit of (two? three? four?) of Employee's personal pets. Individual animals to be covered under this plan must be identified via a medical record within two weeks of their acquisition by the Employee. To facilitate accurate record keeping and inventory management, Employee shall keep records on each personal pet on standard hospital medical charts, record items and veterinary services that Employee/Employer uses or provides on each pet's record, and pay for such items or veterinary services within (15? 30? 45?) days after they are provided or obtained (or alternatively, on a monthly or quarterly basis). Charges for veterinary services for personal pets in excess of (two? three? four?) will be at the practice's retail fees.

2. The following sample contract clause retains most of the above wording but is adjusted to reflect a partially subsidized plan:

Employee is entitled to obtain products such as flea sprays, pet foods, kitty litter, leashes, bandage materials, medications, and vaccines for Employee's personal pets and have diagnostic samples sent to outside laboratories and be charged for these items at Employer's cost plus 10%. Veterinary services such as surgery, anesthesia, in-house diagnostic laboratory work, dentistry, radiographs, hospitalization, fluid therapy, catheterizations, ear irrigations, splints, bandages, and casts performed on a limit of (two? three? four?) of Employee's personal pets performed during non-business hours will be charged to Employee at 30% of Employer's standard fee for such services. When Employee enlists the assistance of a paid staff member to provide veterinary services for Employee's personal pets during the practice's working hours, Employee will be charged 60% of Employer's standard fee for such services. Individual animals to be covered under this plan must be identified via a medical record within two weeks of their acquisition by Employee. To facilitate accurate record keeping and inventory management, Employee shall keep records on each personal pet on standard hospital medical charts, record items and veterinary services that Employee/Employer uses or provides on each pet's record, and pay for such items or veterinary services within (15? 30? 45?) days after they are provided or obtained (or alternatively, on a monthly or quarterly basis). Charges for veterinary services for personal pets in excess of (two? three? four?) will be at the practice's retail fees.

3. The following sample contract clause is for the minimally subsidized/no profit plan:

Employee is entitled to obtain products such as flea sprays, pet foods, kitty litter, leashes, bandage materials, medications, and vaccines for Employee's personal pets and have diagnostic samples sent to outside laboratories and be charged for these items at Employer's cost plus 20%. Veterinary services such as surgery, anesthesia, in-house diagnostic laboratory work, dentistry, radiographs, hospitalization, fluid therapy, catheterizations, ear irrigations, splints, bandages, and casts performed on a limit of (two? three? four?) of Employee's personal pets will be charged to Employee at (70% or 80%) of Employer's standard fee for such services. Individual animals to be covered under this plan must be identified via a medical record within two weeks of

their acquisition by Employee. To facilitate accurate record keeping and inventory management, Employee shall keep records on each personal pet on standard hospital medical charts, record items and veterinary services that Employee/Employer uses or provides on each pet's record, and pay for such items or veterinary services within (15? 30? 45?) days after they are provided or obtained (or alternatively, on a monthly or quarterly basis). Charges for veterinary services for personal pets in excess of (two? three? four?) will be at the practice's retail fees.

PET HEALTH INSURANCE

Some form of insurance is essential if veterinary medicine is to take advantage of the technological gains experienced by the human health care community. Many of the advanced diagnostic and therapeutic procedures used in human medicine are available for companion animals, but delivery of these services is often limited because the costs are perceived to be too high for the average pet owner.

Despite this perception, fees for sophisticated and extensive sick care services for animals often are unrealistically low—a mere 6% to 10% of those for comparable human health care. Many practitioners have learned that for their professional skills and practices to grow and succeed, the cost of quality sick care must be subsidized by income from well care services like annual exams and vaccines, heartworm testing, dewormings, and dentistry. In addition, fees for in-depth diagnostic workups, surgery, and treatment often are discounted to well below market value by compassionate veterinarians whose aim is to avoid euthanasia when owners are unprepared to pay their standard fees.

These reasons, in part, are responsible for the low income earned by many veterinarians. Developing a way to break through the glass ceiling of euthanasia is essential if the profession is ever going to be all that it can be. One way to accomplish that goal is to celebrate and promote the importance and value of the family-pet-veterinarian bond. Another is to understand and promote pet health insurance. And there is nowhere better to begin promoting it than with one's own employees.

RATIONALE FOR PET HEALTH INSURANCE

Risk sharing in the form of pet health insurance enables owners with limited disposable income and/or strong family-pet bonds to access advanced veterinary care with lower out-of-pocket costs. In part, this is because their purchase of pet health insurance essentially requires them to budget in advance for payment of their pets' sick care. Owners with insurance stand to benefit greatly if a serious illness or accident occurs and they pay, for example, $300 in deductibles and copayments to secure $1,000 worth of medical services covered by their pets' insurance carriers. Having insurance actually prompts most people to think as follows: "Since I've already spent the money for the insurance, I expect and deserve some return on that investment. Therefore, I owe it to myself and my beloved Rover to spend another $300 so that I can obtain the $1,000 worth of veterinary services he needs."

REVIEWING THE OBJECTIONS TO INSURANCE

The human health care industry has been under attack because of the explosive rise in costs for health care. The health insurance industry has borne a great deal of the criticism. This is because of its willingness and ability to pay the extraordinary costs associated with saving preemie babies, "diagnosing the impossible," providing organ and bone marrow transplants, treating and rehabilitating accident victims, and providing enormous quantities of care for terminally ill people.

The result of such medical excellence has been that health insurance premiums have risen nearly to the level of house payments, making insurance unaffordable for many Americans. To limit excesses and control costs, "managed care" has been thrust upon the market in the form of HMOs, PPOs, and capitation.

In the midst of the criticism, though, the human health insurance industry has not been credited adequately with the immense financial and technological progress it has fostered within the human health care industry. This country offers the best medical care in the world and has millions of highly compensated health care professionals. That would never have happened without insurance. The same progress is possible in veterinary medicine with the utilization of pet health insurance. The goal is to maximize its benefits while controlling its detriments.

THE COST OF LOST VETERINARY TIME

Veterinarians often spend as much or more time talking with owners about financial costs for veterinary care than they do discussing diagnostic plans and the health risks and benefits of treatment. If this precious veterinary time could be transferred to clients who file their own claims for insurance copayments or to lower-paid claims assistants working for veterinary practices, veterinarians could use that time to explain better and/or more costly alternative treatments to clients. Additionally, they could use the extra time to provide more and higher quality services and/or charge appropriate, nondiscounted fees for the services being provided. This would produce a net financial gain for the profession. Perhaps most importantly, if large percentages of pet owners had pet health insurance, the burnout factor in the profession caused by economically induced euthanasias would be reduced remarkably.

Many veterinarians are reluctant to consider third-party payers as allies in the provision of increased quantities and quality of veterinary care. This is because of their concerns about

- the time required to file insurance claims;

- the need to establish new, claims-oriented billing procedures;

- the possibility of lengthy delays receiving insurance payments;

- the hassles of reconciling differences between amounts billed and amounts paid by insurance, and then having to deal with overpayments or further billing to clients; and

- the complaints they continually hear from physicians about managed care and capitation.

OVERCOMING THE OBJECTIONS TO INSURANCE

The paperwork burden of insurance can be minimized by having owners pay veterinarians when services are rendered and file their pets' insurance claims themselves. This simple process requires that veterinarians merely provide owners with diagnoses and itemized billing statements at the time of treatment—something most already do. Then it is up to the owners to take care of the insurance paperwork.

The processing of claims for complicated cases can be expedited by photocopying pets' medical records and instructing clients to include the copies when they file their claims with the insurance carrier. Moreover, because insurance carriers always are concerned that claims filed within a few months of a policy's initiation date are for pre-existing conditions, medical records also should be provided to owners who file claims within the first six months their insurance policies are in force.

This is how the vast majority of claims are processed by Veterinary Pet Insurance, a company which, until early 1997, was the only pet health insurer in the United States. As of 2002, Veterinary Pet Insurance reports that uncomplicated claims routinely are paid within five to seven working days.[5] Because Veterinary Pet Insurance is the only long-term licensed pet health insurance carrier in the United States and it has used a consistent claims filing and payment system during its 18-year existence, further comments about pet health insurance in this article will refer to methods employed only by that company.

It should be noted that with the expansion of the human animal bond, nearly eight years of economic expansion and affluence in the U.S., and a growing interest in pet health insurance because of successes in Europe, as of September, 1998, *DVM Magazine* reports that at least three pet health insurance companies and one pet health HMO exist in the U.S. market.

In spite of the simplicity of Veterinary Pet Insurance's approach wherein owners file all insurance claims, a small percentage of practitioners have chosen to go the extra mile and file claims for their clients. At the time of discharge, these veterinarians use the company's benefit schedule to estimate their clients' share of the fees owed and bill clients only for the difference. Clients pay that amount, and practices send the claims to the company for direct payment.

When payment from the company arrives, clients either are billed for the difference between what they paid and what their insurance covered or, if they have overpaid, their accounts are credited with the overpayments until the time of their next visit. What the owners of these practices have decided to do is to "walk their talk" about being full-service hospitals. In taking the three to five minutes required to file their clients' insurance claims, an intense bonding develops, keeping these clients from seeking services anywhere else.

Table 7.2. Differences between Pet and Human Health Insurance

Pet Health Insurance	Human Health Insurance
1. Insured owner pays premium costs	Employee benefit or government pays
2. Major owner copay	Zero to some patient copay
3. Insured party files claims	Provider files the vast majority of claims
4. Owner has major involvement decisions	Minimal decisions about costs
5. *When costs or patient suffering are at stake*	
euthanasia is an option	euthanasia is not an option
6. Because of euthanasia, there are virtually no long-term care costs	Because euthanasia is not an option, there are major costs for long-term care
7. Limited intensive care costs	Major intensive care costs (respirators, hemodialysis, supplementary cardiac pumps, etc.)
8. Insignificant liability risks and costs	Major liability risks and costs
9. HIV and AIDS are not cost factors	HIV, AIDS, Hepatitis C, are major cost factors
10. No costs for psychiatric care	Significant psychiatric care costs
11. No suicide treatments	Significant costs for attempted suicides
12. No treatment costs for substance abuse	Major costs to treat substance abuse

CONCERNS ABOUT LOSING CONTROL

Veterinarians worry most about the potential loss of control over their medical decisions. They hear physicians decrying managed care and instantly say, "We want no part of that," forgetting that insurance is what made the human health care industry financially and professionally rewarding. Additionally, doctors always think that they know more about patient medical care than could a bank of computers and epidemiologists assessing medical and financial outcomes of different approaches to treatments. The truth is that, in the long run, the computers and epidemiologists will have the upper hand, because they are objectively evaluating factual data, while doctors will still be comparing subjective clinical impressions and opinions.

Most importantly, though, what most veterinarians fail to recognize are the major differences between pet and human health insurance. Table 7.2 identifies them.

PROVIDING PET INSURANCE FOR VETERINARY EMPLOYEES

Health insurance for employees is a standard benefit in the human health care industry, so physicians are able to provide medical care for their employees as needed and file claims for reimbursement for their services. Physicians thus become the financial beneficiaries of their own employee benefits programs and have no need to discount their services in the process. Why don't veterinarians do the same for the pets belonging to their staff members?

Frequently veterinarians do not recognize the value of insurance for their profession. The best way to experience the usefulness of third-party payment is to provide it as a fringe benefit for staff members. This allows the following advantages:

1. Practice owners can familiarize themselves and their staff with pet health insurance so that they can answer inquiries about the value of insurance with statements like, "Oh yes, we recommend pet health insurance. In fact all of our employees' pets are insured."

2. Employers receive payment for care provided for staff's pets rather than donating or discounting their time, effort, knowledge, drugs, and supplies.

3. Staff members experience the benefits of insurance with their own pets.

4. Staff and doctors become familiar with the benefit schedules for various diagnoses and the simplicity of filing claims.

5. Doctors feel better about scheduling appointments for staff members' animals during standard office hours because they will be paid for their time. They no longer feel that they are "working these people in" between other appointments or at the end of the day, and staff no longer feel that they are imposing.

6. Doctors perform all appropriate diagnostic procedures rather than attempt to save the business and employees money by practicing medicine based initially on treatment response.

7. Doctors are willing to use first-choice drugs for medically ideal time periods instead of economizing with less expensive, second-choice drugs or first-choice drugs for limited time periods.

8. Employees are less tempted to pocket medications when they can submit insurance claims and the insurance company will assist with payments.

9. Staff can seek and afford veterinary care at emergency and specialty clinics when it is needed. Employers no longer need to feel guilt if they are unavailable or unable to provide the best quality of care accessible in the community.

10. Staff members can be referred to specialty and emergency practices without placing those practices in awkward situations in which they may feel that they are expected to discount their fees for staff who work for other veterinarians in the area or in which they are embarrassed because word gets out that they provide discounts for employees of some colleagues but not others.

11. The traditionally low-paid veterinary support staff, who usually are intensely bonded to their pets, are not subject to emotionally and/or financially devastating medical and euthanasia decisions because of economics.

IMPLEMENTING COVERAGE FOR EMPLOYEES

Claims can be handled in one of several ways for employees who have pet-care insurance. The first and most generous choice is to accept the company's coverage as payment in full for all fees owed. This is more costly for employers because it requires them to forego collection of the deductible and any fees not covered by the company's benefit schedule.

A second, somewhat less expensive alternative, is for employers to have employees pay the deductible and accept Veterinary Pet Insurance's benefits as payment in full for all services provided. Under this plan, no employee copayments are required should fees exceed those in the company's established fee schedule. This is similar to the manner in which many physicians handle payments for Medicare patients.

A third and less expensive option for employers is to have employees pay the deductible and any copayments for fees above the established fee schedule.

A fourth and least desirable possibility is for employees to pay for services and submit their bills to the company for reimbursement just as clients do. Though the last option does not particularly enhance the strength of the employer-employee commitment, it still demonstrates value, keeps staff more closely involved in financial decisions, and decreases overutilization.

No matter which option is chosen, practice owners must determine whether or not they wish to place limits on the numbers of pets each staff member can insure at the practice's expense. It may be easier to pay the insurance premiums for no more than two to three pets per household than it is to provide traditional discounts for the first three animals and charge full fees for animals in excess of that threshold.

Pet Health Insurance Summary

As with any insurance program, employers who provide pet health insurance for employees will discover that some years the insurance costs more than the benefits derived from it. Other years it may pay far more than the costs of the discounted veterinary care the practice had traditionally given away to employees. In every year, though, practice owners and their employees will appreciate the peace of mind offered by the expanded veterinary options available to staff.

As mentioned previously, several pet health insurance companies now operate in the United States. Veterinary Pet Insurance, located in Anaheim, CA since 1981, phone 1-800-USA-PETS, grew at a rate of 20% to 30% per year in the early to mid 1990s. However, a $5 million investment by Veterinary Centers of America in 1997 and a $3 million investment by Nationwide Insurance in 1998 have allowed the company to speed its growth. Additionally, strategic alliances with Bayer, Merial, Fort Dodge, Pharmacia-Upjohn, Novartis, Heska, Schering Plough, and Pfizer, all of whom support the company's new comprehensive well-care program, have allowed Veterinary Pet Insurance to more than double its premium growth in 1998 and 1999. A new marketing alliance with Iams, entered into by the parties during the summer of 2002, should continue to speed the company's growth to $100 million annually by the year 2003.

Growth data on the newest pet health insurance entries to the field are not currently available. Nonetheless, practice owners or staff members who are interested in the advantages and flexibility offered by pet health insurance, instead of continuing their current discounted pet care plans, are urged to contact VPI or any other new pet health insurance companies for more information.

Travel and Moving Allowances

Travel Allowances for Associates Seeking Employment

Because of educational debts, minimal cash for travel, and limited time, many veterinary associates and technicians are reluctant to travel long distances in search of employment. This often leads to a surplus of veterinary staff within a 50-mile radius of many veterinary and some veterinary technician schools and shortages in more distant locations.

Employers seeking the best veterinary associates, technicians, and office managers are discovering that by providing travel allowances for job applicants, they can (1) expand the number of candidates, including graduates, from a wider variety of schools; (2) increase the amount of time available to view candidates' medical, surgical, and communication skills; (3) show their practices and more fully introduce their staff to potential applicants; (4) obtain feedback from existing staff members about applicants; (5) engage in direct contract negotiations; and (6) provide opportunities for candidates to investigate housing and visit the community prior to deciding whether or not to accept employment.

Since these financial arrangements generally are in advance and independent of employment contracts, no formal contract clause is provided herein. Instead, employers and applicants should establish financial responsibilities for such arrangements prior to scheduling the visits. Costs to consider include travel and parking (including airfare), car rentals, gasoline, housing, and meals.

MOVING ALLOWANCES FOR NEW EMPLOYEES

In addition to covering job-seeking expenses, employers are becoming more willing to offer moving allowances to new employees located in distant cities or states because of the following: (1) an increasingly competitive job market for quality employees; (2) the large percentage of new graduates with educational debt and insufficient liquid assets to move to distant locations; (3) numerous up-front expenses incurred by employees when moving themselves, their families, their pets, and belongings to new locations; and (4) the desire to obtain an ideal match between their personal and practice philosophies and those of their employees. Additionally, employers gain their employees' allegiance by easing the financial burden during the transition to their new jobs.

As discussed previously, educational debt is an important issue for the majority of new graduates. The national average debt for 2002 graduates was $72,719, an increase of 40% since 1996 and 95% since 1994. Eighty-two percent of graduates had educational debt of $30,000 or greater.[7] In 1997, 62.6% of graduates had debt greater than $40,000;[7] by 2002 that number was 75.9%.

In addition to educational debt, moving expenses incurred by new graduates and their families can be financially and emotionally draining. These usually include searching for housing; transportation costs; security deposits for apartments; initial telephone, utility, and cable television setup fees; and time and financial costs to obtain new drivers' and automobile licenses. In light of the financial stresses on the profession's new graduates, employers are urged to consider incorporating moving allowances into their employment contracts.

Now that this benefit has been discussed with students at numerous veterinary schools and at several regional and national veterinary conventions, there are increasing numbers of offers that include moving allowances in the $500 to $2,000 range. Although such offers are being made by private practitioners, this benefit seems to be much more commonplace among the corporate consolidators such as Veterinary Centers of America, National Pet Care Centers, National Veterinary Associates, and VetSmart. The fact that a recent contract offer made to a young animal science graduate by California-based Foster Farms poultry producer included up to $7,500 for moving expenses shows that the veterinary profession is seriously behind industry with respect to this benefit.[8]

A CONTRACT CLAUSE FOR MOVING ALLOWANCES

A contract clause for moving allowances can read as follows:

Employer will provide Employee with a moving allowance of ($1,000?, $2,000?, $4,000?) (two?) weeks prior to or within (two?) weeks of the commencement of employment for personal expenses incurred moving to a home within a (15? 30? 45? 60?) minute commute of Employer's veterinary practice. Employee accepts and agrees that if Employee resigns from Employer's employment prior to the end of the initial term of this agreement, the moving allowance will be considered an interest-free loan, and Employee will be required either to (1) repay such loan prior to (or within three months of?) termination of employment or (2) agree to have such amount withheld from Employee's final paycheck.

SPEAKING ENGAGEMENTS

Speaking engagements present opportunities for personal, financial, and professional gains for speakers and the veterinary practices at which they are employed. Employees who do public speaking can

- improve their knowledge about a given subject through in-depth preparation and by answering the questions posed by attendees,

- expose the veterinary practices at which they are employed to audiences of potential clients,

- produce supplemental personal income,

- build personal and professional referral networks in the profession and/or community,

- improve self-confidence, and

- develop leadership and public speaking skills.

To prevent financial disputes and scheduling conflicts between speaker employees and their employers, employment agreements should address this issue. Topics to include are:

1. Expenses:

   Employees who retain compensation from speaking engagements should bear the following costs: personal and professional preparation, travel, housing, meals, and supplies. If there is no compensation or if the practice, rather than the individual, is the beneficiary, employers should pay for expenses incurred.

2. Compensation:

   When speakers are compensated and pay the costs associated with their speaking engagements, they should be entitled to retain honoraria from such activities. Conversely, when employers pay all costs, they should receive the honoraria.

3. Notification and subject material:

   Associates should be expected to notify employers about offers for speaking engagements prior to accepting them. This gives employers an opportunity to determine whether the topics or engagements enhance or are detrimental to the associate's provision of veterinary services or the image promoted by the practice.

For example, a conservative veterinary employer with a utilitarian view of animals might not support a young veterinarian's position promoting rights for animals. Conversely, a compassionate and anthropomorphic veterinary employer may not embrace an associate's position that people who cannot afford to provide adequate veterinary care for their animals should not be allowed to own them.

Although freedom of speech is a constitutional right, employers should be able to retain final say over employees' speaking engagements that could subject the employer's business to bad public relations.

4. Time off for presentations:

   Decisions should be made as to the conditions under which employers will grant leaves of absence to fulfill speaking engagements as opposed to the conditions under which employees will be required to use personal vacation time. One could argue that whenever either party arranges a speaking engagement wherein the primary intent is and effect will be to facilitate referrals of cases to employers, employers will provide excused time off with compensation.

The best example of this occurs when recently hired specialists speak at their local veterinary association meetings. If honoraria are provided under these circumstances and employees used some of employers' lecture notes or Kodachrome slides or created presentations on company time, it could be argued that honoraria should be paid to the employer. However, anyone who has presented lecture materials knows that for every hour of speaking time, speakers probably will have 10 to 25 hours of preparation. Because of this, it is likely that employees will have devoted more off-the-job personal time to their presentations than they will have used on-the-job company time.

Without specific agreements to the contrary, honoraria in such cases probably should be paid to employers, if presentations were created during the employee's scheduled work time, and to the employees if the lectures were created primarily during off-the-job night and week end time periods.

A CONTRACT CLAUSE FOR SPEAKING ENGAGEMENTS

A contract clause for employees who incur the costs and retain compensation associated with speaking engagements could read:

Employee may engage in veterinary-related teaching, speaking, or research activities provided that the time for such activities is on a schedule acceptable to the Employer and provided that engagements are not in conflict with or detrimental to Employee's provision of veterinary services or the image of the Employer's veterinary practice. Employer must be notified of such invitations and approve them prior to the time Employee accepts them.

In situations where Employee bears the majority of the costs of preparation and presentation and creates the majority of such speaker programs during non-work time, Employee will be entitled to retain honoraria and reimbursements associated with expenses incurred for these engagements. In the event Employer bears the costs of Employee's efforts to create such speaker programs, including the provision of the majority of the time required to generate such presentations and payment of costs associated with presenting them, Employer shall be entitled to receive speaker honoraria and reimbursement associated with expenses incurred for these engagements.

UNIFORM ALLOWANCES AND REQUIREMENTS

Originally, uniforms were worn by veterinarians and support staff to keep clean and protect themselves from contracting zoonotic diseases or being injured by aggressive animals. Wearing appropriate apparel when providing professional services has many other advantages, however, such as

- strengthening one's professional appearance, thereby increasing clients' perception of value.

- providing a consistent appearance among staff, further enhancing a professional look.

- enhancing the perception of authority, which can be particularly helpful to younger veterinarians and, thus, increase the likelihood that clients will follow their medical and surgical recommendations.

- enabling clients to differentiate between doctors, technicians, receptionists, and office managers.

To heighten employees' awareness of uniform expenses and the importance of job appearances, employers are advised to include this information in employment contracts or personnel policy manuals. Standards for the wearing of uniforms in the workplace should be set, and the dollar amount of uniform allowances should be stated. The following points should be incorporated:

- Employees are required to use uniform allowances only for the purchase of uniforms.

- Employees must conform to employer's standards and policies regarding the wearing of uniforms.

- Employers (or employees) are responsible for cleaning and maintaining their uniforms.

• Employees who exceed uniform allowances or who damage their uniforms needlessly shall have such excesses deducted from their compensation.

Uniform attire that employers should consider includes white lab coats, coveralls, surgical tops and bottoms, embroidered smocks, and name tags. For maximal visibility, name tags should be worn on the right side of the chest, rather than the left, so they are readable as employees shake hands with clients.

A CONTRACT CLAUSE FOR UNIFORM ALLOWANCES AND REQUIREMENTS

A contract clause regarding uniforms could read:

> *An annual uniform allowance of $ will be provided to Employee by Employer. Employee agrees to spend the allowance only for veterinary uniforms. Employee agrees to conform to Employer's standards and policies regarding the wearing of uniforms during Employee's scheduled work time, and be responsible for the cleaning and maintenance of such uniforms. Careless destruction of or damage to uniforms by Employee shall allow Employer the option of deducting expenses incurred in replacing such uniforms from Employee's pay.*

USE OF AUTOMOBILES

The use and/or misuse of business vehicles is an issue that poses serious problems for veterinary practices and about which little has been written. To avoid strife, owners and employees of ambulatory practices are encouraged to identify and address the issues involving the use of these vehicles at the commencement of employment. Doing so can help prevent severe financial losses, preserve good interpersonal and business relationships, provide reliable services for clients without time-consuming delays, and avoid legal battles.

A large animal practitioner in South Central Pennsylvania mandates that his associates who are on emergency call take a business vehicle home at the end of the workday.[9] His position is that clients who require after-hours emergency care for their animals receive faster responses when his associates have fully stocked business vehicles readily available at their homes. For example, an associate living 10 miles west of the office was able to respond to an emergency milk fever patient belonging to an owner residing 15 miles west of the office without first having to drive to the practice, thereby saving valuable time and expense.

The vehicular issues to be addressed before employment agreements are signed include:

1. Provision of insurance for vehicles that are readily available for employees' use: Employers should be responsible for insuring all vehicles owned by the business regardless of who uses them.

2. Compensation to be paid to employees for the costs of their automobile insurance when these vehicles are used for their employers' business purposes: Employees should secure such insurance via policies obtained through their own insurance companies. Coverage levels should be at least equal to that carried on vehicles owned by the practice. Employers can reimburse employees for insurance costs based on percentage usage of the vehicle for business purposes or as a component of a mileage allowance. Coverage levels in excess of those fixed by the practice should be the responsibility of the employees. Employees should be required to provide copies of policies and paid insurance premium receipts to their employers prior to the use of an employee's vehicle for business purposes.

3. Mileage compensation provided for employees who use their own vehicles for business travel: This allowance should cover the depreciation of the employee's vehicle, insurance, general maintenance,

licenses, gasoline, repairs, and lost-opportunity costs.

4. The operation and maintenance of vehicles in a condition acceptable to employers: Regardless of whether vehicles are owned by the practice or its employees, employees should ensure that (a) vehicles are supplied with gasoline and medical supplies at all times; (b) oil and oil filter are changed every 3,500 to 7,500 miles, depending on the driving environment and recommendations of the vehicles' manufacturer; (c) tires and tire pressure are checked monthly, and tires are rotated every 10,000 miles and replaced every 35,000 to 75,000 miles; (d) engines are tuned every 35,000 to 45,000 miles or as recommended by the vehicle's manufacturer; (e) repairs are attended to as soon as possible; and (f) vehicles' external and internal condition is presentable to clients and colleagues.[10]

5. Conformance with traffic laws and the wearing of seatbelts: Employees must remember that their actions represent their employers and, thus, laws should be obeyed regardless of circumstances.

6. Policies regarding business vehicles being used for business purposes only: It is usually impossible to limit all use of vehicles to business purposes. If some personal use of the business vehicle is acceptable, employers are advised to determine the acceptable number of miles, who pays for expenses incurred for personal use, and who keeps track of miles and expenses and how.

7. Availability of vehicles for emergency calls: To expedite the provision of emergency care, employers are encouraged to allow employees to take business vehicles home when receiving calls. This is good for business and a valuable perquisite for employees.

8. Consequences of vehicle mistreatment: Though all ambulatory veterinarians know how to drive, employers typically find that some are harder on vehicles than others. Employees need to understand that vehicles are a major expense for their employers and that mistreating vehicles decreases their reliability, increases employees' propensity for accidents and traffic violations, increases maintenance expenses, and will result in termination of their employment if they refuse to apply good driving habits while on business. Because of these factors, contracts should address damage to vehicles and increased insurance premiums caused by employee negligence or poor driving records.

9. The duty for employers to provide safe, properly maintained vehicles: Employees who anticipate considerable travel during their employment should inspect the business vehicles they will be expected to drive prior to accepting employment. If, in their judgment, the vehicle(s) is/are unsafe and their employers are unresponsive to their requests for repairs or replacement vehicles, they may want to seek employment elsewhere.

MILEAGE COMPENSATION FOR EMPLOYEES DRIVING THEIR OWN VEHICLES

Employees who use their personal vehicles for business purposes should be reimbursed by their employers for vehicle depreciation, insurance, general maintenance, licenses, gasoline, and lost-opportunity costs on the money they have invested in the vehicle. The following is an example illustrating how an employee with a one-year contract could calculate mileage costs:

Example: The vehicle costs $20,000. The employee drives it 25,000 miles/year, and 80% of that time is for business purposes (20,000 miles).

1. If the vehicle depreciation is approximately $4,500 per year, the resale value

at the end of the year is $15,500. Thus, the cost to the owner is $4,500 for the year.

2. The insurance, general maintenance, repairs, and licenses cost about $2,500 per year.

3. Gasoline expenses are determined by multiplying the price per gallon times the anticipated volume of gasoline used for the 25,000 miles. For example, 25,000 miles ÷ 18 mpg = 1,389 gallons per year times $1.70/gallon = $2,361.

4. The lost-opportunity cost, which is what the employee could have earned investing the money tied up in the cost of the vehicle in a secure mutual fund at 10% interest, i.e., $20,000 x 10% = $2,000.

The sum of the business portions for depreciation, insurance, general maintenance, licenses, gasoline, and lost-opportunity costs is $4,500 + $2,500 + $2,361 + $2,000 = $11,361. However, since 80% of the vehicle's use is for business purposes, one must multiply the $11,361 x 80% = $9,088 and then divide by the 20,000 business miles/year to determine that the cost per business mile is $0.45.

Employers may prefer that employees obtain their gasoline from the employer's pump, using the employer's credit card, or from specified fuel companies or service stations and then submit receipts for reimbursement. When the gas has been paid for in this manner, employees don't need to include the gasoline expense in the mileage compensation rate when calculating the per-mile cost. Without gasoline, the per-mile compensation rate falls to $0.34 per mile.

It is apparent from this exercise that, because of the high cost of depreciation, it could cost less per mile to operate used, low-mileage, less-expensive vehicles than it would to operate new, rapidly depreciating ones. This assumes, however, that the vehicle owner experiences no major expenses for repairs.

A CONTRACT CLAUSE FOR EMPLOYEES' USE OF EMPLOYER'S VEHICLES

The following contract clause addresses employee use of employer vehicles for business purposes:

Employer will provide insurance for Employer-owned vehicles at such dollar limits of coverage as Employer may from time to time establish. Gasoline required in connection with business use of Employer's vehicle shall be obtained from (Employer's pump?; specified service stations, i.e., Mobil?; via Employer's credit card?). Upon provision of appropriate gasoline receipts within one month of incurred expense, Employee will be reimbursed by Employer.

Employee is responsible for operating Employer's vehicle(s) in a manner that preserves its/their function and value and is acceptable to Employer. (Employee?, Employer?) is responsible for keeping vehicles supplied with gasoline and medical and surgical supplies at all times; ensuring that the vehicle is scheduled for oil changes and lubrications every (3,500?, 5,000?, 7,500?) miles; checking tires and tire pressure monthly, assuring that tires are rotated every (10,000?) miles; and informing Employer when replacements are needed, e.g., every (35,000?, 40,000?) miles; making appointments for engine tuneups every (30,000?, 50,000?, 75,000?) miles; attending to or seeing to it that repairs are made as soon as possible after the need arises; and maintaining the vehicle's external and internal condition so that it is presentable to clients. Damages to Employer's vehicle(s) up to a maximum of ($500? $1,000?, $1,500?) caused by Employee's negligence or inattentive driving not covered by Employer's insurance shall be the responsibility of Employee. Should Employee's driving or accident record lead to increases in Employer's auto insurance premiums, Employee will be held responsible for such increases.

In the event that Employee incurs and pays authorized vehicle expenses,

Employee will be reimbursed within one month of the provision of receipts.

It is Employer's policy that all occupants wear seatbelts and that Employee obey traffic laws regardless of circumstances. Employer's vehicles will be used for veterinary business purposes only and will be left at (Employer's practice site?, Employee's home?) when Employee is not on employment-related business. Employees who fail to comply with one or more of the vehicle policies established herein may be terminated for cause.

A CONTRACT CLAUSE FOR EMPLOYEES' USE OF THEIR OWN VEHICLES

If employees use their own automobiles for business-related activities, the following contract clause should be included in their employment agreements:

Employee will use Employee's own vehicle while providing services for Employer. Employee shall purchase liability insurance for said vehicle equal to or greater than that carried on business vehicles owned by Employer. Employer will reimburse Employee for (collision?, comprehensive,? and liability?) insurance expenses incurred on a per-mile basis depending on the percentage of time the vehicle is used for business purposes. Coverage in excess of the levels fixed by the practice will be the responsibility of the Employee. Employee must provide Employer with a certificate verifying the existence of insurance for Employee's vehicle prior to use for business purposes.

Employer will provide Employee with ($0.365, i.e., the amount allowed by the IRS? or $0.45, representing the previously calculated expense to the Employee?) per mile to cover all employee vehicle expenses including but not limited to vehicle depreciation, insurance, general maintenance, repairs, licenses, gasoline, and lost-opportunity costs. Employee agrees to submit detailed mileage reports to

Employer justifying the number of miles driven by the last day of each month for reimbursement by the 15th of the subsequent month. (Alternate language might state, "Upon provision of receipts verifying Employee's vehicle expenses, Employer will reimburse Employee within 10 work days for legitimate business use of Employee's vehicle at the rate of [$0.365, i.e., the amount allowed by the IRS? or $0.45, representing the previously calculated expense to the Employee?] per mile.")

Employee agrees to comply with Employer's veterinary business policies regarding the use of Employee's vehicle while serving the business interests of Employer by assuring that all occupants wear seatbelts and by obeying traffic laws regardless of circumstances. Employees who fail to comply with one or more of Employer's vehicle policies set forth herein may be terminated for cause.

HEALTH CLUB MEMBERSHIPS

Employers who provide opportunities for staff members to use employer-funded health club memberships as signing bonuses, Christmas gifts, or as a standard component of the benefits package can attract and retain health-conscious employees in a competitive job market and show employees that they are interested in their mental and physical well-being. Employees benefit by saving money, having a location at which they can socialize with fellow employees and other people outside the work environment, and having an outlet to reduce stress.

Health clubs can provide numerous services, including[11]

- personal trainers, who help individuals plan and accomplish fitness goals and use the facilities;

- nutritional consultants;

- aerobics classes;

- cardiovascular rooms, containing stationary bikes, stair masters, and treadmills;
- workout rooms, containing circuit machines and free weights;
- indoor/outdoor pools and running tracks;
- spas, whirlpools, saunas, and steam rooms;
- racquetball and tennis courts; and
- outdoor sun decks.

In determining the health club with which to affiliate, employers should check the types of services available, the individual and group rates, and the numbers and locations of facilities. It is best to consider health clubs with multiple locations because employees may prefer to exercise near their homes rather than near the practice. National-based clubs enable employees who travel distances for vacations or continuing education seminars to have access to health clubs at multiple destinations.

When considering the provision of health club memberships as an employment benefit, employers are advised to consult with their certified public accountants to ensure that there are no negative tax consequences for either party and to review the following options:

1. Standard benefit:

   Employers provide employees with access to employer's group health club membership after completion of the orientation and training period. Upon termination of employment, or if employees no longer care to belong, employers discontinue paying the additional membership dues.

2. Optional benefit:

   Employees interested in health club memberships can elect to forfeit certain compensation benefits, for example, two sick days per year, to participate in employer's health club. This salary savings will be applied toward employer's cost for employee's annual health club membership. If the dues are greater than the value of the employee's sick day(s), employers pay the difference. Giving this benefit option enables employers to offer every employee the benefit but only provide it to parties who are interested enough to contribute to its cost; encourages employees to stay physically fit and use fewer sick days each year; and provides different benefits for different employees.

3. Signing bonus:

   Employers provide new employees with access to employer's health club for one year as a signing bonus. Employees who value the membership and wish to continue a membership start paying the second year.

4. Holiday bonus:

   Rather than cash holiday bonuses, employers provide employees with the use of a health club membership for as long a period as the employees are employed at the practice, or on a quarterly, semiannual, or annual basis.

A CONTRACT CLAUSE FOR HEALTH CLUB MEMBERSHIPS

The following clause provides for the use of the employer's health club membership as a standard benefit to all employees:

To enhance Employee's physical and mental health, upon completion of the (60?, 90? day) orientation and training period, Employer will pay all costs to allow for Employee's use of Employer's health club membership at (name of club) for the remainder of the term of this Agreement or until Employee elects to discontinue such usage.

The following is a sample contract clause for health club memberships provided as an optional benefit to employees.

To enhance Employee's physical and mental health, upon completion of the (60?, 90? day) orientation and training period, Employee shall have the option of forfeiting (two?) sick days and apply-

ing this potential compensation toward the use of Employer's health club membership at (name of club). If dues are greater than the value of the Employee's (two?) sick days' compensation, Employer will pay the difference for the term of this Agreement or until Employee elects to discontinue the use of such club.

The following is a contract clause for the use of the employer's health club membership provided as a signing bonus to new employees.

To enhance Employee's physical and mental health and as a signing bonus to the Employee, Employer will pay the cost of Employee's use of Employer's health club membership at (name of club) for the term of this Agreement or until Employee elects to discontinue such membership.

CHILDCARE

If practice owners were to advertise, "Wanted, veterinary associates and support staff with children," one can only imagine what would happen to the number of job applicants. In 1980, 9.5% of veterinarians were women; by 1994, that percentage had increased to 28.7%. If things continue to progress at this rate, the number of female veterinarians will equal the number of male veterinarians by the year 2004.[12]

Only one contract in the authors' retrospective study included a provision for childcare benefits. The increasing number of women entering the veterinary profession is heightening the need for employer assistance with childcare. Childcare benefits in the form of childcare spending accounts, on-site childcare programs, and alliances with operators of childcare programs in the community soon may begin to appear in veterinary employment agreements and personnel policy manuals. Practice owners may well find that such provisions can provide leverage in hiring and retaining employees.

CHILDCARE SPENDING ACCOUNTS

Section 129 of the Internal Revenue Code states that employees can deposit a maximum of $2,500 per year of pretax wages into an employer-administered childcare spending account, thus allowing the use of pretax dollars to pay for childcare expenses.[13] If the childcare expenses ultimately exceed the money allocated to the childcare accounts, employees pay the difference from taxable, take-home income. Any extra money in the accounts at the end of the year, however, is forfeited to the employer.[14] Married couples filing joint tax returns may have one spouse place a maximum of $5,000 per year from wages into such an account.[10]

For example, a married employee works for an accounting firm in Plymouth Meeting, PA. This employee allocates $100 per week from her paycheck to a childcare spending account, totaling $5,000 annually. At the end of each month, the firm disburses the childcare funds to the employee. In the Plymouth Meeting area, weekly childcare expenses range from $120 to $150 per week, surpassing the $100 weekly allocation. The employee pays the $20 to $50 difference from her taxable, take-home income. Though the employee still has out-of-pocket childcare expenses at a taxable income rate of 30%, between FICA, medicare, federal and state taxes, this family saves $1,500.[11]

Certain restrictions apply in utilizing childcare spending accounts. First, the accounts only cover costs incurred in caring for children under the age of 13 or persons of any age who are physically or mentally handicapped. Second, the accounts are available only to those employees who need childcare while working. Third, an employee's spouse must be working as well. Fourth, childcare must be provided in state-licensed facilities. Finally, childcare expenses cannot exceed either the employee's or the spouse's income.[15]

ON-SITE OR NEAR-SITE PROGRAMS

Above and beyond childcare spending accounts, practice owners might consider establishing a state-certified program on or near their veterinary practices. Such programs can be funded by the employees' childcare accounts. Of course, this entails a commitment on the part of the practice owner to set up, oversee, and hire a director for such a facility.

On-site or near-site day care programs are feasible when practices have available space within or near their veterinary facilities. For example, the owner of a tire plant in Alabama established a childcare center in a three-bedroom house near the factory. The seven-day-a-week childcare center is funded by the employees in need of childcare.[16]

Employer-provided childcare programs are beneficial both to veterinary employers and employees. For employers, it enables quality personnel to work instead of staying home to care for children. Furthermore, employees are more readily available to work when called upon to substitute on relatively short notice. Employees benefit in that quality, dependable childcare is readily available, and transportation time and costs are minimized.

Standards for childcare programs are determined by state and local laws. Programs at veterinary practices may be exempt from state laws if only a few children are involved (usually up to six) and if the programs are located on the veterinary practice site. Most likely there will be several different types of programs regulated in your state.

As an example, there are four types of state-certified childcare programs in Pennsylvania: daycare centers, which provide care for 7 or more children; group daycare homes, delivering services for 7 to 12 children; family daycare homes, which provide care within state-certified family residences; and nursery schools, which are housed at part-time preschool facilities.

Pennsylvania veterinary practices that provide care for fewer than six children, then, would not qualify as daycare centers or group daycare homes. Neither would they qualify as family daycare homes or nursery school daycare centers. Thus, veterinary practices with childcare programs on the premises caring for no more than six children are not regulated by the state of Pennsylvania.[17] Nationwide, most veterinary practices that provide childcare will have fewer than six children and, therefore, like Pennsylvania, state regulations may not apply.

CREATING A DAYCARE PROGRAM

When creating programs, employers need to assess the number of children likely to participate to determine whether the program will be governed by state regulations and local zoning laws. Even if the program is exempt from state regulations, it is advisable to comply with state standards of care to minimize the potential for liability. If childcare programs deviate from state guidelines, they should meet at least some minimal criteria.

The first criterion is that daycare staff members be 18 years of age or older, have no criminal record, and have at least a high school, but preferably a college, diploma. Ideally, these individuals have a minimum of six months experience working with children, are first-aid certified, participate in annual fire-safety courses, and have annual physical exams.

A director appointed to manage the program collects fees; pays expenses; hires, supervises, and fires staff; plans daily activities and meal schedules for the children; and ensures that facilities are properly maintained. The director and staff members provide the children with activities that stimulate social, intellectual, emotional, and physical growth. The children are supervised at all times. Physical punishment or abusive language by child care employees is forbidden.

Appropriate staff:child ratios are strongly encouraged. Most states determine such ratios by the ages of the children. For example, in Pennsylvania, childcare centers must meet the following staff:child ratios:

- Infants (birth to 12 months)— a ratio of 1:4.

- Young toddlers (13 months to 24 months)—ratio of 1:5.

- Older toddlers (25 months to 36 months)— a ratio of 1:6.

- Preschoolers (37 months to entry into first grade)—a ratio of 1:10.

- Young school age children (first to third grade)— a ratio of 1:12.

- Older school age children (9 to 15 years old)—ratio of 1:15.[18]

Signed written agreements between parents and the childcare facility must be kept for each child. Included in these documents would be participation fees; time of payment; program services provided; parental responsibilities; names of individuals to whom the children can be released; the hours that the program will operate; emergency contact names; and the name, address, and telephone number of the child's physician.

Childcare staff must maintain facilities in a manner that minimizes health and safety risks to the children. Facilities should follow state guidelines strictly to ensure the children's safety and to limit liability.

To minimize program costs, parents can provide daily food and beverages for their children.[19] Parents can deliver food to directors or daycare staff at the time children are brought to the programs. For example, if a child is fed breakfast at home and stays at the program from 8:00 a.m. until 4:00 p.m., the parents would provide a mid-morning snack, lunch, and mid-afternoon snack. Moreover, parents can provide books, toys, and games for their children. To further ease the financial burden, the veterinary hospitals can provide first-aid supplies.

Before enrollment, children must have medical examinations and proof of immunizations for childhood diseases. Copies of these medical records should be kept on file at the child care facility. To limit liability, parents must be notified immediately if their children are injured or become sick. Telephone numbers for the nearest hospital, ambulance, police and fire departments, and poison control centers should be posted near the phones.

It is essential for practice owners to obtain comprehensive general liability insurance that covers their childcare programs and associated employees. Standard hospital liability packages do not cover such programs, so a consultation with one's insurance agent is mandatory.

Finally, children must be forbidden from visiting with clients' animals to eliminate the possibility of animal bites or transmittal of zoonotic diseases such as roundworms, hookworms, and giardia.

ALLIANCES WITH CHILDCARE PROGRAMS IN THE COMMUNITY

Rather than provide an on-site childcare program, employers may opt to establish alliances with operators of existing childcare programs in the community. If employers research and form alliances with quality childcare programs, employees save time and money. Moreover, since such alliances potentially provide the childcare facility with the business of multiple families, the facility operators may be more likely to accommodate employees' specific needs.

Veterinary employers should designate one employee to select the childcare program. This designee first obtains background information about employees' children, such as their ages and special medical needs. After reviewing the checklist for selecting a childcare program (Figure 7.1), the designee identifies the childcare programs in the community and interviews program operators to complete the checklist. The results are presented to partici-

1. Staff members

   ____treat children with respect and patience
   ____are able to meet children's developmental and emotional needs
   ____take time to discuss children's status and progress with parents
   ____practice good personal hygiene
   ____have previous experience or training working with children
   ____are present on a consistent basis, so that children see the same faces every day and feel secure

2. Facilities

   ____safe indoor and outdoor areas and equipment
   ____orderly, clean play areas
   ____airy rooms with bright colors
   ____sanitary bathrooms and diaper changing areas

3. Health and safety

   ____comfortable, stable temperatures during the summers and winters
   ____rounded table corners and other furniture safety features
   ____nontoxic play materials
   ____first aid kits
   ____healthy snacks and/or meals
   ____clean kitchen areas
   ____staff wash hands after using the restrooms and before meals and snacks
   ____separate cribs for infants and separate cots/mats for others
   ____cleaning materials and medicines are kept out of reach of children
   ____toys periodically sanitized, particularly with very young children

4. Program

   ____proper child:staff ratios   ____supervised rest time
   ____organized programs of activities   ____minimal, supervised TV
   ____adequate play materials   ____stories read
   ____sufficient educational materials   ____creative play

5. General

   ____a license or registration certificate from the appropriate state department
   ____rules clearly explained
   ____good behavior encouraged
   ____children allowed to get dirty naturally through play
   ____no children looking excluded
   ____lots of laughing, caring, and sharing
   ____other parents visiting
   ____HAPPY CHILDREN

   Ask these questions:
   - May I drop in anytime?
   - May I participate in program planning?
   - May I take part in special events and trips?
   - Will the hours during which the facility is open fulfill my needs as a working parent?
   - What are the hourly, daily, and monthly fees?
   - What does this include?
   - Is there a reduction in fee if my child is out sick?

Figure 7.1. A checklist for choosing a daycare program

- What happens if my child gets sick or injured at the center?
- Are the care givers trained in child development?
- What are the hiring procedures?
- How long have most staff members worked here?
- May I contact staff references?
- Is there a parents' group or program?
- Are there restrictions regarding who may pick up my child?

Ask yourself:
- Is the center conveniently located?
- Is it affordable?
- Do I feel comfortable with the care givers?
- Do I feel good watching my child play at this center?
- Does the center provide the "right fit" for my child and myself?

Set up a trial day when your child can join activities while you observe. And, finally, after your child begins attending:

_____drop in unannounced and visit regularly
_____leave emergency contact information with the care giver
_____set up two or three backup plans in case of your child's or your own illness

Figure 7.1. A checklist for choosing a daycare program (cont.)

pants, and a childcare program is selected. In the event that children's ages and needs vary, two programs might be chosen.

EMPLOYEE HOUSING

Employers who provide housing in lieu of a higher salary save money for themselves and their employees. Pursuant to Section 119 of the Internal Revenue Code, the value of housing is excluded from employees' gross incomes.[20] Consequently, employers make lower payments for social security, medicare, worker's compensation, and federal and state unemployment taxes, and employees pay lower social security, medicare, and federal and state taxes.

According to Section 119, housing is excluded from gross income only when three requirements are met: the housing is furnished on the business premises; the employer needs the employee to live onsite for the benefit of the practice; and onsite living is a condition of employment.[17]

Aside from paying less taxes, there are other benefits to employers having veterinarians live onsite. Such employees can attend to emergencies and hospitalized patients during the evenings and weekends. Live-in employees also are potentially available when on-call doctors need assistance with emergencies. And finally, employees' presence at the practice during evening hours improves security.

Additional savings for live-in employees include reductions in housing and transportation costs. This is particularly important to new graduates who have large educational debts and limited cash flow or liquid assets. It is a great help to them to avoid up-front housing expenses incurred when moving to new job locations, such as security deposits and initial telephone and utility setup fees, and to have no commuting costs.

On the other hand, housing employees can become problematic if they are irresponsible or not trustworthy. Employers who do not choose their live-in employees wisely face consequences similar to those encountered by landlords who house irresponsible tenants. To avoid untoward consequences, employers are advised to enter into written lease agreements with live-in employees.

Leases

Leases are established to minimize conflicts between parties. With this in mind, employers must ensure that leases address certain issues.

Leases must state that housing is a condition of employment; when employment is terminated, so is the lease agreement. Leases should specify the employer's (landlord's) and the employee's responsibilities. Written documentation clearly and specifically defining both parties' duties minimizes the potential for liability and ill will between parties.

To further minimize conflicts, leases should stipulate that both parties, together, complete a housing inspection checklist before employees move in and after they move out of the living quarters (Figure 7.2). Furthermore, leases should state that employers will comply with federal, state, and local housing laws. Employers also may wish to retain a security deposit as collateral in case employees damage the property. Finally, leases should indicate which party bears insurance costs such as fire, liability, accident, and theft insurance.

Employment Contracts and Job Descriptions

In addition to establishing lease agreements, the employment contract should include a clause explaining the housing benefit and job description, thereby accomplishing two objectives. First, employers can substantiate their tax breaks to the IRS. Second, by linking terms of employment with the terms of the lease agreement, employers safeguard themselves against wrongful eviction suits if they evict employees upon termination of employment.

A contract clause addressing these issues could read as follows:

Housing is furnished to Employee on the business premises of the Employer as a condition of employment during the term of this Agreement. In the event employment is terminated for any reason, the lease is terminated, and Employee must surrender the living quarters in the original condition immediately.

The contract also can state that misuse of the living quarters and/or conduct of the employee not in keeping with employer's business polices is/are grounds for termination of employment. This reinforces the benefit as a condition of employment and emphasizes to employees the consequences of such actions.

A CONTRACT CLAUSE FOR HOUSING

Employer and Employee agree that as a condition of employment, Employee shall reside in the apartment on Employer's premises so that Employee can be responsible for (1) providing evening and weekend observation and treatment of hospitalized patients, (2) overseeing the security of the building and safety of hospitalized patients, and (3) providing emergency care for patients when Employee is on emergency call or assistance for other doctors when they are on call.

Loans for New Employees

Because approximately three-quarters of new graduates have educational debt and, in many cases, insufficient liquid assets to enable them to move to distant job locations, employers often find it necessary to offer moving allowances or salary advances to attract top-quality candidates. It would be great if employers could help pay off the educational loans of young veterinarians they hire, but such payments cannot be made without being considered income to the

Employee's Name_____

Employer's Name_____

Description	Move-In Condition	Move-Out Condition
KITCHEN		
Light Fixtures		
Walls & Ceilings		
Cupboards		
Counter Surfaces		
Floor Coverings		
Sinks		
Faucets		
Garbage Disposal		
Stove & Oven (broiler pans, grills, etc.)		
Microwave Oven		
Range Hood-Fan/Light		
Refrigerator		
Dishwasher		
Sockets & Switches		
DINING ROOM		
Light Fixtures		
Walls & Ceilings		
Floor Coverings		
Sockets & Switches		
Window Blinds & Screens		
LIVING ROOM		
Walls & Ceilings		
Floor Coverings		
Sockets and Switches		
Window Blinds and Screens		
Doors		

Figure 7.2. Sample housing inspection checklist

Description	Move-In Condition	Move-Out Condition
BATHROOM		
Light Fixtures		
Walls & Ceilings		
Floor Coverings		
Cabinets		
Counter Surfaces		
Tub or Shower Enclosure		
Sinks		
Faucets		
Toilet		
Plumbing		
Doors		
Sockets & Switches		
BEDROOM #1		
Light Fixtures		
Walls & Ceilings		
Floor Coverings		
Window Blinds & Screens		
Closet Doors		
Doors		
Sockets & Switches		
BEDROOM #2		
Light Fixtures		
Walls & Ceilings		
Floor Coverings		
Window Blinds & Screens		
Closet Doors		
Doors		
Sockets & Switches		
MISCELLANEOUS		
Air Conditioning/Heating Equipment		

Figure 7.2. Sample housing inspection checklist (cont.)

Description	Move-In Condition	Move-Out Condition
Air Conditioning Filters		
Hot Water Heater		
Patio/Balcony		

Date of Move-In_____Date of Move-Out_____

Employee's Signature_____Employee's Signature_____

Employer's Signature_____Employer's Signature_____

Figure 7.2. Sample housing inspection checklist (cont.)

recipients. An alternative way to appeal to highly desirable veterinary candidates, office managers and, perhaps, veterinary technicians is to offer them short-term loans that enable them to accept jobs that otherwise would be financially impossible to accept.

The need for an advance on salary occurs, in part, because employees typically do not receive their first paychecks until two to four weeks after starting their new jobs. Short-term loans enable them to finance the up-front expenses associated with jobs in new locations, such as searching for housing, relocation costs, security deposits for apartments, deposits for phone and utilities; and time and financial costs required to acquire new auto and drivers licenses.

A story with a happy ending involves a first-year graduate from Mississippi State Veterinary Medical School who had no cash reserves because of the expenses he incurred during veterinary school and his wedding immediately after graduation. An employer in South Carolina offered him full-time employment, but he needed help financially to afford the move from Mississippi to South Carolina.

Rather than a salary advance, the employer made a $5,000 loan via a promissory note. This formalized agreement provided the employer financial security while enabling her associate to meet his financial responsibilities.

The repayment agreement in this situation entailed applying the quarterly production reconciliation compensation (see Chapter 3) in excess of the employee's base salary toward payment of the debt. If there was no surplus compensation at the end of two consecutive quarters, the associate was required to pay $1,000 towards the debt out of his base salary. Fortunately, with this as an incentive, the associate generated sufficient income in excess of his base salary to repay the loan in full within the first 24 months of employment. Had he not done so, he would have had to authorize his employer to deduct payments directly from his monthly salary checks or receive his base compensation on schedule but make payments back to his employer on a monthly basis.

There are numerous advantages to providing new employees with loans. For employers, offering loans can

- expand the number of viable candidates, including graduates from a wider variety of schools.

- persuade quality applicants to accept employment.

- promote loyalty from employees hired.

Additionally, employers who are over-joyed with their choices have the option of forgiving these loans and, in effect, converting them to bonuses for worthy employees.

Loans are advantageous to employees because they

- ease the financial burden created when moving from distant locations.

- enable employees to settle into their new locations with fewer difficulties and diminished stress.

- can be repaid with monthly or quarterly production reconciliation compensation, thus avoiding the pain of writing checks to employers while worrying about whether they will have sufficient funds to cover payments that are due.

The negative possibilities for employers who provide loans include

- nonpayments from employees with poor financial management skills.

- nonpayments due to a death, disability, resignation, or unexpected hardship experienced by an employee.

- a negative impact on an employer-employee relationship because an employer is aware of an employee's lifestyle and resents nonpayment of the loan.

- termination of employment prior to completion of the loan repayment.

- complaints or lawsuits for discrimination from other employees who were not offered equivalent loan benefits.

Because of the potential negative consequences when furnishing loans to new employees, employers are urged to offer this benefit equitably and to use formal loan agreements to formalize the process and protect themselves.

Written Loan Agreements

Employers providing loans for new employees are urged to use promissory notes. These are signed documents promising employers/lenders the repayment of a specific sum of money. Issues to be addressed in such notes include:

1. Loan amounts: Loans for new employees typically range from $1,000 to $5,000. To comply with IRS rules, employers must deduct payroll taxes from these direct loan repayments by employers because forgiveness of debt in this fashion constitutes income to the employee.

2. Interest rates: Interest rate options include: (a) no interest if repaid in full within (three?, four?, six?) months of the commencement of employment, provided that any portion not repaid within the specified time period shall become due in monthly installments thereafter with interest payable on the unpaid balance at a rate of 6% per year or (b) interest to be paid on outstanding balances at a more realistic 8% to 12% per year, commencing with the first monthly installment.

3. Repayment terms: To ease the pain of the first few months of tight budgets, repayment could start the second, third, or fourth month after the commencement of employment. Providing a short grace period like this enables employees to use their monthly salaries to pay current bills while saving for their upcoming monthly loan installments. The repayment term could range from as low as three months for small loans to as long as two to three years for bigger ones.

4. Repayment plans: Repayment options include (a) authorization for employers to deduct installments from payroll checks, (b) consents for employers deducting installments from monthly or quarterly production reconciliation bonuses, (c) employees receiving formal monthly billing from employers and making timely payments, or (d) an informal arrangement wherein employees voluntarily repay as much as they can on a monthly basis.

5. Delinquent payments: If employers do not receive payments from employees within 10 days of the monthly due date, a surcharge of 5% of the amount due can be added as a delinquency fee, just as banks do with mortgages.

6. Defaults: Borrowers should be considered in default if they fail to pay any part of the principal or interest when due and if continuance of such failure persists for 30 days. In these situations the entire balance should be due immediately.

7. Termination of employment prior to completion of repayment: To protect employers in these situations, contracts or promissory notes can stipulate that employers have the right to withhold unpaid debt from employees' final paychecks. This sounds like the perfect answer, but employers should be aware that this constitutes garnishment of wages and may be used only for its psychological rather than its legal value. In states where garnishment is allowed, wages may be withheld in this manner only with a court order. In other states, garnishment of wages is prohibited. Thus, veterinarians who provide loans for associates are urged to contact local legal counsel before invoking this remedy.

A SAMPLE PROMISSORY NOTE

,200__

1. For Value Received, (Employee's name), of (Employee's home address), hereinafter referred to as "Borrower," promises to pay to the order of (Employer or Veterinary Practice Name) of (Employer's Address), hereinafter referred to as "Lender," the principal sum of ($1,000.00?, $5,000.00?).

2. During the term of this Note, the interest rate shall be (6%?, 8?, 10%?, 11%?, 12%) each year. The interest rate shall be effective commencing the (first?, second?, third?, sixth?) month of employment and until full payment of the Note.

3. Commencing on the_____day of 200__, and continuing on the_____day

of each month thereafter, Borrower shall pay Lender installments of principal and interest in the sum of ($250?, $500?) until_____,200__, when the full amount of unpaid principal and all accrued interest shall be due and payable. Borrower reserves the right to make prepayments of principal in whole or in part at any time without penalty.

4. Should Lender not receive any payment within 10 days of the due date, Borrower shall pay Lender an additional 5% of any such payment owed as a delinquency payment. The failure of Borrower to pay any part of the principal or interest on this Note when due and payable and the continuance of such failure for 30 days shall constitute a default by Borrower, in which case the entire balance is due and payable immediately.

5. In the event Borrower's employment is terminated prior to completion of repayment, Lender has the right to withhold any monies due on the note from Borrower's final paycheck. If the loan is greater than the final paycheck, the balance is due and payable immediately.

6. This Note may be changed or amended only by an agreement in writing signed by the party against whom enforcement of any waiver, change, modification, or discharge is sought.

7. Borrower agrees to pay all costs and expenses, including, without limitation, attorneys' fees at any time paid or incurred by Lender in collecting this indebtedness or any part thereof.

8. If any clause, sentence, part, or provision of this Note is for any reason invalid, no other clause, sentence, part, or provision shall be affected or deemed invalid thereby.

9. This Note shall be construed and enforced in accordance with, and the rights of the parties shall be governed by, the laws of the State/Commonwealth of _____

Date _____

Lender's Signature_____

Address _____

(City, State)_____

Borrower's Signature _____

Address _____

*(City, State)*_____

Conclusion

There are many options to improving the overall compensation package for employed professionals. Some of these are tax-free benefits, many create tax-deductible expenses for employers without producing taxable income for employees, and others simply show a great deal of care and concern for the personal and financial success of one's employees. If the growing shortage of veterinarians in the United States continues, including some or all of these benefits may provide ways for employers to improve the likelihood of acquiring their number one candidate.

References

1. Wilson J, Nemoy JD: Retrospective study of veterinary employment contracts. Yardley, PA, 1987-1998. Because of the nature of local MVAs, variable timing of their dues payment requirements, relatively low cost, and lack or reporting of such payments, it is possible and likely that employers paid local VMA dues at a higher percentage than indicated by the contracts reviewed by the authors.

2. Digest of Veterinary Practice Acts. *AVMA Membership Directory and Resource Manual.* Schaumberg, IL, pp 304,312, 1996.

3. Title 21 CFR Statute 1301.24.

4. Eubanks D: Veterinarians at risk. *Intervet* 31(1):9, Fall 1995.

5. Personal contact with Dr. Jack Stephens, President, Veterinary Pet Insurance, ph. 800-USA-PETS, during July of 1998.

6. Wise KJ: Employment, starting salaries, and educational indebtedness of 1998. *JAVMA*: 214(4):488-490, 1999.

7. Gehrke B: The information exchange, employment, starting salaries, and educational indebtedness of 1997 graduates of US veterinary medical colleges. *JAVMA*: 211(12): 1520, 1997 and *JAVMA*: 220(2): 179-181, 2002.

8. Personal advice and consultation with Catherine Cowling, June 1998.

9. Ott J: Personal consultation, Greencastle, PA, 1996.

10. Stuber R: Personal consultation, Annville, PA, 1996.

11. Kanzinger B: Personal consultation, Oxford Valley, PA, 1996.

12. Gehrke B: Information exchange. Gender redistribution in the veterinary medical profession. *JAVMA_*208(8): 1254, 1996.

13. Internal Revenue Code, §129.

14. Fegley B: Personal communication, Fegley & Associates, Plymouth, PA, 1997.

15. *Introduction to Group Insurance*: USA, Dearborn Financial Publishing, Inc, 1993, p 89.

16. Shellenbarger S: Jo Browning built a child-care agenda into a factory's plan. *Wall St J*:1997.

17. Laumer C: Personal communication, Dept Public Welfare, PA, 1997.

18. *Child Care Is Everybody's Business. A Guide for Parents Selecting Child Care.* Dept Public Welfare, Philadelphia, PA, 1997.

19. Prior M: Personal communication with long term operator of a home day care center, Maplewood, NJ, 1997.

20. Internal Revenue Code, §119 (7222.015).

Chapter 8

RETIREMENT BENEFITS

By Alan Fishman, CLU, CFP®

During the 1960s, 70s, and 80s, the American workforce enjoyed a generous retirement plan package, the federal government's social security program was secure, and an inflationary period brought extra dollars to those who sold their homes to supplement existing savings in retirement. As we approach the 21ˢᵗ century, it is an entirely different scenario. So what has changed?

Today, many employer-funded retirement plans have been replaced with employee-funded programs, thus shifting the cost of retirement from employers to employees. Demographic changes have put great pressure on the social security system's ability to deliver promised benefits. And home sales no longer generate the hefty profits seen only a decade ago. Moreover, as advancements in medical care have improved the quality of our lives, people find themselves living longer into retirement, with increasingly costly investments for health care. The good news is that a healthy 62 year old is likely to live to age 85. The bad news is that living a third of one's life in retirement has forced people to begin saving sooner and reconsider the extent to which their savings need to be increased to retire comfortably.

SOURCES OF RETIREMENT INCOME

To retire comfortably, most financial planners agree that one's annual income in retirement will need to approximate 55% to 70% of the retiree's preretirement income. One of the major issues young veterinarians face today is to plan for and determine the source of that retirement savings.

Today, there are three primary sources of retirement income: social security, personal savings and investments, and corporate or individual retirement plans. A fourth source, cash value life insurance, can be a significant contributor if the death benefit for which the coverage was purchased is no longer needed. A fifth source, money from family inheritances, often is unavailable and almost always is unpredictable. Refer to Figure 8.1 for a comparison of how sources of retirement income are projected to change over time.

With social security, a common misconception is that payroll taxes contributed today by employees and employers are set aside to fund the contributing worker's future retirement. In reality, these contributions are benefiting the workers in retire-

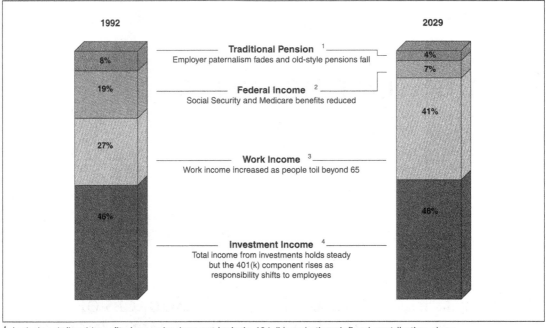

¹ Includes defined-benefit plans only; does not include 401 (k) and other defined-contribution plans.
² Assumes 50% cut in Social Security and Medicare/Medicaid benefits by 2009.
³ Assumes no increase in real wages.
⁴ Includes interest earned on all capital, including defined-contribution plans, annuities, IRAs, and market value of rent on owner-occupied residences.
FORTUNE estimates based on data calculated by Laurence Kotlikoff and Alan J. Auerbach for EBRI and Merrill Lynch.

FORTUNE   August 19, 1996"

Figure 8.1. How you'll pay for retirement

ment now, and there is a major concern with that. Between 1990 and 2030, the number of Americans over age 65 is expected to double, yet the working population is expected to grow by only 25%. When today's baby boomers begin to retire in the 21st century, the workforce therefore may be unable to support this mass exodus to retirement.

Assume for the moment, however, that the social security system remains strong and is capable of delivering on its promise. The higher one's preretirement income, the less that person's social security benefit will contribute as a percentage of total income in retirement. Moreover, much of today's social security benefit is likely to be received as taxable income. Depending on one's postretirement income, as much as 85% of that income could be subject to fed-eral income taxes. With social security likely to contribute a limited percentage of one's retirement income, only personal savings or inheritance, individual or corporate retirement plans, and/or cash value life insurance remain from the original five options.

OBSTACLES TO SAVING

With a heightened awareness of the need to save and the proliferation of new personal finance magazines on the market, it is reasonable to assume that Americans would take the necessary steps to plan for a comfortable retirement. Unfortunately, this is not true. According to a June 1990 study prepared by the United States Department of Health and Human Services, for every 100 people beginning their careers, the following situation exists at age 65: 25 are dead, 20 have annual incomes of less than $6,000, 51 have annual incomes between $6,000 and $35,000, and only 4 have annual incomes in excess of $35,000.

Why is this? According to the Organization for Economic Cooperation and Development, Americans on average save only 4.6% of their after-tax income (1993). This compares unfavorably to other nations: Italy at 16.8%, Japan at 15%, France at 14.1%, Germany at 12.3%, United Kingdom at 12.2%,

and Canada at 9.2%. As a rule of thumb, Americans need to save somewhere in the neighborhood of 10% to 15% of their salaries each year to meet their retirement income objectives. The exact percentage depends on the factors illustrated in Table 8.1.

There are many theories as to why it is so difficult for Americans to save. The most common reasons given include procrastination and the desire to maintain an expensive lifestyle, or "keeping up with the Jones." With the myriad products and services available in our society, from $1,000 big-screen TVs, to $40,000 sport utility vehicles, to

Table 8.1. Retirement? Go Figure

Workers covered by pensions don't have to save as much for retirement as workers who aren't. Here's how much of your salary you might have to save each year to have an old-age income equal to 80% of your final pay, assuming you live until 90 and start your fund from scratch.

Earnings	To retire at 65, save this percent of salary starting at:*			
	Age 25	35	45	55
$30,000				
With Pension]	0.7%	0.5%	0%**	0%**
Without Pension]]	8.5%	13.5%	23.4%	51.0%
$60,000				
With Pension]	1.9%	2.7%	4.1%	7.2%
Without Pension]]	9.8%	15.7%	28.0%	63.5%
$100,000				
With Pension]	3.0%	4.8%	8.2%	17.8%
Without Pension]]	10.9%	17.8%	32.1%	74.1%
$150,000				
With Pension]	3.6%	5.8%	10.3%	23.1%
Without Pension]]	11.4%	18.8%	34.2%	79.5%

* Assuming 3.5% inflation, a 7.5% after-tax return on investments, and social security at 1% less than inflation.

] Traditional pension at 50% of final salary with cost-of-living increase.

** Pension and social security cover you in full.

]] Including plans like 401(k)s. Includes any contributions your business or employer makes.

Source: *Newsweek*, December 16, 1996, p.54

$120 sneakers, and $4-per-pound prewashed lettuce, temptations are great. Establishing the discipline to save is difficult. In one's 20s, retirement is a distant consideration. When people enter their 30s, family obligations are paramount. As the mid life 40s approach, college costs for children gut the budget. In the 50s, the need to catch up may be so great that consideration of retirement is postponed. And in the 60s it is too late.

As shown by the profile of two individuals and their saving habits in Table 8.2, procrastination brings with it a hefty price, even without the cumulative detriment of inflation. Over the past 20 years, consumer prices have increased on average 6% per year, eroding close to two thirds of the dollar's purchasing power. To ensure a comfortable retirement, people need to keep up with inflation just to stay even.

Saving for retirement is no easy task given the myriad expenses that families incur, but one thing is clear. With social security likely to account for a relatively small percentage of a retiree's postretirement income, and given that many people are unable to save considerable amounts on their own, the probability that veterinarians will retire comfortably may depend on whether they choose to adopt a good retirement plan.

RETIREMENT PLANS

Retirement plans, often referred to as *qualified plans*, are programs that provide for tax-deductible contributions and tax-deferred growth on accumulated balances. These plans adhere to strict minimum IRS and Department of Labor guidelines, benefiting all employees equally. In essence this means that practice owners cannot discriminate in favor of themselves or a selected few employees. For employees, the funds afford the opportunity for contributions and tax-deferred growth. Benefits to practice owners include the following business advantages:

- attract qualified veterinarians and other employees
- reward loyal employees
- motivate employees to stay with an employer on a long-term basis
- provide retirement security to practice owners and employees

The tax advantages to practice owners and participants include the following:

- contributions are tax deductible when made
- money accumulates tax deferred until it is withdrawn at retirement
- participants are not taxed when the money is contributed, only when it is distributed from the plan

Tax-deductible contributions and tax-deferred growth are the two major reasons to implement a retirement plan. Tax-deductible contributions are treated like all other practice expenses. They are deducted from earned income, which means the government is picking up the costs for a portion of the contribution.

Consider this example: A corporate veterinary practitioner with a net income of $50,000 will pay approximately $15,500 in federal income taxes (assuming an S Corporation status in which profits "flow through" to a practice owner who is in the 31% bracket). With a retirement contribution of $20,000, net income drops to $30,000 and federal income taxes decrease to $9,300 ($30,000 x 31%). In short, a contribution of $20,000 will help reduce taxes in excess of $6000! The real cost, then, to put $20,000 into a retirement plan is only $13,800 (the $20,000 contributed less the $6200 in tax savings). In essence, the government contributed $6200 of the $20,000!

Once money has been contributed to the plan, there are no federal, state, or local income taxes assessed on the money's growth via capital gains, interest, or dividends. Generally speaking, such advantages are not available to other types of invest-

Table 8.2. The Price of Procrastination

The Earlier Compounding Begins, the More Your Money Can Grow

Age	Cumulative Investment of Investor #1	Total Value at 10% Annual Return	Cumulative Investment of Investor #2	Total Value at 10% Annual Return
36	$2,000	$2,200		
37	4,000	4,620		
38	6,000	7,282		
39	8,000	10,210		
40	10,000	13,431		
41	12,000	16,974		
42	14,000	20,872		
43	16,000	25,159		
44	18,000	29,875		
45	20,000	35,062		
46		38,569	$2,000	$2,200
47		42,425	4,000	4,620
48		46,668	6,000	7,282
49		51,335	8,000	10,210
50		56,468	10,000	13,431
51		62,115	12,000	16,974
52		68,327	14,000	20,872
53		75,159	16,000	25,159
54		82,675	18,000	29,875
55		90,943	20,000	35,062
56		100,037	22,000	40,769
57		110,041	24,000	47,045
58		121,045	26,000	53,950
59		133,149	28,000	61,545
60		146,464	30,000	69,899
61		161,110	32,000	79,089
62		177,222	34,000	89,198
63		194,944	36,000	100,318
64		214,438	38,000	112,550
65		235,882	40,000	126,005
	$20,000	$235,882	$40,000	$126,005

Even if you invested twice as much for twice as long, you can never catch up! That's the price you may pay if you procrastinate starting your IRA.

ments. Income earned or gains realized outside a retirement plan are taxed annually. Consider the following example, which dramatizes the benefits of tax-deferred investing and highlights the differences between retirement plan contributions and bonuses.

James Abbott, VMD is the sole shareholder of Optimal Care Veterinary Hospital. The practice has just experienced a second successive good financial year and he is considering a year-end bonus of $20,000 to himself. He expects that the practice will have sufficient cash flow in the future to continue such bonuses until he is ready for retirement. Discounting the fact that if he implemented a corporate retirement plan he'd need to contribute for other employees in his practice, and focusing solely on the difference to Dr. Abbott, here is how the numbers stack up:

Assuming the entire balance in the plan were distributed in Year 1 of retirement (an unlikely scenario which would place the professional in the highest tax bracket) and a 36% tax bracket (again an unlikely scenario if we assume one's tax bracket will be lower in retirement), the after-tax balance of $632,613 would far exceed the $508,828 accumulated on bonuses. Not factored into this example is the temptation to spend a bonus on incidentals during one's life. Unlike a retirement plan that places strict rules on the withdrawal of contributed money prior to age 59½, a bonus has no such restriction and, therefore, is a more likely source to tap when money is needed.

Tax-deductible contributions and tax-deferred growth are common to all qualified retirement plans. There are many types of plans from which to choose, though, each with its own set of rules,

	Money Placed in a Retirement Plan	Money Paid as a Bonus
Amount contributed	$20,000	$20,000
Taxes—assuming 31%	0	6,200
Balance to invest	$20,000	$13,800
Return on investment assumed	8% gross	5.52% net after taxes
Accumulation—20 years	$988,458	$508,828
Net of taxes at time of withdrawal assuming 36% tax rate	$632,613	probably already spent

A bonus of $20,000 will be subject to taxes. Assuming an annual tax bracket of 31%, and ignoring state and local taxes which would only further dramatize the difference, Dr. Abbott would receive a check for $13,800. If that money were invested at an 8% rate of return, he'd need to pay taxes on the earnings, resulting in a net interest rate of 5.52%. If, however, the $20,000 were instead contributed to a retirement plan, the entire $20,000 would go to work. Earnings on the money would grow tax deferred until they were withdrawn.

advantages, and disadvantages.

Types of Plans

Retirement plans generally fall into two categories, defined contribution or defined benefit. A defined contribution plan specifies the contribution to be made in the program, e.g., Dr. Jasper decides that the practice will contribute a percentage of each person's salary to the plan. Alternatively, a defined benefit plan defines the benefit at retirement, e.g., in Dr. Henkels' practice, eligible employees retire on a percentage of their final year's salary irrespective of the contribution needed to fund this requirement.

Defined contribution plans include profit sharing plans, money purchase pension plans, and 401(k) programs. (Note: profit sharing and pension plans for self-employed professionals are sometimes referred to as *KEOGH Plans*).

A simplified employee pension plan, or SEP, is a popular type of retirement plan and is similar in many respects to a profit sharing plan. It is neither a defined contribution nor defined benefit plan, but is governed by many of the same rules that apply to an individual retirement account (IRA).

The plan design that is most appropriate for a particular veterinary practice depends on certain factors, including

- identifying the primary beneficiaries,

- the extent to which these primary beneficiaries wish to benefit,

- the practice's cash flow, and

- the ages and salaries of employees.

The best choice is identified only after considering these issues. The various types of plans are detailed further below and are illustrated by a hypothetical veterinary practice situation. Refer to Figure 8.2 for a family tree of retirement plans.

PROFIT SHARING PLANS

Profit sharing plans are the most popular type of retirement plans. In contrast to pension plans, contributions to such plans are not mandatory. This means that practice owners can make maximum contributions in good years and skip or decrease contributions in years when cash flow is down. IRS rules require that overall tax-deductible contributions cannot exceed 25% of covered payroll, with individual maximums capped at 100% of pay or $40,000 (2003 limit), whichever is less. Consider this example:

Dr. Fisher is thinking of implementing a profit sharing plan for the practice. Total practice salaries for all eligible employees equal $200,000. Dr. Fisher's salary is projected to be $80,000 for the current year. What is the most she can contribute to the profit sharing plan? Assuming the practice is incorporated, the maximum contribution for all eligible employees is $50,000 ($200,000 x 25%), with no more than $40,000 allocated to Dr. Fisher's personal account.

While the 25% limit on total plan contributions is true of all profit sharing plans, the allocation among eligible employees will vary predicated on the type of profit sharing plan chosen. The following discussion considers each type in more detail.

TRADITIONAL PROFIT SHARING PLANS

These plans divide employers' annual contributions among participants as a uniform percentage of pay. They treat all employees identically, with no favorable treatment for practice owners or other professionals.

INTEGRATED PROFIT SHARING PLANS

Integrated plans allow more of the employer's contribution to be directed to those whose earnings exceed a minimum amount, called the integration level, not to exceed the current year's Social Security Taxable Wage Base ($87,000 in 2003). In favoring those whose salaries exceed this integration level, this plan design benefits owners and other highly compensated professionals more than others in the practice.

AGE-WEIGHTED PROFIT SHARING PLANS

These plans allow employers to allocate more of the practice's contribution to older employees who are closer to retirement age and less to younger employees who have more time to save for retirement. They

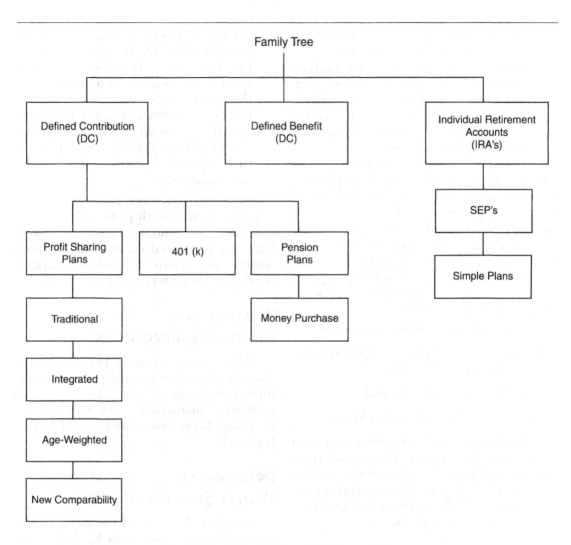

Figure 8.2. A Family Tree of Retirement Plans

work well in practices whose owners are older than the workforce. They may not be ideal, though, for practices with owners of disparate ages, e.g., owners whose ages are 62 and 38, who would like to receive equal contributions to their retirement plans.

NEW COMPARABILITY PROFIT SHARING PLANS

This relatively new plan design gives employers the flexibility to define groups of employees and to allocate contributions differently to each group provided that it can be "definitely determinable" under IRS rules. This differs slightly from the age-weighted plans above in that contributions are based on salary, age, and group classification in this type of plan. For example, one practice can decide to place owners in Group 1 and all other employees in Group 2. Another practice can decide to place senior practitioners in Group 1, junior practitioners in Group 2, technicians and senior receptionists in Group 3, and veterinary assistants and kennel or stable help in Group 4.

Most of the plans in existence today fall into the traditional and integrated profit sharing groups, Types 1 and 2 above. Plan Types 3 and 4, where applicable, may materially impact participant contributions by allocating a larger portion of annual profit sharing contributions to those most responsible for the success of the business. It is important to note, however, that there are rules in determining the allocation to participants under plan Types 3 and 4. Although contributions are predicated on salary, age, and job classification, the IRS and Department of Labor impose additional guidelines on the extent to which plans can allocate contributions among their participants. This is done so that plans cannot unfairly discriminate against certain participants or groups of employees.

To understand the four types of profit sharing plans, it is appropriate to discuss a hypothetical practice and consider their options via a case example.

A Case Study

Dr. Katz, whose practice is incorporated, wishes to implement a retirement plan for himself and his employees. Because he knows that business expenses and the practice's net income are likely to fluctuate each year, though, he does not want to be committed to contributing to the plan on an annual basis. He wants to contribute when profits permit. He also wishes to maximize contributions to himself. A census of employees and their ages and salaries follows in Example 8.1.

An age-weighted plan would appear to benefit Dr. Katz most. After all, he is older than his employees. And although Ms. Nelson is 52, her salary is considerably lower than Dr. Katz's and, therefore, should not materially affect the allocated contributions. Let's look at the available options in Example 8.2.

The traditional plan allocates a uniform 25% of each participant's salary to the plan. The integrated plan has increased Dr. Katz's contribution slightly, since his salary is greater than those of the other employees; all other contributions have been reduced. As can be seen, there is little difference between these two types of plans. Dr. Katz's contribution as a percentage of the total contribution only increased from 37% to 39%.

With the third type of plan, though, the age-weighted plan, Dr. Katz's percentage increases from 39% to a whopping 63%! Dr. Katz was able to allocate close to 43% of his salary to his account (and reach the maximum $40,000 in 2003), approximately 49% to Ms. Nelson, and much less to the others. Why were Dr. Katz and Ms. Nelson able to allocate more? In addition to salary, the age-weighted plan allows the calculation of contributions to be based on age. Since Ms. Nelson and Dr. Katz are older and closer to retirement than the other employees, their contributions are favorably affected.

If Dr. Katz wished to reduce the practice's overall contribution to the plan, he could do

Name	Age	Position	Salary
Dr. Katz	59	older professional	$95,000
Dr. Fox	35	younger professional	$65,000
Ms. Jones	26	veterinary technician	$26,000
Ms. Alan	25	veterinary technician	$24,000
Ms. Smith	22	veterinary assistant	$20,000
Ms. Nelson	52	receptionist	$25,000
			$255,000

Example 8.1. Census of Employees

	Traditional	Integrated	Age-weighted	New Comparability
Dr. Katz (59)	$23,750	$24,943	$40,000	$40,000
Dr. Fox (35)	16,250	16,659	7,914	3,250
Ms. Jones (26)	6,500	6,062	1,519	1,300
Ms. Alan (25)	6,000	5,595	1,292	1,200
Ms. Smith (22)	5,000	4,663	843	1,000
Ms. Nelson (52)	6,250	5,828	12,182	1,250
Totals	63,750	$63,750	$63,750	$48,000
% to Dr. Katz	37%	39%	63%	83%

Example 8.2. Profit Sharing Plan Comparison
(Class 1 in new comparability plan includes Dr. Katz only)

so by choosing the fourth type of plan, the new comparability plan. With this plan, Dr. Katz is able to place employees in classes based on the title of their positions in the practice, thus benefitting those employees in Class 1. If he were to place himself in Class 1 and all others in Class 2, he could contribute close to 43% of his pay to the plan (83% of the total), with only a 5% contribution for all others, including Ms. Nelson.

The new comparability plan design affords practice owners a great deal of flexibility, assuming the group classifications selected are properly set up so that the plan passes IRS-established testing guidelines. If Dr. Katz wishes to reward all veterinarians by including both himself and Dr. Fox in Class 1, though, and all others in Class 2, contributions would be calculated as shown in Example 8.3.

As can be seen through these hypotheticals, considerable flexibility exists in retirement plans for those practitioners who become educated on this subject and plan for their retirement as well as that of their staff.

	Traditional	Integrated	Age-weighted	New Comparability
Dr. Katz (59)	$23,750	$24,943	$40,000	$35,031
Dr. Fox (35)	16,250	16,659	7,914	23,969
Ms. Jones (26)	6,500	6,062	1,519	1,300
Ms. Alan (25)	6,000	5,595	1,292	1,200
Ms. Smith (22)	5,000	4,663	843	1,000
Ms. Nelson (52)	6,250	5,828	12,182	1,250
Totals	63,750	$63,750	$63,750	$63,750
% to Class 1	63%	65%	75%	93%

Example 8.3. Profit Sharing Plan Comparison
(Class 1 in new comparability plan includes Drs. Katz and Fox)

ADDITIONAL TERMS AND CONCEPTS

No discussion of profit sharing plans would be complete without addressing several additional terms common to all plans. They are as follows:

- eligibility: Generally speaking, owners may exclude employees under the age of 21 and/or anyone whose term of service is less than one year. Under certain circumstances, owners may exclude employees with less than two years of service; refer to the vesting explanation below for details.

- full time versus part time: Full-time employees are those who work in excess of 1000 hours a year; part timers are those who work less. Generally, part timers can be excluded from retirement plans.

- vesting: The vested portion of retirement savings is that portion of the business's contribution to the participant that is paid to an employee at termination.

When eligibility is restricted to employees who have at least one year of service, there are two vesting schedules commonly used, the graded vest and the cliff vest. With a graded vesting schedule, 20% of each participant's balance vests with the employee after three years of service, 40% after four years, and so on until the employee is 100% vested in Year 7. With a cliff vesting schedule, no portion of the employee's balance is vested until the conclusion of five years of service, when vesting is 100%.

Vesting schedules can be more favorable than this but cannot be more restrictive. Upon termination of employment, only the vested portion of each participant's balance is paid to the employee. Any nonvested portion can be reallocated to remaining participants

(a nice reward for long-term employees) or used to offset employer costs such as employer contributions and/or administrative costs.

For owners who decide to use the two-year eligibility rule, all contributions immediately vest with the employees, i.e., there is no vesting schedule.

- top-heavy plans: When account balances for certain key employees total more than 60% of a plan's total account balance, the plan is deemed top heavy. In such cases, employers may be required to contribute additional amounts to employees. Also, vesting is accelerated so that the graded schedule vests entirely in six years instead of seven, and the cliff schedule entirely vests in three years rather than five.

SIMPLIFIED EMPLOYEE PENSION PLANS (SEPs)

Despite the descriptive name of this retirement plan type, a simplified employee pension plan (SEP) is not a pension plan. In fact, it more closely resembles a profit sharing plan. Like the types previously discussed, employers are permitted to make nondiscriminatory contributions on behalf of their employees. Unlike the plans above, contributions are made to each employee's IRA. From the employer's perspective, there are advantages and disadvantages.

First, the advantages: If employers wish to restrict participation in the program, they can do so by excluding employees not employed by the practice three out of five years.

The disadvantages: Part timers, those who earn only the indexed amount of $450 a year in 2003, cannot be excluded, and all contributions immediately vest with the employee from day one! This type of plan is well suited for consultants/solo practitioners with few or no employees or small practices looking for simple plans with no administrative costs.

Pension Plans

Pension plans generally provide for either a fixed or defined contribution during one's working years, or a fixed benefit at retirement. The money purchase is an example of the first type; the defined benefit plan is an example of the second type.

Money Purchase Plans

Up until 2002, money purchase plans were a popular choice for practice owners wanting higher contribution limits than those offered with profit sharing plans. While profit sharing plans permitted maximum contributions equal to 15% of covered practice payroll, money purchase pension plans allowed maximum contributions equal to 25% of covered payroll. Though the pension plan offered higher limits, the trade-off was flexibility. Once the formula, or percentage of pay, was established under a pension plan (i.e., a practice decides to contribute 8% of employee compensation each year into the plan), the contribution was required to be made each year.

In 2002, though, new pension legislation eliminated the main advantage the pension plan held over the profit sharing plan. The Economic Growth and Tax Relief Reconciliation Act of 2001, known as "EGTRRA", increased the maximum contribution limit for profit sharing plans from 15% to 25%. Therefore, veterinarians looking for maximum contributions of 25% need not subject themselves to the mandatory contributions required under a pension plan. Both plans offer the same maximum contribution of 25% of covered payroll but only the profit sharing plan design provides the flexibility in contributions. Those veterinarian-owners with existing pension plans may wish to consider the benefits of converting their plan design to a profit sharing plan. For veterinarian-owners seeking to adopt a new retirement plan, a profit sharing plan is now the better choice.

Defined Benefit Plans

With defined benefit plans, employers can specify the benefit each participant will receive at retirement. Benefits at retirement can be based on the following actuarially determined approaches: fixed dollar amount, percentage of salary, or length of service. Benefits cannot exceed the lesser of 100% of compensation or $160,000 (2003). Disadvantages include the following:

- cost – particularly as "nonowner" participants approach retirement

- liability – employer is contractually obligated to provide the guaranteed retirement benefits

- complexity – administration, in addition to reporting and disclosure, is more complicated

Defined benefit plans are most suitable for stable, well-established professional practices that wish to favor older or highly compensated owners and employees. These are the only plans that permit annual deductions in excess of $40,000 per person.

Readers are encouraged to refer to Tables 8.3 and 8.4 for a comparison of retirement plans summarized above.

The 401(k)

The retirement plan programs discussed up until now have one common thread: contributions are made by the employer. In contrast, 401(k) programs are savings plans that permit employees the opportunity to make elective salary deferral contributions.

Participants generally can contribute up to 100% of their salaries to a maximum of $12,000 as of 2003 (this limit will increase $1,000/year to a maximum of $15,000 in 2006. And those age 50 and older can generally save more). Similar to profit sharing plans, eligibility generally is limited to employees age 21 and older who have one year or more of employment with the practice. Though practice owners can make the

Table 8.3. Retirement Plan Comparison - Basic Differences

	Defined Contribution							Defined Benefit
	Profit Sharing				Pension Plans		SEP	
	Traditional	Integrated	Age Weighted	New Comparability	Traditional	Integrated	SEP	Defined Benefit
Flexible Contributions	✓	✓	✓	✓			✓	
Predictable Retirement Benefits								✓
Favors Older Employees			✓	✓				✓
Favors Younger Employees	✓	✓			✓	✓	✓	
Plan Design Easy to Explain	✓				✓		✓	
Administrative Costs	Low	Low	Moderate	Moderate	Low	Low	None	High

Table 8.4. Retirement Plan Comparison - Limits, Exclusions & Features

	Defined Contribution		SEP	Defined Benefit
	Profit Sharing Plans	Pension Plans	SEP	Defined Benefit
Maximum Contributions - Practice	25% of eligible payroll	25% of eligible payroll	25% of eligible payroll	#1
Maximum Contributions - Employee	100% of salary, max $40,000		25% to $40,000 #2	#1
Can exclude those . . .	Under age 21 & employed under 1,000 hours/year		Not employed 3/5 years & earning less than $450/year	Same as profit sharing & pension plans
Vesting Permitted	Yes		No	Yes
Loans Allowed	Yes		No	Yes

#1 The annual defined benefit limit for 2003 is $160,000. This represents the maximum annual payout for retirement, in today's dollars. The annual contribution is determined by an actuary and is based on salary, age, investment performance, and years of service to normal retirement.

#2 As is the case with all plan designs, individual compensation is not defined the same for corporate practices as it is for non-corporate practices (i.e., self-employed individuals and partnerships). Employee and owner compensation in a corporate entity is generally defined by their W-2 earnings. For non-corporate entities, only employee compensation is defined by W-2 earnings: owner and partner compensation, on which contributions to a plan are based, is determined differently and is beyond the scope of the book. Self-employed veterinarians or partners in a veterinary practice should seek assistance from tax professionals with expertise in these areas.

eligibility requirements more favorable by eliminating these conditions, they generally cannot make eligibility more restrictive (by increasing the minimum age beyond age 21 or increasing the service requirement beyond one year).

In essence, with the 401(k), employees are permitted to save on a pretax basis. Like other plans discussed earlier, contributions grow tax deferred until retirement. These programs are well suited for larger practices that employ several veterinarians and numerous support staff.

In addition to employee contributions, many 401(k) programs incorporate the following two components:

- an employer match: Employers can assist employees who wish to save for retirement by matching a portion of the employee's 401(k) contribution. Though this is not not required, matching is a good idea since it motivates employees to participate. As discussed below, employers generally benefit most when employee participation is high.

- an employer profit sharing contribution: In addition to a match, employers can make profit sharing contributions in profitable years to the benefit of all eligible employees.

Employee-contributed money in 401(k) plans always is 100% vested with the employees. Employer-contributed money, via the employer match or a profit sharing contribution above, is subject to the same vesting rules discussed earlier in the chapter.

Although the 401(k) is an increasingly popular program, this plan design shifts the burden of saving to the participants, essentially from an employer-pay-all to an employee-pay-all retirement plan. With corporate downsizing the norm for the past 10 years, many large employers have scrapped the more traditional defined benefit plans in favor of 401(k) plans, in which the primary responsibility for contributions rests with the employee. Consider this statistic from the United States Department of Labor's Pension and Welfare Benefits Administration: In 1984, there were 165,000 defined benefit plans and only 17,000 401(k)s. In 1992, there were 89,000 defined benefit plans and 140,000 401(k)s!

Getting Started

The first step in determining the viability of a 401(k) program is to determine the interest level among employees (Figures 8.3 and 8.4). It is a mistake to implement this type of retirement program in practices where little interest exists because, in general, employers cannot benefit from 401(k) plans unless their employees participate in the plans.

To understand the mechanics of the 401(k), two separate groups are defined, these being the highly compensated (HC) employees and the non-highly compensated (NHC) employees. For 2003, HC employees include employees and family members owning in excess of 5% of the practice, or those earning more than $90,000 in salary in 2002. NHC employees include everyone else.

To ensure that HC employees do not unfairly benefit from their 401(k) plans, there are rules that limit how much they may contribute from their annual salaries. The average deferral of the HC group may

If the average deferral percentage among NHC is:	Then the average deferral percentage for HC may not exceed:
0% to 2%	200% of the NHC%
2% to 8%	2 percentage points more
8% or more	125% of the NHC%

401 (k) Plan
Employee Survey

Dear Employee:

We are exploring the possibility of implementing an exciting new employee benefit — a 401(k) plan. It is a salary savings plan that:

✓ Allows you to make tax-deductible contributions

✓ Earns tax-deferred interest on your contributions

✓ Permits access to your funds before retirement for "financial hardship"

✓ Includes many other attractive features

We want you to help us determine if this benefit would be worthwhile to offer. Would you take a minute to answer these few questions? There is no obligation. This is only a preliminary survey.

Name:_____Date of Birth:___/___/___

What is your approximate annual salary? $_____

Would you be interested in this new tax-deductible savings plan?

Yes_____   No_____

If you answered "Yes", what percentage of your salary or dollars per month would you consider contributing?

% of salary _____% OR $_____per month
  (1% - 100% maximum)

Figure 8.3. 401(k) plan employee survey

The 401(k) Plan

Q. What tax advantage does the 401(k) salary savings plan offer me?

A. You receive two major advantages. Your contributions are made with before-tax dollars, thus decreasing your taxable income, and your investment earnings accumulate free of taxes until you withdraw your funds.

Q. Is there a maximum amount that I can contribute?

A. The maximum dollar amount that you are able to defer is $12,000 per calendar year (2003 limit), not to exceed 100% of your income. Those age 50 and older may save more.

Q. Once I've invested my money, can I withdraw it?

A. 401(k) allows you to withdraw your funds for "financial hardship", at termination of employment, at disability, retirement (as early as 55) or at age 59½. In addition, loans may be available with no penalty for premature distribution. Repayment of both principal and interest is made to YOUR account.

Q. Is a 401(k) contribution better than a regular savings?

A. Yes. Because your contribution is made with before-tax dollars, your spendable income actually increases by the amount of the tax savings.

Q. Is a 401(k) contribution better than an IRA?

A. Yes, IRA annual contributions are limited to only $3,000, loans are not available, and penalty-free distributions are not permitted prior to age 59 ½.

Q. How much money can I accumulate?

A. Your 401(k) contributions can accumulate substantially. For example, if you save $2,000 per year for 20 years, your account will grow to $95,696.09 (assuming an 8% return on your savings). Not only do you contribute with before-tax dollars, but you pay no tax on the growth until the money is withdrawn.

Q. What salary is used for my W-2 form?

A. Your W-2 form reports your income less your before-tax 401(k) contribution.

Q. What happens if I leave my job?

A. If you terminate employment, you take 100% of the "vested" portion of your 401(k) account. This may be rolled over into a new 401(k) or into an IRA rollover account.

TAX SAVINGS . . .

	With 401(k)	Without 401(k)
Taxable income	$25,000	$25,000
401(k) contribution	$1,000	$0
Net taxable income	$24,000	$25,000
Taxes due (28%)	$5,599	$5,799
Tax savings	$200	$0

WHY WAIT . . .

	Starting Age	Ending Age	Total Contribution	Years Contributed	Value At Age 65
Chris	23	33	12,000	10	236,224
Mike	35	65	36,000	30	150,030

Each contributes $100 a month, but for different periods
Chris starts at 23 and contributes for 10 years
Mike starts at 35 and contributes for 30 years
Assumes investments earn 8% annual return

Figure 8.4. Eight frequently asked questions asked about the 401(k) plan

exceed the average deferral of the NHC group by only a small increment, as shown in the box on page 298.

Suppose that a practice with 10 employees includes 2 HC employees and 8 NHC employees. If all 8 NHC employees were to contribute the same 6% of salary to the 401(k) program, the average deferral among NHC employees would be 6%; the maximum average deferral then for the two HC employees would be 8% (2 percentage points more). Now suppose only four of the eight NHC employees decide to participate and contribute 6% of their salaries, then the average deferral among NHC employees would be only 3% (24% total deferrals divided by the 8 NHC employees), and the maximum deferral for the two HC employees would be 5%.

Some employees will decide not to participate due to a shortage of personal finances, lack of interest, and/or because they have not been adequately educated about the program's features and advantages. If interest cannot be generated in a 401(k) plan, an employer can decide to match contributions and hope that this will motivate employees to contribute at higher levels.

A match of 50% of employee contributions with a 6% maximum is common. Matches of 100% of, for example, the first 3% of participant contributions should be avoided. This type of match motivates employees to contribute only 3% of earnings to take advantage of the entire match. An alternative like the "50% to 6% match" will accomplish the same 3% net match but will motivate participants to withhold at the higher 6% level rather than the lower 3%.

Finally, if there is a vesting schedule on these voluntary matches and there are forfeitures due to employees terminating employment before being fully vested, employers can use those forfeitures to offset future matches or administrative costs.

If a voluntary match is not enough to generate interest in the 401(k), employers will need to consider two alternatives. First, prac-

tices can avoid discrimination testing if they adopt either one of two safe-harbor provisions in their 401(k) plans that became available in 1999. These require that employers match a portion of an employee's contribution or make a nonelective contribution for all eligible employees. Second, employers can consider adopting either one of two types of savings programs collectively referred to as *SIMPLE plans*. Unlike the voluntary match discussed previously, required employer contributions to these two alternatives vest with employees immediately, as discussed later in the chapter.

PROGRAM TYPES

401(k) programs are offered through mutual fund families, stock brokerage houses, banks, and insurance companies. They are typically sold through an intermediary, i.e., by a stockbroker, insurance agent, or other investment professional specializing in the retirement plan market. In sorting through the various programs, they can be differentiated by the parties involved and the investment options included.

Investment, record keeping, and administrative personnel oversee the plans. In most 401(k) programs, the investment, record keeping, and administrative functions are handled under one roof. This is economical, facilitates better communication, and ensures timely participant statements. Other investment institutions combine the investment and record keeping functions of the 401(k) and are administered separately. Administrative services in this case include responsibility for the discrimination tests and governmental forms.

Investments also will differentiate one program from another. Though individual stocks can be used as an investment option, most 401(k)s use mutual funds. For many small plans, offering mutual funds affords employers a level of diversification not easily achieved with a portfolio of individual stocks and bonds.

Programs offer either (1) their own stable of investments, known as a *single fund family approach*, or (2) investments from several fund families, called the *multiple fund family approach*. Those which offer their own stable of funds include mutual fund families large enough to offer a 401(k) program, such as Putnam, Massachusetts Financial Services, Vanguard, Fidelity, and American Fund Families. For reference, this group, will be titled type "A."

Programs offering investments from multiple fund families are available through large life insurance companies, banks, and stock brokerage firms. In addition to offering their own in-house funds, these programs offer investments from other mutual fund families considered to be among the strongest in the industry, i.e., Nationwide, Transamerica, Principal Financial, Aetna, Merrill Lynch, and Salomon Smith Barney. This group will be called type "B."

Which program is most suitable will depend on an employer's budget and objectives. Funds in all programs (Types A and B) include an investment expense to manage the funds. The multiple fund family approach, Type B, typically assesses an additional fee based on the value of the assets in the program. These asset fees can range from .50% to 1.25% and are often paid by the participants.

In some Type B programs, typically marketed to businesses with fewer than 20 employees and/or less than $30,000 in annual contributions, the asset fee is assessed partially to subsidize the annual administrative and record keeping charges. Other Type B programs include the asset fee to cover the expense of including popular funds from other families as investment choices. Still others use a portion of the asset fee to pay commissions to salespeople who market the program. If practice owners wish to own recognizable investments, or if employee participation in the 401(k) would be lacking without popular offerings, practice owners may wish to restrict their search to Type B plans.

Loads and Surrender Charges

Loads and surrender charges, in addition to investments, differ among programs. Loads and/or charges come in two varieties:

- front end: assessed as a percentage of the contribution

- back end: commonly referred to as *surrender charges*, this load is assessed as a percentage of the amount withdrawn. Surrender charges are typically assessed, especially with smaller programs, to recoup setup costs and other initial expenses (including commissions to brokers) when programs are terminated in the first several years.

Program providers generally do not assess any front-end or back-end loads when plan assets exceed $1,000,000. This would be the case, perhaps, with large practices whose 401(k)s have been in existence for several years. Some providers aggressively seek the small business market and waive all front-end and back-end loads when annual contributions are expected to be greater than a minimum amount such as $50,000.

As to back-end loads, there are two types: (1) those assessed to plan participants when employees withdraw from the program and (2) those assessed to the practice only when the program is terminated. The latter is less restrictive. Back-end loads are highest in Year 1 and decline each year until they are eliminated, typically in five to seven years. Practice owners selecting 401(k) programs need to know how penalties are assessed. For example, is the five- to seven-year surrender period based on the contract origination date of the entire plan or the date of each contribution? The former is less restrictive, since contributions made in Year 4 of a six-year schedule would have only a two-year surrender charge remaining, and contributions made after six years would have no surrender charge.

PROGRAM FEATURES

Today's good 401(k) programs boast the following generous features:

- 8 to 20 investment options

- quarterly participant statements

- quarterly newsletters

- an 800 phone number for participants to use to obtain daily investment balances and/or transfer funds between accounts

An additional feature that varies among plans is the preparation of the Form 5500. This is an informational tax return required by the IRS each year. Some programs furnish practice owners with all of the information they'll need to complete the form, and others assist them in the process. Veterinary professionals should stick with those programs that complete Form 5500 on a "signature-ready" basis, which means forms are completed with all of the necessary details and lack only the signature of the business owner before they are mailed to the IRS.

Administration costs vary among programs. Some programs base their annual administration costs on the number of eligible employees, others on the number that participate. For veterinary practices with high participation levels, the difference is minimal. For practices with low participation levels, in which the number of participants is considerably fewer than the number eligible, the difference in fees can be considerable. In such cases, owners may wish to restrict their searches to those programs that charge by the participant.

Administration costs vary based on level of service and plan features. Less expensive programs generally offer standardized prototype plan documents only and may restrict the options available under the plan, i.e., eligibility, loans, vesting schedules, and contribution flexibility. Consider the following disparity in cost among top 401(k) programs:

- Program 1: $1800 flat fee for practices with up to 50 eligible employees, plus $300 for Form 5500 preparation.

- Program 2: $1000 base fee, plus $16 for each participant. Add $200 for Form 5500 preparation.

- Program 3: $15 for each participant, with a minimum charge of $750. Preparation of the Form 5500 is included.

- Program 4: $1250 base fee plus $18 for each participant. Signature-ready Form 5500 is included.

With individual limits increased under EGTRRA, a new plan design is now being marketed that may hold terrific benefits for solo practitioners (and spouses) with no employees or partners with no employees. Veterinarians looking for higher contribution limits and greater deductions than those offered with a SEP may look to adopt a combination Solo 401(k) and profit sharing plan. The veterinarian can defer 100% of compensation to a maximum of $12,000 (2003 limit) under the Solo 401(k) and contribute up to an additional 25% of compensation under the profit sharing plan, with a combined $40,000 maximum (2003 limits) under both programs. Here is an example. A veterinary consultant earns $80,000 a year. She can defer $12,000 under the 401(k) and contribute an additional $20,000 under the profit sharing plan, for a total contribution of $32,000! Though the combination plan offers greater contribution limits when compared to the SEP, there are administrative costs that need to be considered. Since discrimination testing is not needed under the Solo 401(k), though, these costs are generally much less than those charged with a traditional 401(k).

SIMPLE PLANS

Though the 401(k) has become a popular retirement program, it does have its drawbacks. Strict discrimination rules often limit the extent to which HC employees can save. Also, employees tend to be dissatisfied with employers who do not match any portion of their contributions. Because of these drawbacks, the Small Business Job Protection Act of 1996 introduced two new retirement programs, called the *SIMPLE IRA* and *SIMPLE 401(k)*. For veterinary practices with low employee participation in 401(k) programs, practice owners who wish to contribute maximum amounts may consider either of the SIMPLE plans. The popularity of these plans will depend on whether the required costs (i.e., matches or nonelective contributions) are offset by the promised flexibility in the program.

The maximum tax deferral under the SIMPLE Plans is $8,000 ($4000 less than the 2003 401(k) limit of $12,000). When employers adhere to several predetermined conditions, though, discrimination tests and top-heavy requirements are waived. The most restrictive of these conditions requires employers to make 100% matching contributions of up to 3% of employee compensation or contribute 2% of compensation for all eligible employees. In other words, employers can choose to match up to 3% of compensation for only those employees who decide to participate or, like a profit sharing contribution, contribute 2% of compensation for all eligible employees (regardless of participation).

Although the SIMPLE IRA and SIMPLE 401(k) are fairly similar, there are several differences worth noting. The SIMPLE 401(k) will permit loans to participants; the SIMPLE IRA will not. Aside from this one disadvantage, however, the SIMPLE IRA provides more flexibility for the veterinary practice owner. Consider the following advantages of the SIMPLE IRA versus the SIMPLE 401(k):

- minimal or no administrative costs

- fewer administrative responsibilities in the form of IRS filings, qualifications, and Form 5500s

- withdrawal flexibility: Although there is a 25% tax penalty for withdrawals during the first two years, withdrawals from SIMPLE IRAs can be made at any time for any reason. Withdrawals from SIMPLE 401(k)s can be made only for death, disability, hardship, or separation from service. A 10% tax penalty for premature withdrawals applies to both for most distributions made prior to age 59½.

- investment flexibility: Employees participating in SIMPLE IRAs generally can select the financial institution in which contributions are invested. With a SIMPLE 401(k), employee contributions must be made to the program's preselected investment options, similar to traditional 401(k)s.

- more fiduciary protection for the employer: With the SIMPLE IRA, much of the fiduciary responsibility is with the financial institution in which the investment is made. With the SIMPLE 401(k), more of the responsibility is with the plan sponsor, or the employer.

- more flexibility with matched contributions: The SIMPLE IRA allows for reduced employer-matched contributions—1% of compensation instead of the regular 3%—in no more than 2 out of any 5 years.

Figure 8.5 highlights the factors involved in deciding between the SIMPLE IRA and the traditional 401(k). Depending on the workforce demographics, company budget, and the objectives of the employer, one plan design usually is more suitable than the other. When analyzing this type of situation, the following issues are considered:

1. Contributing desired amounts: When employers are not interested in participating in the 401(k) or if they do not need to contribute maximum amounts to supplement existing retirement savings, the need to pass discrimination tests is irrelevant. In such cases there may be no

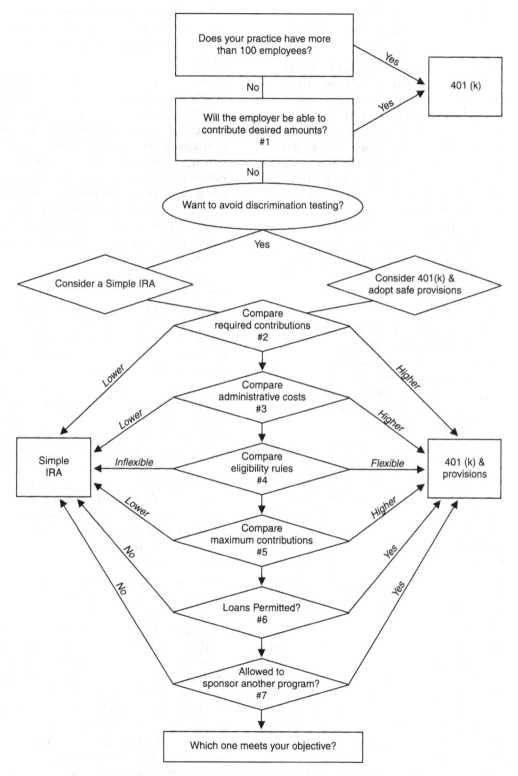

Figure 8.5. Simple IRA vs. Traditional 401(k)

need to adhere to the restrictions in SIMPLE IRAs, and traditional 401(k)s may be the better choice.

If, however, a 401(k) represents the main source of retirement savings for the employer, interest among NHC employees will need to be determined. If interest is strong, the traditional 401(k) again may be the better choice. If employee interest is weak, but a voluntary match will motivate employees to participate at high levels, the traditional 401(k) may again be the better choice. (Recall that an employer can provide a vesting schedule on the match so that employees who terminate employment prior to becoming fully vested will need to return portions of employer-contributed money to the plan.)

If the voluntary match is not sufficient, employers have two choices: select a traditional 401(k) and adopt one of the two safe-harbor provisions available in 1999, or select a SIMPLE IRA. In either case, the required contributions vest immediately with the employee.

2. Comparing required contributions and resulting benefits: Beginning in 1999, employers can avoid discrimination testing under traditional 401(k)s if they comply with one of the following two safe-harbor provisions: provide for matching contributions equal to 100% of the first 3% of compensation and 50% on deferrals between 3% and 5% (equal to a 4% match), or provide a 3% of compensation nonelective contribution for eligible employees.

With SIMPLE IRAs, discrimination testing is automatically waived because the employer has elected to match 100% of the first 3% of compensation or contribute 2% of compensation for all eligible employees. In comparison, the required contribution with the traditional 401(k) is slightly higher than that required with a SIMPLE IRA (4% versus 3% match or 3% versus 2% non-elective contribution).

Though the required contributions in both scenarios appear to be costly, consider the following hypothetical example.

A veterinary owner has 12 eligible employees and is interested in adopting a qualified plan. She has distributed the survey form and determined that only four employees are interested in participating. A match is less costly than a nonelective contribution for all eligible employees since the match is made for only the four participants who elect to receive this benefit. Alternatively, a nonelective contribution must be made for all eligible employees.

3. Assessing administration costs: If the cost of administering the plan is an issue, a SIMPLE IRA may be the better choice. Administrative costs with a traditional 401(k) will generally include a base fee and a per-participant charge; costs for a SIMPLE IRA are modest.

4. Evaluating eligibility rules: Eligibility under SIMPLE IRAs is based on compensation, i.e., employees earning a minimum of $5,000 in annual compensation are eligible. Eligibility under a traditional 401(k) is based on hours worked, and those who work less than 1000 hours in a plan year generally can be excluded from participation. Although the basis on which each program determines eligibility is different, the main issue concerns flexibility.

With the SIMPLE IRA, there are few options with eligibility. Employers can include a service requirement of up to two years. Eligibility under a traditional 401(k) can be inclusive or restrictive. This means the employer can decide to include or exclude employees who work fewer than 1000 hours in a plan year or, alternatively, exclude a class of employees (as long as certain coverage tests are met). If all employees are full timers, though, and therefore earn in excess of $5,000, there is little difference in eligibility under the two programs. If employers have significant populations of part-timers, and their objective is to limit benefits and, thus, employer costs, they will need to review the eligibility rules for each program. If a practice's part timers are likely to earn in excess of the $5,000 threshold but work fewer than 1,000 hours, the traditional 401(k) may be the better choice.

5. Comparing maximum contributions: With SIMPLE IRAs, participants are permitted to defer 100% of their compensation to a maximum of $8,000, without regard to participation levels. With traditional 401(k) plans, maximum deferrals are $12,000 in 2003, approximately 50% higher. Unless a safe-harbor provision is adopted in a traditional 401(k), though, this $12,000 threshold is not guaranteed. As a result, HC employees may have difficulty contributing desired amounts if participation among NHC employees is low. Reaching the $8,000 maximum income deferral with the SIMPLE IRA is predicated solely on a participant's interest in saving for retirement. Reaching the $12,000 limit with the traditional 401(k) is based on other factors not easily controlled by participants.

6. Considering loans to participants: Loans to participants can be an important provision in retirement plans. Employees sometimes feel more comfortable contributing amounts to savings plans if they know they have access to their balances without penalty. When employers wish to offer plans with loan features, traditional 401(k)s are the only option because loans are not available with SIMPLE IRAs.

7. Contrasts with other employer-sponsored retirement plans: With SIMPLE IRAs, practices cannot sponsor additional qualified plans. If profits permit and veterinary practice owners are interested in making maximum contributions to a plan, a traditional 401(k) plan (with safe harbor provisions) coupled with a profit sharing plan provides good options. If, however, there is no interest in sponsoring ancillary programs and employee tax deferrals are the primary motivation for adopting a plan, the condition prohibiting additional qualified plans when implementing SIMPLE IRA plans is irrelevant. Finally, the SIMPLE IRA restricts additional qualified retirement plans only. Employers could, for example, supplement SIMPLE IRAs with nonqualified deferred compensation programs.

Though similar in some respects, there are cost and flexibility differences between SIMPLE IRAs and traditional 401(k)s. 401(k) programs may provide more flexible plan designs (more so now with the safe harbor provision), but administrative costs are higher. Only time will tell whether the SIMPLE IRA proves to be a popular alternative to the traditional 401(k).

SELECTING A BROKER

Selecting the right retirement plan for a veterinary practice is not easy (see Figures 8.6 and 8.7 for forms that can be used to compare different programs). Although various plan designs have been outlined above, selecting a broker to help with the process is essential. A broker's responsibilities will include the following: (1) helping to select the most appropriate plan design, (2) educating employees, (3) monitoring the program's investment performance, and (4) assisting practice owners with adherence to strict plan regulations. Good brokers are objective, knowledgeable about all types of plans, and able to provide the ancillary services typical of well-coordinated retirement plans.

Some brokers sell one program, while others represent several programs. The latter group may be more objective and better able to match a specific program with a particular practice. Good brokers continually screen the most popular programs, i.e., those offered by mutual fund families, stock brokerage firms, banks, and life insurance

Retirement Plan Survey

Profit Sharing Offered?	Standard	#1	#2	#3
✓ Type design (#1)				
✓ $ contributed - last year				
✓ $ contributed - previous year				
✓ Eligibility	1 year			
✓ Vesting (#2)	graded			

#1 traditional (TRA), integrated (INT), age-weighted (AGE) or new comparability (COMP)

#2 graded — (20% vested in 3 years, 40% in 4 years, 60% in 5 years, 80% in 6 years, 100% in 7 years) or cliff — (0% vested for 4 years, 100% in year 5?)

Figure 8.6. A retirement plan survey form

companies, and recommend only those that meet high standards. Typically these include turnkey programs boasting excellent investment performance and offering superior administrative and record keeping functions.

Determining the broker's emphasis, or different strengths, is essential. Investment knowledge is important, but most brokers can present programs with favorable investment performances. It is important to determine whether or not they understand retirement plan design and how programs can be tailored to benefit the practice owners. 401(k) plans can be administrative nightmares for brokers whose only strengths are investments.

Ancillary services also are important. Brokers should be able to address retirement planning issues with practice owners and determine whether annual personal and retirement savings are sufficient to retire comfortably. With respect to 401(k)s, brokers need to educate employees as to how they can and should make informed decisions. Because of this, it is critical that the brokers be interested in conducting periodic semi-

nars on topics of interest such as investment basics, risk tolerance, and asset allocation. If employees are well educated, they will be more likely to participate in 401(k) programs, properly allocate their investments among several options, and be less likely to panic with market fluctuations.

In addition to the above responsibilities, good brokers step in to answer questions and resolve problems when they arise. This can include handling new employees with questions on participation or rollovers of plans they may have acquired while working for other employers or advising departing employees with questions on distributions. Furthermore, brokers may need to counsel employees on differences between 401(k) loans and home equity loans. When investments fail to perform sufficiently to meet expected benchmarks, when participants' statements are not received on a timely basis, or the plan's administration is considered subpar, good brokers will be there to resolve issues and/or suggest alternative programs. Even turnkey programs require some monitoring. In short, good brokers are needed to help practice owners focus on the

401 (k) Plan Survey

	Standard	#1	#2	#3
✓ Eligibility	1 year wait			
✓ Match	50% to 60%			
✓ Vesting (#1)	graded			
✓ No. of investment options	8 - 20			
✓ Identify investments (#2)				
✓ Who pays administration?	Employer			
✓ Test Problems? (#3)				

#1 vesting: graded — (20% vested in 3 years, 40% in 4 years, 60% in 5 years, 80% in 6 years, 100% in 7 years) or cliff — (0% vested for 4 years, 100% in year 5.)

#2 use reverse side to summarize 1-, 3- and 5-year investment performance

#3 test problems: are highly compensated employees limited in what they can contribute?

Figure 8.7. A 401(k) plan survey form

practice of veterinary medicine. It is worthwhile to invest considerable effort in choosing a good one.

SOME EXAMPLES

To better appreciate the differences among plans, several hypothetical practices are presented herein, each with its own population of employees, cash flow picture, and objectives.

Practice 1: Susan Kramer, DVM, is a consultant who specializes in cardiology. She works for multiple referring veterinary practices and is incorporated. As an independent contractor, she is responsible for paying her own income taxes and benefits, and therefore is ineligible to participate in any of the plans offered by the practices for whom she consults. She has no employees and is interested in beginning her own qualified plan. Susan has two choices. Assume Susan earns $130,000. She can start a sim-

plified pension plan, or SEP, in which she can contribute a maximum of 25% of her earned income, or $32,500. What if she is nearing retirement and knows she hasn't saved nearly enough to retire comfortably? What if her spouse has a terrific job but with a small company without a retirement plan? If she wants to contribute more and receive a greater deduction, she can adopt a combination 401(k) and profit sharing plan. Though there are some administrative costs, she can contribute $12,000 (2003 limit) under the Solo 401(k) and contribute up to an additional 25% of earned income (2003 limit), to the profit sharing plan, not to exceed a total of $40,000 (2003 limit). In this case, her contribution increases from the $32,500 allowed in the SEP to $40,000 allowed in the combination plan.

Practice 2: Bart Simpson, DVM, has recently attended a seminar on the advantages of a retirement program and believes this would be a terrific benefit to offer his employees. He would also like to include his wife, a veterinary technician with the practice, who works approximately 750 hours a year and earns $9,000. Initially, Bart considered a 401(k). While he could modify the eligibility rules to allow his wife to participate (typically employees who work fewer than 1000 hours in a plan year can be excluded), there are three other employees who work under 1000 hours who would then become eligible to participate. With a traditional 401(k), Bart understands that his ability to contribute is based largely on the average deferral of his employees. Since these three employees have expressed no desire to participate, Bart believes the traditional 401(k) may not be his best choice. With a SIMPLE IRA, though, Bart can contribute the $8,000 maximum amount and not be concerned if others participate. Although the part timers are eligible, based on their minimum compensation of $5,000, the fact that they do not participate is not a problem. In fact, although Bart is required to contribute on behalf of his staff to avoid discrimination testing, his choice to match 3% of compensation will not be costly since only a few of his employees seem interested in the plan. In addition, Bart's wife can contribute a maximum $8,000 of her $9,000 salary.

Practice 3: Jack Wilson, DVM, is a veterinary practice owner who for many years has managed a small but popular practice in North Central Wisconsin. For various reasons, Jack has never gotten around to implementing a retirement plan. He believes this year is different. A veterinary colleague who for many years was his only competition, has decided to retire. As a result, Jack suddenly finds his practice booming. He meets with his accountant, who suggests a type of retirement plan that will afford him the opportunity to catch up for missed years.

Jack's best choice probably will be a defined benefit plan. Jack is considerably older than the two employees with whom he works, and a defined benefit plan will allow for larger contributions to be allocated to Jack. Although contributions are mandatory, Jack will be able to contribute amounts far in excess of those he'd be able to contribute under a profit sharing plan. If the mandatory contributions are a problem, an age-weighted profit sharing plan may work. Although total practice contributions are limited to a maximum of 25% of covered payroll, contributions are still based on age and will therefore benefit Jack the most.

Practice 4: Andrew Silvers, VMD, and Amy L. Johnson, VMD, friendly competitors for years, decide to merge their practices. As individual practitioners, they never benefited from retirement plans and feel that now is a good time to begin. Since Andrew is 32 and Amy is 41, an age-based plan would not benefit each equally. In fact, Andrew and Amy wish to benefit all employees of the practice equally, as the two believe much of their success is due to the talent, long-term loyalty, and experience of the staff. The best choice for them probably is a traditional profit sharing plan. With this type, the practice will make contributions for each employee, including the two owners, representing the same percentage of each worker's salary. As income and profits in the practice fluctuate, they can alter their contributions from year to year.

Practice 5: A large cat clinic in Texas is considering a retirement plan. Roberta Simmons, DVM and Cathy Richards, DVM have shied away from initiating a plan in the past because of the financial commitment needed to benefit the other employees. Although an age-weighted profit sharing plan may appear to make the most sense, Drs. Simmons and Richards employ an older veterinary technician who may unfairly benefit due to her age.

Not wanting to ruffle any feathers, the owners would like to design a plan so that contributions are targeted by salary, age and, more importantly, by position or class of employee. In this way, they can reward those most responsible for the growth and success of the practice. Best choice: a new comparability profit sharing plan. With this type of plan, the doctors can target contributions to the specifications outlined above. For example, the following would be considered permissible classes of employees: class 1 for owner-veterinarians, class 2 for employee-veterinarians, class 3 for veterinary technicians, class 4 for receptionists, and class 5 for veterinary assistants.

Practice 6: Animal Care Center, Inc., a large veterinary hospital in Iowa, is considering a retirement plan. While recognizing the benefits of a retirement plan, the hospital has recently incorporated, and cash flow is a concern. Robert Hovers, DVM, needs to recruit top talent and is interested in a plan that will allow associate veterinarians the opportunity to contribute portions of their paychecks to a retirement plan. To motivate the workforce to participate, he is willing to match a small percentage of their contribution. To encourage and reward long-term employment, he would like the corporation's matching contribution to vest on a graded basis. His best choice is a 401(k) program with a modest employer match.

RETIREMENT PLANS: A FINAL THOUGHT

Graduating veterinary students, interns, residents, and support staff members need not become experts in the finer details of the retirement plan process. Nonetheless, to best serve their interests, they should bring a reasonable understanding of retirement plan concepts to the interview and job selection process. This places them in a much better position to make an intelligent job choice. Confronted with several veterinary practices that claim to offer generous pension or profit sharing plans, for example, job applicants can obtain a wealth of information by asking only the following three questions:

1. What type of plan is offered?

2. What is the vesting schedule (or how many years of employment are needed for me to fully vest)?

3. What kind of money has this employer contributed in recent years?

For veterinary practice owners, a better understanding of the concepts outlined in this chapter will assure that the most appropriate plan design is selected to meet practice objectives. In the final analysis, a competitive retirement plan program can and will help practice owners attract, hire, motivate, and retain their talented employees.

Chapter 9

RESTRICTIVE COVENANTS

By James F. Wilson, DVM, JD and Jeffrey D. Nemoy, DVM, JD

Restrictive covenants are contractual provisions that limit the geographic area and time in which former employees can work at jobs similar to those they held previously. Restrictive covenants protect veterinary employers against employees competing for clients, disclosing trade secrets, and using mailing lists and other confidential information. Moreover, they clearly define employers' expectations of employees' professional activities following employment. Readers should be aware that for situations following employment, the terms *restrictive covenant, noncompete clause*, and *covenant not to compete* are used interchangeably.

During the past decade, the authors have reviewed hundreds of oral contracts and over 600 written contracts. Although practice owners sometimes believe that they have an oral covenant not to compete with their associate veterinarians, proving the terms and existence of such agreements is virtually impossible. Because of the ambiguities associated with oral covenants, the results of the retrospective study reported in this chapter pertain only to written contracts.

Over 91% of the veterinary employment contracts reviewed for this study contain restrictive covenant clauses.[1] This chapter explains the reasons for including restrictive covenants in veterinary agreements, pro-vides information about state statutes that govern what is permissible in many states, discusses the legal limitations of restrictive covenants, and supplies sample contract clauses. Although the primary focus is on restrictive covenants in employment agreements, restrictive covenants in sales of businesses and partnership interests also are covered.

Because local laws differ and legal precedents change, employers should have local legal counsel review all sample contract clauses before including them in their own veterinary employment agreements.

ANTITRUST ISSUES

Restrictive covenants are a form of trade restraint because they limit the freedom of veterinary associates, practice managers, and veterinary business sellers to practice their profession. One might suspect, then, that such clauses violate the Federal Sherman Antitrust Act and/or state antitrust laws. For a more complete understanding of the antitrust laws in the United States, readers are encouraged to review Chapter 7 of *Law and Ethics of the Veterinary Profession*.[2] Otherwise, the basic principles in this complicated area of the law follow.

THE SHERMAN ANTITRUST ACT

The Sherman Antitrust Act was enacted in 1890. Sections 1 and 2 of this federal law provide that

Every contract, combination in the form of a trust or otherwise, or conspiracy in restraint of trade or commerce among the several states, or with foreign nations, is declared to be illegal. Every person who shall make any contract or engage in any combination or conspiracy hereby declared to be illegal shall be deemed guilty of a felony and, on conviction thereof, shall be punished by fine not exceeding one million dollars, or, if any person, one hundred thousand dollars, or by imprisonment not exceeding three years, or by both said punishments, in the discretion of the court.[3]

The only substantive changes to this act in the past 100 years are those that have increased the fines and criminal penalties.

RESTRAINTS OF TRADE

The Sherman Act clearly states that every contract that restrains trade is illegal. If this were to be interpreted literally, many business agreements would be banned. To circumvent this, the Supreme Court has held that only those contracts, combinations, and conspiracies that *unreasonably* restrain trade are prohibited.[4] This judicial limitation in turn has led to what is known as the *rule of reason*. Under this rule, when evaluating the reasonableness of a restraint, courts consider a variety of market factors such as the nature of the restraint and its effect, market conditions, and the history of the restraint.[5]

THE PER SE RULE

A major corollary of the rule of reason is the *per se rule*. The Supreme Court has held that certain practices are so plainly anticompetitive that they are conclusively presumed to be illegal without the need to examine market factors or business reasons for their existence.[6] Per se illegality is limited to those activities that lack any redeeming virtue and have no purpose except to stifle competition. Included in the per se category are agreements between competitors whose only purpose is to fix prices (upward, downward, or remaining the same), allocate territory or divide markets, limit production, and boycott third parties.[7] Over the years, courts interpreting the Sherman Antitrust Act have determined that restrictive covenants in employment agreements are not a per se violation but must be evaluated under a rule of reason standard.

THE RULE OF REASON

If a business activity is held not to be a per se restraint of trade, it still does not necessarily mean that that procedure or practice is legal. The court must determine the reasonableness of any restraint in which the business is involved. The burden of proof in such cases is on the party challenging the business practices to show that the practices at issue are unreasonable.[8] Consequently, there are no ready answers regarding the legality or illegality of business practices that are not classified as illegal per se. Instead, the courts interpret cases on an individual basis as they arise.

OTHER ISSUES

A careful review of the Sherman Act shows that four basic requirements must be met in order to successfully litigate a claim under that law:

- There must be at least two people acting in concert.

- The restraint must involve trade or commerce.

- The restraint must involve interstate commerce.

- The restraint must be unreasonable.[9]

A Contract, Combination, or Conspiracy

The first requirement of a Sherman Act violation is the presence of a contract, a combination, or a conspiracy. A contract is a legally enforceable agreement between parties. A combination is the union of two or more previously independent persons. A conspiracy is a combination of two or more people planning and acting together secretly, especially for an unlawful or harmful purpose. In this case that purpose is to restrain trade. This first element is easily met in cases of a restrictive covenant because a formal contract exists.

Trade or Commerce

The second requirement, trade or commerce, also is fairly easy to prove. The landmark *Goldfarb* v. *Virginia Bar* case held that the practice of a profession was indeed trade or commerce and, therefore, for at least some purposes, federal antitrust laws will be applied to members of the "learned" professions.[10]

Interstate Commerce

The third requirement, interstate commerce, can be more questionable because the practice of veterinary medicine is predominantly a local activity.[11] The two key requirements under the Sherman Act are that either the actual or potential effect of the restraint on interstate commerce be adverse and substantial.

In most cases it is not difficult to prove that the practice of veterinary medicine has a substantial effect on interstate commerce. Among the factors the courts review is the amount of revenue that flows into and out of the veterinary practice from interstate transactions. The courts do not specify any particular amount of money that must change hands, but decide cases on an individual basis. Practitioners near state borders or those who provide services at dog, cat, and/or livestock shows or racetracks, where many of the animals move interstate, can affect interstate commerce sufficiently to satisfy this requirement.

Another often significant factor is the volume of supplies and equipment shipped to the practice from out of state. Since the sale and movement of most biologicals, drugs, hospital supplies, equipment, computer systems, diagnostic blood tests, telephonic consultations, and/or transfers of records involving diagnostic ECGs and images occur via interstate commerce, practitioners always are at risk that courts will hold that one or more of these activities substantially involves interstate commerce.

Other considerations are the number of patients practitioners treat that have moved or will be moving interstate. And do the practitioners and staff travel interstate? Ancillary to these questions are two more concerns: (1) Do the veterinarians have practices that serve clients in more than one state? and (2) Do the practice owners spend money on interstate travel for business purposes? Receiving referrals from adjacent states, attending continuing education seminars or veterinary meetings out of state, issuing health certificates for interstate movement of animals, and making ambulatory calls in more than one state all could be significant.

An Unreasonable Restraint

The fourth requirement that must be present in order to successfully challenge a violation under Section One of the Sherman Act is the presence of an unreasonable restraint of trade or commerce.

Since covenants not to compete do not fall under the United States Supreme Court's definition of an unreasonable restraint of trade (like price fixing), they must be analyzed under the court's "rule of reason" standard of review. This rule requires courts to fully evaluate the reasonableness of covenants not to compete. Although this discussion involves only federal law applications of the rule of reason, state law applications closely parallel the federal precedents.

The primary factors that the Federal Trade Commission or the courts consider when determining the reasonableness of restrictive covenants include the practitioner-employer's need for protection, the hardship experienced by the employee, and the effect the restraint has or will have on the public. These and other factors will be discussed in more detail later in this chapter.

THE PREVALENCE OF RESTRICTIVE COVENANTS IN VETERINARY EMPLOYMENT CONTRACTS

Restrictive covenant agreements generally are viewed with disfavor by courts. For example, in *Bishop* v. *Lakeland Animal Hospital*, the Appellate Court of Illinois held that restrictive covenants were to be closely scrutinized.[12] Bishop, the employee, entered into an employment agreement that contained a restrictive covenant with Lakeland Animal Hospital. After working for Lakeland less than one year, Bishop was terminated without cause.

At issue was whether the restrictive covenant was enforceable even though Bishop was terminated without cause. The trial court dismissed Bishop's complaint, stating that the contract terms were clear and the restrictive covenant was valid. The Appellate Court reversed the trial court ruling concerning the restrictive covenant.

The Appellate Court held that restrictive covenants are disfavored and are not enforceable when employees are terminated without cause. Moreover, the contract language was ambiguous. The terms of the contract stated that the restrictive covenant was triggered when employment was terminated for any cause. "Any cause" could have been interpreted as no cause or as the existence of some cause. When a contract is ambiguous and susceptible to more than one meaning, it must be construed against the drafter of the contract, which in this case was Lakeland. Since the contract consisted of ambiguous language, the restrictive covenant was unenforceable.

Although restrictive covenants are disfavored by most courts, they are commonplace in veterinary employment contracts, and well-drafted agreements usually are enforced. The authors' study of several hundred veterinary employment contracts across the United States, the oldest of which was signed in 1987 and the newest in 1997, revealed that 97% of the contracts included restrictive covenants. Among these covenants, time and geographic limitations varied remarkably (Tables 9.1 and 9.2). These

Table 9.1. Percentage of 225 Employment Contracts That Included Restrictive Covenant Clauses

Restrictive Covenants	All	Male	Female	Small Animal	Equine	Large Animal	Mixed
Percentage	92	88	93	90	100	92	100

Table 9.2. Average Time Periods and Geographic Areas of Restrictive Covenants

Restrictive Covenants	All	Male	Female	Small Animal	Equine	Large Animal	Mixed
Lowest years	0.6	0.8	0.6	0.6	1	1	1
Highest years	5	5	5	5	3	5	6
Median years	3	3	3	3	3	3	2
Lowest miles	2.5	2.5	3	2.5	10	5	5
Highest miles	100	75	100	100	50	35	45
Median miles	10	10	10	10	25	16.5	20

variations are likely due to (1) the difficulty in ascertaining the kinds of restraints necessary to protect employers without placing undue hardships on employees; (2) the lack of a scientific basis for the distances selected by many employers; and (3) the limited number of precedents establishing what courts, rather than practice owners, consider an appropriate balance between protection for employers and the rights of employees to engage in reasonable competition with their former employers.

THE NEED FOR RESTRICTIVE COVENANTS

Restrictive covenants are necessary when protectable interests are at risk. Courts have long held that practice owners have a right to protect tangible and intangible interests. Intangible interests are related to goodwill and include practice goodwill, professional goodwill, and client goodwill. *Practice goodwill* is the practice's reputation within the community and among colleagues and staff. *Professional goodwill* refers to the depth and breadth of doctor-client-patient relationships, which are strengthened by a veterinarian's personal traits such as professional competence, attendance at continuing education seminars, compassion and empathy, interactions and communications with clients and patients, time-management skills, consistency in follow-up calls, and specialized training. Together, professional goodwill and practice goodwill form *client goodwill*, or the reputation among a practice's clientele.[13]

Protectable tangible interests include trade secrets and confidential information, such as medical records and client lists. A trade secret, as defined in the Restatement of Torts, is:

> Any formula, pattern, device or compilation of information which is used in one's business, and which gives him an opportunity to obtain an advantage over competitors who do not know or use it.

It may be a formula for a chemical compound, a process of manufacturing, treating or preserving materials, a pattern for a machine or other device, or a list of customers.[14]

The AVMA endorses tangible interests as a protectable asset. The AVMA Principles of Veterinary Medical Ethics state that "the records of a veterinary facility are the sole property of that facility, and when a veterinarian leaves salaried employment therein, the departing veterinarian shall not copy, remove, or make any subsequent use of those records."[15]

To illustrate protectable interests, let's look at an example. Dr. Apprentice works three years for Dr. Mentor without a written employment contract and without discussing a restrictive covenant clause. Dr. Apprentice learns a great deal under Dr. M's guidance and has access to a clientele provided by Dr. M upon which he develops his skills as a veterinarian. Dr. A consistently provides quality medicine and surgical techniques, has excellent bedside manners, and makes follow-up calls to the clients he sees. Dr. A has created great professional goodwill which, in turn, strengthens the practice goodwill and the client goodwill. Furthermore, Dr. Apprentice has gained access to and has developed confidential information about his patients and, through his familiarity with the operation of the computer system, has access to the client list. After three years of employment, Dr. A quits working for Dr. Mentor and establishes his own practice a half-mile away. Several hundred clients who have entrusted the care of their animals to Dr. A while he was employed by Dr. M follow him to his new practice.

Dr. M's interests are at risk upon the occurrence of any of the following events: (1) Dr. A leaves the practice and starts a new practice or goes to work for another practice within Dr. M's trade area; (2) the practice owner(s) decide to put the practice up for sale; or (3) the practice partnership or corporation dissolves.

In this case, Dr. Mentor could have protected his goodwill, trade secrets, and confidential information if he had had Dr. Apprentice sign an employment contract that included a reasonable restrictive covenant clause. Because he did not, he likely will lose a considerable portion of the practice's clientele and goodwill. Also, if he were to try to sell the practice, he undoubtedly would find that it had lost a major portion of its value.

Another reason for restrictive covenants is that at the time of the sale of a practice or partnership interest, or in a corporate dissolution, the restrictive covenant of a departing owner is a valued asset to be sold to a purchaser. Without restrictive covenants attached to the sale, sellers can start practices near the original businesses and retain much of their goodwill. Only if sellers promise to refrain from competing with buyers can the buyers protect the value of the goodwill being sold.[16]

This is demonstrated in the case *Durio* v. *Johnson* in which both parties were partners of a veterinary practice.[17] Upon dissolution of the partnership, Durio and Johnson entered into an agreement that contained a restrictive covenant. The covenant stated that Durio could not practice veterinary medicine within or be associated with anyone practicing veterinary medicine within a radius of 10 miles of the practice for a period of 10 years from the date of the agreement. Breaching the covenant, Durio practiced veterinary medicine in the area within the 10-year time limit. The court enforced the covenant after concluding that goodwill exists in professional practices and that Johnson's newly purchased goodwill was protectable.

FREQUENTLY ENCOUNTERED PROBLEMS

Amid the differences among employment contracts are common problems encountered with the drafting and interpretation of restrictive covenants.

1. Employers intentionally or unwittingly overdraft time periods, distances, and/or liquidated damages in noncompete agreements in an effort to maximize their protection. This discourages potential employees from considering or accepting jobs that could ultimately result in a breach of covenant. These employers also may intend that a highly restrictive covenant will discourage colleagues with practices inside the restricted areas from offering positions to their present or former associates. Their colleagues may fear negative repercussions between themselves and the veterinary practice owner who is trying to enforce the covenant as well as damage to their reputations within the general veterinary community. Additionally, local colleagues may fear that job applicants will be legally prohibited from accepting jobs being offered or, if their breach of a restrictive covenant is challenged after they are hired, from completing the term of employment to which they agreed.

2. Employers often include restrictive covenants in employment contracts in states where the statutes are unenforceable, i.e., California, Montana, Alabama, Oklahoma, and North Dakota (see subsequent discussion in this chapter). They do this either because they are ignorant of state laws or they are trying to bluff naive veterinary associates into believing that the clauses are enforceable.

3. Employers usually have greater financial reserves and access to legal counsel than employees have. Because of this, they are able to secure temporary restraining orders prohibiting violations of restrictive covenants, and thus obtain unfair advantage over employees who lack the time and money needed to challenge the enforcement of unreasonable covenants.

4. Employers who require that employees sign excessive restrictive covenants, such as 50 miles and 5 years, and are unwilling to negotiate anything more reasonable exhibit a lack of self-confidence and a

controlling attitude that discourages applicants from accepting employment.

5. Employers who are unwilling to negotiate reasonable covenants set the stage for hard feelings between themselves and associates whose employment has been terminated. Additionally, the ensuing legal challenges usually create an environment in which the primary winners will be the attorneys and expert witnesses hired by each side rather than the employers or employees.

6. Some employees sign unreasonable covenants without contemplating their legal effect and/or enforceability and without ever planning to honor them. When their employment is terminated, they simply ignore the clauses and compete. This puts the former employers in a position of having to ignore the breaches and waive their rights under the contracts or pursue legal actions to preserve their rights. Employers faced with such challenges also must contemplate the risk that a decision not to enforce the contract will lead to a precedent whereby a court could hold that they have waived their rights to enforce the covenant against future challenges.

7. Experience has shown that many young veterinarians who sign these covenants do so because they do not expect to stay in the area in which they are working. Then, because of financial reasons, or because they fall in love and wish to marry someone in the community, they suddenly discover that they have no viable employment option other than to continue working for their current employers. This can put a huge emotional and monetary stress on a newly married couple.

A hypothetical example involves a young veterinarian who accepts a job on Martha's Vineyard, an island off the coast of Massachusetts. The veterinarian never expects to stay on the Vineyard but ends up marrying one of her clients. When the employment relationship with her employer sours, she discovers that the distance in her restrictive covenant prevents her from obtaining work as a veterinarian anywhere else on the island.

8. Employees naively sign noncompete clauses without plotting the distance boundaries on the map, only to discover too late that the number of miles in the contract extend far beyond the distance they had anticipated. Usually this is because such covenants represent air miles, i.e., distances that are far greater than those imposed by surface miles. When a compass is applied to a map to determine the actual boundaries, ex-employees discover that the distance radii are just long enough to preclude them from working for every desirable practice in the area. In some cases, had the radii been shortened by a half mile, their options for employment would have doubled.

It is apparent from this list of potential problems that restrictive covenants can pose difficulties if they are ill researched and unclearly stated. The remainder of this chapter will expand upon these issues and provide sample clauses that can be used in noncompete agreements to meet the needs of employers and employees.

A CONTRACT CLAUSE FOR INTANGIBLE INTERESTS: GOODWILL

The following contract language is designed to substantiate and protect employers' goodwill:

The parties agree that the Employer's business is local in scope and that the Employer would suffer serious damage and loss of goodwill if, upon termination of this employment agreement, Employee competes with the Employer by providing veterinary services for clients who reside within the practice's trade area or currently are regular clients of the Employer. It is understood that the restrictive covenant contained in this Agreement is necessitated because of the time, effort, and resources required to develop and maintain the Employer's business.

A CONTRACT CLAUSE FOR TANGIBLE INTERESTS: TRADE SECRETS AND CONFIDENTIAL INFORMATION

The following sample contract language is intended to protect Employers' tangible interests:

Employee agrees that Employee will not, during or at any time after the termination or expiration of this agreement, disclose to any person, firm, corporation or other party, any of the following: the names or addresses of past or present clients of Employer; client or patient records; information about Employer's financial affairs; information about Employer's management or medical systems and personnel or medical policy and procedures manuals; or any confidential reports, fee schedules, trade secrets, or other information or documents that may be used in any way to injure, damage, or interfere with the Employer's business and professional methods and operations.

All business and medical records, including treatment forms, laboratory results, radiographs, phone logs, appointment books, telephone and address books, mailing lists, and computer software programs and data created before or amended during the term of this contract are the property of the Employer, and not the Employee. Employee agrees that such materials, as well as continuing education materials and reference works, shall not be removed from Employer's place of business without Employer's express consent, and that such removal will be grounds for immediate dismissal. Upon termination of the Employee's employment under this agreement, the Employee shall return to the Employer all client and patient records (whether furnished by the Employer or prepared by the Employee in the course of employment), and the Employee shall neither make nor retain copies of any of such records in anticipation of nor after such termination.

STATE LAWS

State statutes regarding restrictive covenants vary, and the laws that exist are in a constant state of flux. Thus, when drafting restrictive covenants for employment contracts, readers must refer to pertinent state statutes (Appendix III) and check with local legal counsel for the current status of the laws.[18]

To illustrate the differences among state statutes, California, Montana, Oklahoma, North Dakota, and Alabama all prohibit the enforcement of restrictive covenants associated with employment contracts but all, except Alabama, permit such covenants in contracts for the purchase or sale of professional businesses. The laws employed by these jurisdictions generally read: "Except as provided in this chapter, every contract by which anyone is restrained from engaging in a lawful profession, trade or business of any kind is to that extent void except in the case of the sale of goodwill where the buyer carries on a like business." [19-23]

The Alabama statute has special rules for professionals. It states, "every contract by which anyone is restrained from exercising a lawful profession, trade or business of any kind...[is to] that extent void...(1) "Professionals are subject to general statutory prohibitions against covenants not to compete; (2) exceptions to the general rule, including the exception for sale of goodwill of business, are not available to professionals."[22]

The Alabama Supreme Court applied this law to veterinarians in *Friddle* v. *Raymond*.[24] In that case, Friddle and Raymond, both licensed veterinarians, entered into a partnership. Five years later, Friddle purchased Raymond's 50% share of the partnership. Their sales agreement contained a restrictive covenant which prohibited Raymond from competing with Friddle within six miles of the practice for three years. Raymond practiced veterinary medicine within the restricted territory and time. Friddle filed suit, seeking declaratory relief. The Circuit Court held the restrictive covenant unenforceable. The Alabama Supreme Court affirmed.

The Alabama Supreme Court first determined that veterinarians were included in the group defined as professionals. According to Alabama law, professionals were not bound by noncompete clauses, and no exceptions applied. Since both Friddle and Raymond were professionals, they were subject to the general rule prohibiting restrictive covenants.

Other states enforce what the laws call "reasonable" restrictive covenants. For example, Wisconsin law states:

> A covenant...not to compete with his employer or principal...within a specified territory and during a specified time is lawful and enforceable only if the restrictions imposed are reasonably necessary for the protection of the employer or principal. Any such restrictive covenant imposing an unreasonable restraint is illegal, void and unenforceable even as to so much of the covenant or performance as would be a reasonable restraint.[25]

Even though the statute allows for reasonable restrictive covenants in employment agreements, it makes it clear that covenants which are unreasonable are void and unenforceable.

South Dakota not only enforces restrictive covenants in employment contracts but also clearly defines what is reasonable.

> An employee may agree at the time of his employment or at any time during his employment (not to compete) for any period not exceeding two years from the date of termination of the agreement and not to solicit existing customers...within a specified county, first or second class municipality or other specified area for any period not exceeding two years from the date of termination of the agreement, if the employer continues to carry on a like business therein.[26]

Prior to 1990, employees bound by noncompetition agreements in Florida rarely prevailed in their attempts to prevent injunctions prohibiting their competition or to invalidate their covenants. That all changed, however, when Florida Statute §542.12 was passed into law in 1990. As amended, this law provided that a presumption of irreparable harm arises only when employers can establish employees' use of specific trade secrets or customer lists or direct solicitation of existing customers.[27] In all other situations, employers must prove irreparable harm before they will be allowed to obtain injunctive relief, i.e., be able to enjoin a former employee from violating the restrictive covenant. An injury is considered to be irreparable if it cannot adequately be compensated by monetary damages.[28]

A *Florida Bar Journal* article describing the effects of this changed Florida law indicates that this amendment will preclude employers from enforcing noncompetition agreements without regard to their reasonableness and for the sake of prohibiting fair competition. It should, nonetheless, still allow employers to protect their legitimate business interests.[29]

Because the laws do vary widely among states, it is imperative to check the relevant state statutes (Appendix III). Much of the information provided is from the 1996 *Restrictive Covenant Survey* completed by The Health Care Group. If interested in updated material, write to The Health Care Group at 140 W. Germantown Pike, Suite 200, Plymouth Meeting, PA 19462 or call 610-828-3888.

Legal Limits of Restrictive Covenants

Reasonableness of Restrictive Covenants

Even though most courts hold that client goodwill is an interest that is protectable by restrictive covenants, courts will not enforce such covenants unless they are reasonable. Courts take a balancing approach in assessing a restrictive covenant's reasonableness, including:

- the relationships among covenantees (employers/buyers) and covenantors (employees/sellers);

- the scope of activity restricted;

- the time limitation;

- the geographic restraint; and

- the adequacy of consideration.

Each component of the noncompete clause then is assessed as being reasonable if it is no greater than required for the protection of the employer, does not impose undue hardship on the employee, and is not injurious to the public. Subsequent discussion focuses on each component.[12, 29]

The *Florida Bar Journal* article quoted previously elaborates even more on the factors courts consider when determining the reasonableness of noncompetition agreements.[29] Among those listed are:

- the time and area of the restriction,

- the nature of the employee's duties,

- the existence of trade secrets or confidential information,

- the employer's need to protect customers and goodwill,

- the employer's investment in training and education of the employee,

- unique skills possessed by employees,

- the oppressive effects of the restriction on the employee,

- the ability of the employee to obtain other employment, and

- the pretermination activities of the employee.[29]

RELATIONSHIPS AMONG COVENANTEES AND COVENANTORS

To determine a covenant's reasonableness, courts consider the relationship between covenantees (the parties to whom covenants are made) and covenantors (parties who promise not to compete). In agreements for practice sales, partnership formations or dissolutions, or corporate stock sales, courts tend to consider that both parties have equal bargaining power. The courts view restrictive covenants among parties entering into sales of practice interests as accurate manifestations of both parties' intentions. Furthermore, because consideration has been provided for the covenant, they usually enforce these covenants as drafted. In such cases, restrictive covenants usually involve greater distances and time periods than would be acceptable with employment contracts, e.g., 10 miles instead of 6, and 5 years as opposed to 3.

When analyzing employment agreements, however, courts usually deem that employers have greater bargaining power than employees. Courts are more skeptical with regard to restrictive covenants between employers and employees[12] and thus are more likely to ensure that they meet the requirements of reasonableness before enforcing them.

PROTECTABLE INTERESTS AND THE SCOPE OF ACTIVITY RESTRICTED

When reviewing restrictive covenants, courts infer that the restricted activity is limited to the fields of veterinary services provided by the employers' practices. Thus, for example, agreements that restrict "the practice of veterinary medicine" when an employee was engaged only in feline or equine medicine may be deemed to be overly broad. Since the employer's practice did not encompass dogs or cows, it can be argued that the employer had no protectable interest in those species.

Therefore, instead of using the all-inclusive "practice of veterinary medicine" restriction, it may be necessary to draft noncompete agreements that limit the restriction only to the type of veterinary services provided by the employer's practice. For example, if employers provide services only to small animals, prohibiting former employees from practicing on large animals is overly broad and probably unenforceable. After all, employers whose practices do not treat large animals have no protectable interest and suffer no detriment from this type of competition. Similarly, veterinarians employed at mixed animal practices that never treat horses should not, upon leaving, be prohibited from practicing equine medicine, while associates who leave exclusively large animal practices should not be prohibited from accepting employment in a practice providing veterinary care only to dogs and cats.

Another issue regarding protectable interests has to do with employers trying to protect their businesses from competition in the form of services not currently offered by their practices. An example involved a dairy practitioner in Pennsylvania who became angry because the veterinarian he had employed as a large animal practitioner resigned and opened a small animal practice in the same medium-sized town in which his dairy practice was located. The dairy practitioner wanted the restrictive covenant enforced. When his attorney asked if his former employee was competing with him for any of his large animal clients, his answer was, "No, but I am planning to open a small animal practice sometime this year and now she's stealing all that business. Don't they teach ethics in school anymore?"

This employer was even more upset when his attorney informed him that even though his former associate was practicing veterinary medicine within his trade area, she really was not competing with him. This is because she was not treating any of the animals owned by the clients she saw while she was working for him in his large animal practice. Furthermore, his plans for opening a small animal practice did not constitute a protectable interest unless the associate had gained and relied upon or used confidential information acquired through her employment with him. When asked if the two of them had discussed the opportunities of opening a small animal practice, his reply was, "No, not really, because I was just beginning to think about expanding my practice into the small animal sector." Unfortunately for the dairy practitioner, the law usually does not protect the mere thinking about expanding one's business into new areas unless employees use confidential information gained via their employment to compete unreasonably with their employers.

To prevent challenges based upon "protectable interests," employers should minimize hardships and enhance the reasonableness and enforceability of their covenants. Employers are encouraged to add clauses to their restrictive covenants that allow former employees to engage in the following noncompetitive activities even within the established radii and time restrictions:

1. In communities where nonprofit humane society or animal control spay and neuter clinics do not compete unreasonably with small animal practice owners, small animal clinicians who leave daytime private practices should be allowed to work at such facilities.

2. Noncompete clauses for exclusively large, small, or exotic animal practices or species-specific facilities should not be drafted so broadly as to prohibit employees from practicing on species of animals never treated by their employers' practices.

3. Veterinarians who work full or part time for routine daytime practices should be allowed to work at nighttime/weekend emergency clinics that generally are

open for business when their former employers' facilities are closed.

4. Veterinarians who work full or part time at emergency clinics should not be prohibited from working as relief veterinarians within the radii wherein they agree not to compete as emergency clinicians.

5. Employees leaving full or part time positions in private practices should be allowed to pursue employment or careers as relief veterinarians within the restricted trade areas provided they work only short stints of time at multiple veterinary practices.

6. Practitioners who leave private veterinary practice should not be prohibited from working for state or federal animal health agencies or university teaching hospitals that do not provide competing services for existing clients.

An example of the principle articulated in point Number 6 can be found in *Tench* v. *Weaver*, wherein the Wyoming Supreme Court reversed a trial court decision and found that Tench's exit from private practice and subsequent employment at the United States Department of Agriculture did not violate the restrictive covenant he had signed.[30] The covenant language stated that "Dr. Tench shall not engage in the practice of Veterinary Science or medicine, nor render any services as a Veterinarian for compensation, in the county of Albany, Wyoming, for a full period of five (5) years." Soon after termination of employment, Tench began working for the United States Department of Agriculture and participated in the government's program for disease eradication in Albany County.

After analyzing the Wyoming statute, it was concluded that such government work did not constitute the "practice of veterinary medicine." The Court also concluded that although Tench had agreed not to "render any services as a veterinarian for compensation," his employment with the government did not violate the agreement. This was partly because Tench received a fixed salary and clients were not charged for his services. The Court refused to conclude that the salary constituted "compensation for veterinary services."

Most notably, the Court stated that the employer had the burden of proof to show that the contract was fair and the restrictive covenant reasonable and necessary to protect the employer. The Court held that the employer did not uphold this burden of proof and, therefore, Tench had not violated the restrictive covenant.

TIME LIMITATIONS

Courts determine the reasonableness of time limits on a case-by-case basis. When analyzing reasonableness, courts have held that a duration is judicious "only if it is no longer than necessary for the employer to put a new [individual] on the job and for the new employee to have a reasonable opportunity to demonstrate his effectiveness to the customers."[12]

"Putting new [individuals] on the job" means locating and interviewing candidates, hiring them, allowing them sufficient time to quit their previous jobs and move to the new practice, introducing these associates to the clientele, and integrating them into the practice. In some cases this process is completed within a few months, while in others it requires a year or longer.

The meaning of "reasonable opportunity" is more difficult to ascertain. Rather than defining it, courts rely on the principle that time restraints are reasonable if they are no longer than necessary to protect employers, do not impose undue hardship on former employees, and are not injurious to the public.[12]

In general, time restraints should be related to the length of employment. Long-term employees have opportunities to provide services for an increasing percentage of the practice's clientele. They also have time to develop stronger bonds with the practice's clientele, strengthening the practice's goodwill in the process. In fact, developing and advancing this goodwill is part of what they are being paid to do. Thus, the longer employees work at practices, the more goodwill employers have to protect.

The result is that unless associate veterinarians are incompetent, competition by these long-term employees poses an increased threat to the employers' goodwill and necessitates longer time restraints. On the other hand, short-term employees routinely have weaker or no bonds with clientele. Consequently, the damage to employers' protectable goodwill is more tenuous, allowing for shorter time restraints to fulfill employers' needs for protection.

In addition to employment length, courts consider the frequency with which the employees have contact with the clientele. In *Spring Harbor Veterinary Associates v. Schackter*, the Wisconsin Court of Appeals stated:

> The reasonableness of the time period depends upon the period of time required to obliterate in the minds of the [employer's]...customers the identification formed during the period of the [employee's]...employment. If an employee's contacts are regular and frequent, a shorter time period may be more reasonable than a longer one. Where the contacts are sporadic and at longer intervals, a longer time period may be reasonable. The reasonableness of the time period depends upon the facts of the particular case.[31]

Although time period reasonableness is examined on a case-by-case basis, a guideline the authors have developed and promoted after years of experience in veterinary practice and the review of numerous legal cases is for general practitioners who work one full year to be expected to promise not to compete for one year postemployment. This time period is reasonable and, unless prohibited by state law, should be legally enforceable. If associates work for employers two years, two-year restrictive covenants seem fair and reasonable. In many states, employers entering into restrictive

covenant agreements with time restraints greater than two years risk unfavorable rulings by the courts.

For example, the South Dakota statute prohibits outright restrictive covenants limiting activity for more than two years after termination of employment.[25] The Georgia statute states that "in an employment contract, reasonable duration would be 2 years in the case of an agreement not to compete after termination."[32] This two-year restriction was enforced in a 1997 Georgia Court of Appeals decision which upheld a two-year, five-mile radius veterinary non-compete clause.[33]

Since courts determine the reasonableness of time restraints on a case-by-case basis, it is difficult to ascertain what is "reasonable" beyond two years. States like Arizona, New Hampshire, and Virginia have precedents enforcing time periods as long as five years.[34-36] However, with respect to these clauses in employment contracts, the legal trend clearly seems to be away from the enforcement of such extended time periods.

For example, in *Hopper v. All Pet Animal Clinic, Inc.*, Hopper, a veterinarian, commenced employment at All Pet Animal Clinic under a contract which included a restrictive covenant prohibiting Hopper from practicing veterinary medicine within a restricted area for a period of three years.[37] Employment was terminated, and soon thereafter Hopper purchased and operated a veterinary practice within the restricted time period. The trial court determined that the time limitation was reasonable.

The Supreme Court of Wyoming disagreed. It found no reasonable basis for the three-year restrictive covenant. An expert witness at the trial revealed that in Wyoming and nationwide 70% of clients visited a veterinary practice more than once a year and the other 30% visited at least once a year. The employer confirmed this data by testifying that the average client sought veterinary care from All Pet one and one-half times a year. In light of these figures, the Court determined that new veterinarians could demonstrate their skills to clients within one year. Furthermore, All Pet presented no evidence showing that clients needed to make multiple visits in order for its doctors to establish influence over the clientele. Thus, the Court concluded that a one-year restrictive covenant would reasonably protect All Pet.

Four situations spark exceptions to the above guidelines regarding time:

- agreements with short-term associates;

- contracts with veterinary specialists (e.g., ophthalmologists, dermatologists, and other "ologists");

- agreements tied to the sale of businesses, and

- partnership, limited liability company, or corporate formations and dissolutions.

SHORT-TERM EMPLOYEES

Legal challenges to the enforcement of restrictive covenants and serious ill will between employees and employers occur when employment is terminated within three to six months of its commencement and employers nevertheless attempt to enforce the restrictive covenants contained in the contracts. Employees argue that their term of employment has been too short for them to have bonded with the practice's clientele, and thus their departure and practice elsewhere will cause no or only minimal damage. Furthermore, they believe their early exit poses far greater hardship for them than it does for their employers.

What these associate veterinarians do not consider is the time and costs required of employers to search for and select, hire, and train new veterinarians. It is quite a financial drain if the employer has just concluded this process, only to have to start over, with the added burden of a former associate working at a competing practice within the restricted radius.

Employers thus can argue that employees who tender early resignations ought to suffer some negative consequences for such action because of the costs and time required to locate replacements. Employees can argue that early termination of their employment by their employers places them at risk if they have rented an apartment or purchased a home but now cannot work within a 20- to 60-minute commute of that residence.

A CONTRACT CLAUSE FOR SHORT-TERM EMPLOYEES

The following clause assures that restrictive covenants for short-term employees are reasonable and minimizes the hardships incurred by each party:

*In the event that Employee's employment under this Agreement is terminated by Employer without cause within (four?, six?) months of its inception, Employee will not be bound by the **time and distance** terms of the restrictive covenant set forth in this Agreement. However, should Employee resign at any time during the term of this Agreement, the restrictive covenant shall be enforced as written.*

This clause exempts employees from the time and distance provisions of the covenant if they are fired without cause. It keeps intact, however, the covenant's prohibitions against the use of confidential information, the solicitation of existing clients, or the solicitation of fellow employees. Furthermore, it offers protection to employers in situations where employees are tempted to or elect to resign because they find jobs with better hours, salaries, staff, or benefits inside the restricted zones. Finally, the contract's definition of the term *for cause* should be referenced or restated in this clause to eliminate the possibility of ambiguity (see definition of *for cause* in Chapter 3).

An exception to these general rules would be in cases where employers provide loans, signing bonuses, or relocation expenses for employees, and the newly hired employees appear to have used such financial assistance simply to help offset their moving expenses. In such cases, resignations within the first few months should be presumed to have been in bad faith, requiring that the breachers go forward with evidence proving that this was not the case.

A clause to cover situations like this follows:

> If Employer has provided Employee with a loan, a signing bonus or the reimbursement of moving expenses, and such Employee resigns within (three?, four?) months of the commencement of the Agreement, and accepts employment at any of the above-exempted veterinary establishments, it shall be presumed that Employee acted in bad faith, in which case the above exceptions to this restrictive covenant shall be null and void.

Specialists

Contracting with veterinary specialists poses multiple, unique concerns. Because veterinary specialists are in short supply, practices can be harmed if these employees compete after leaving. Damage is greatest when employers have invested heavily in salaries, office space, equipment, and staff to build their specialty practices. Damages are incurred because

- it often takes one to two years to locate replacement specialists and allow sufficient time for them to finish their training, complete their existing commitments, and pass their qualifying or certification boards.

- the equipment and staff training required for specialists to pursue their specialties can cost employers as little as a few thousand dollars for dermatologists and animal behaviorists to tens of thousands of dollars for ophthalmologists, surgeons, radiologists, and critical care personnel.

- whereas generalists usually see patients belonging to 2,000 to 3,000 individual

small animal owners per year, specialists may see patients belonging to only 600 to 1,000 clients per year, referred by a mere 20 to 50 veterinary colleagues. This low number of "veterinary referral clients" makes it much easier and less expensive for locally popular specialists to start and grow new practices and/or transfer their goodwill to different locations than it is for generalists.

Thus restrictive covenants for specialists need to be enforced for longer time periods than they are for generalists. Unfortunately, however, while longer time restraints protect employers, they often are disadvantageous to the public. Because there may be only one or two specialists in any given specialty in a certain community, public access to other specialists may not be readily available. Additionally, depriving clients of access to the specialists who have handled their animals and requiring or merely allowing generalists in the practice to proceed with services for them may not be in the best interest of the animals.

One such case involved the attempted enforcement of a restrictive covenant against an oncologist in a large southwestern city. For simplicity, he will be titled "Dr. SW." The specialist maintained that owners and patients of his that were undergoing complicated chemotherapy treatments would suffer serious negative consequences if they were denied access to his expertise after his departure. The general practitioner owner of the practice at which Dr. SW worked maintained that other doctors at the practice could manage these cases without harm to the patients just as well as Dr. SW could.

Another case, in Arizona, involved a noncompete agreement for a board-certified human orthopedic surgeon.[38] This surgeon left his practice and, according to his contract, was not supposed to compete within a certain restricted area. He breached his contract by practicing in that area. The court subsequently modified the restrictive covenant so that the orthopedic surgeon was allowed to treat former patients seeking emergency services related to his prior care at hospitals within the restricted area. This was upheld in order to provide the surgeon's patients with continuity of medical care, in spite of the fact there were many other orthopedic surgeons in the area who could have provided the same specialty service. This case provides a good example of a court's action to accommodate the needs of the public while enforcing a contractual agreement.

Because of these clashes between the rights of practice owners to protect their goodwill and the rights of the public to receive veterinary care from the only specialist in the community, feuding parties and courts must consider carefully the benefits to employers versus the detriments to employees and the public before deciding how best to resolve such disputes.

A CONTRACT CLAUSE FOR SPECIALISTS

In the event Employee ceases to be employed by Employer, Employee and Employer agree that some patients attended by Employee (especially patients receiving chemotherapy or with complex surgical or internal medicine problems) will need ongoing veterinary care under the supervision of a specialist with skills similar to those possessed by Employee. Thus, should Employee no longer be employed by Employer's practice, Employer and Employee agree to review the medical status of those patients afflicted with complex, ongoing (name of specialty) problems. If the parties conclude that staff at Employer's veterinary practice are not sufficiently trained and/or experienced to provide competent ongoing veterinary services for these specified patients, Employer agrees that Employee can continue serving owners of those animals, and only those, at Employee's home, at another veterinary practice within the above-defined

radius, or by referring them to another veterinarian with sufficient specialty training so that appropriate and competent specialty veterinary care can be provided. Should the Employer and Employee disagree as to the need for ongoing care being delivered by a specialist, the client, in agreement with the attending veterinarian who provided the majority of the patient's care, shall be the party entitled to make the decision. If the client and the attending veterinarian cannot agree, then the client shall have the final decision.

TIME RESTRICTIONS FOR SPECIALISTS

After weighing the previous issues, it seems reasonable that veterinary specialists who work only one year in communities where other similar specialists reside be expected to sign two-year restrictive covenants. Although this could be harmful to the public, such detriment can be minimized by permitting the specialists to provide ongoing services to a narrow group of patients identified at the time of their departure whose health care requires their special expertise until the existing medical conditions are stable. If these specialists complete more than one and a half years of employment, then three-year restrictive covenants seem fair, provided that they be allowed to service the same selected group of patients in need of ongoing care set forth previously.

However, in communities where no similar specialists reside, it may be reasonable to enforce only one-year restraints for one year of employment and two years for two years of employment. Lastly, and much to the chagrin of employers who have invested heavily in hiring and promoting a unique specialist, there may be situations where the detriment to the public is so great and state law precedents so clear that these restrictive covenants should not be enforced at all.

Defining Clients of Specialists

With respect to generalists, the word *clients* means animal owners and caretakers. With respect to specialists, the word takes on additional meanings. This is because referrals of complicated cases from general practitioners constitute the majority of the cases attended by specialists.

For specialists to build their practices and succeed, it is as important for them to please the veterinarians who refer cases to them as it is to satisfy the needs of their patients and the owners whose animals they care for. This requires, among other things, that they

- provide competent and compassionate veterinary services,

- respond to requests for information from referring veterinarians on a timely basis, provide referring veterinarians with punctual referral reports or letters,

- keep fees for services within the estimates they gave to their referring doctors,

- send cases back to their referring doctors as soon as it is medically appropriate, and

- not perform procedures or administer or sell medications or biologicals that routinely are part of the care provided by the generalists.

As discussed previously, specialists who are highly regarded in their veterinary communities can create booming practices with as few as 50 to 100 referring veterinary practices as their "clients." Because of this, the term *client* needs to be defined differently in their restrictive covenants than it is in the contracts of generalists. In fact, it also may be critical to define the term *referring veterinary practice*, since these are the clients of most specialists.

A Sample Definition of *Client*

Definition of Terms: As used in this Agreement, "clients" shall include any person or entity that, directly or indirectly, through one or more intermediaries, owns or controls the medical decision making for an animal that received veterinary care from the Employer business during the term of Employee's employment with the Employer. The term referring veterinarian(s) shall mean any person or entity that owns, is employed by, works as an independent contractor for, or manages a veterinary practice or possesses a veterinary degree and/or a veterinary license and who referred a client attended by the Employee during the term of the Employee's employment with the Employer. The term solicit means all communications or advertising directed intentionally to specific individuals for the purpose of obtaining their employment or business, but does not include press releases, mass advertising, or professional listings in telephone books.

Practice Sale Restrictions

The issues and precedents involving the enforcement of restrictive covenants linked to sales of veterinary sole proprietorships, partnership interests, shares of stock, limited liability companies, and limited liability partnerships deal with different points and require entirely different thought processes.

First of all, it is assumed that the parties involved in sales and purchase transactions involving ownership interests have reasonably equal bargaining power.

Secondly, when buyers purchase the interests of veterinarians who have been owners, the values of the practices being sold are highly dependent on the existence of promises by sellers not to compete after the sale. Without such promises, buyers cannot justify paying, nor can they afford to pay, the high prices required to purchase a veterinary practice. For example, Dr. Charisma sells her three-doctor practice grossing $1 million for $800,000 and within one to two years starts a new practice within the trade radius of the practice she sold. There is a high likelihood that the competition from her presence in the community, and that of an additional competing practice in the trade area, will impact the buyer's income so severely that the buyer will no longer be able to run a profitable practice.

Thirdly, practice owners usually are charismatic, entrepreneurial, active, and well known within their communities, and/or have been present at their practices for periods of time long enough to form strong bonds with their clients. Because these bonds usually have been developed over many years, it requires longer than the standard one- to two-year covenants found in employment contracts to sever such bonds. Lastly, buyers purchasing practices usually pay tens and often hundreds of thousands of dollars of consideration in exchange for sellers' covenants not to compete.

Because of these reasons, five-year restrictions are common with respect to sales of practices, and courts tend to enforce these covenants as drafted. In *Griffin* v. *Hunt*, the Oklahoma Supreme Court upheld the validity of a five-year restrictive covenant.[39] A widow and her daughter inherited a veterinary facility from their veterinarian husband/father. They arranged with a veterinarian, Griffin, to practice at the facility. Four years later, the widow made an agreement with Hunt, a recent veterinary graduate, to buy the facility. Hunt stated that he would purchase the practice only if Griffin agreed not to compete. Hunt and Griffin entered into a written restrictive covenant whereby Griffin agreed not to compete in the area for five years in exchange for $1.00 and other valuable consideration. About six months later, Griffin began to practice within the prohibited area. Hunt brought suit to enforce the restrictive covenant.

The trial court applied the Oklahoma statute allowing the enforcement of restrictive covenants in conjunction with the sale of a business. The trial court upheld the validity of the restrictive covenant and rejected Griffin's argument that he was not part of the sale negotiations and received no consideration therefrom. It also found that the Hunt/Griffin restrictive covenant agreement was not a mere courtesy on Griffin's part, but a vital reason as to why Hunt agreed to buy the practice. The Supreme Court of Oklahoma affirmed the trial court opinion granting a permanent injunction against Dr. Griffin's practice of veterinary medicine in the restricted area for five years.

While courts are more likely to uphold restrictive covenants in buy-sell agreements, they will evaluate closely whether the contract truly concerns the sale of goodwill. In *Boggs* v. *Couturier*, Boggs and Couturier entered into a veterinary partnership agreement.[40] The agreement included a restrictive covenant that would be triggered should one partner decide to end the partnership. After several years, Couturier elected to leave the partnership and received reimbursement for his capital investment. Boggs sought to enforce the restrictive covenant.

At the time of this case, Michigan law allowed restrictive covenant agreements only pursuant to buy-sell agreements. Thus, at issue was whether the restrictive covenant in this partnership agreement was protected. The Michigan Court of Appeals held that since all the goodwill remained with the veterinarian who had started the veterinary practice seven years before the junior partner bought in, and the partnership agreement gave the senior partner the privilege of remaining in the present location and conducting the business even if the partnership was dissolved, there was no goodwill linked to the junior partner's participation in the partnership which could be transferred. Thus, the buy-sell agreement and its restrictive covenant was not afforded any statutory protection and it was not enforced. It should be noted that Michigan law changed in 1985 and allowed for the enforcement of reasonable restrictive covenants even in employment contracts.

An example involving a restrictive covenant tied to the lease of a piece of real estate can be found in the Ohio case *Marysville Animal Care Center* v. *Andreas*.[41] Andreas, the owner of a small animal hospital, leased his land and capital improvements (building and personal property) to Sullivan. The lease agreement contained a restrictive covenant which prohibited Sullivan from engaging in a small animal practice within a 15-mile radius of the leased premises for a period of 5 years from the lease termination date. The owners of Marysville Animal Care Center were concerned that if Sullivan left the practice site and opened a practice within the restricted area, other veterinarians would be discouraged from leasing the site. The trial court held and the Ohio Court of Appeals affirmed that the restrictive covenant was unreasonable and unenforceable.

The Appellate Court stated that a restrictive covenant was enforceable if the restraint was no greater than necessary to protect the employer, did not impose undue hardship on the employee, and was not injurious to the public. The Court then concluded that Andreas' concern with enforcing the restrictive covenant was to protect the value of the real estate as rental property, not to protect his interest in the practice's goodwill. Thus, the Court determined that since the restraint protected only an unprotectable interest in the real estate, it was unenforceable.

Additional issues that buyers and sellers of practices must consider when purchasing or selling include

- the presence, absence, and current status and terms of the employment contracts sellers have with existing associates,

- the presence or absence of noncompete clauses in such employment contracts,

- whether the terms and obligations under such contracts inure to the buyers at the time of the sale, and

- whether the buyers will have the right to terminate and/or negotiate new contracts with the employers' associate veterinarians and support staff after their purchases.

If sellers have long-term or highly regarded clinicians working without employment contracts, buyers run the risk of purchasing such practices only to have those employees leave and compete with them at a nearby practice. As with competition from sellers, this could pose serious financial consequences for buyers. Of course, buyers of practices also could inherit unhappy, unmotivated, or undesirable doctors with binding contracts, which could prove to be equally problematic.

As discussed previously, practice *goodwill* is the practice's reputation within the community and among the staff. *Professional goodwill* refers to the doctor-client-patient relationship, strengthened by veterinarians' personal traits. Together, professional goodwill and practice goodwill form *client goodwill*, or the reputation among a practice's clientele. Buyers who purchase practices lacking contracts with existing staff members are not really purchasing the client goodwill being valued during the course of the practice appraisal or the client goodwill they have anticipated. Thus, such practices may be overvalued.

Considerable protection is offered when practices being purchased contain employment contracts with noncompete clauses; however, where a valued practice manager or one or more popular and established associates do not have contracts with covenants, the sales value of the practice must be adjusted downward accordingly. What this really means is that it is critical for sellers to establish contracts with associate veterinarians and practice managers containing reasonable and, thus, enforceable restrictive covenants well before sales of their practices are undertaken.

PROTECTING A TRADE OR "CATCHMENT" AREA

Anyone who owns a veterinary practice is aware that the majority of one's customers tend to live within a given distance of the business's location. This is known as the practice's trade or "catchment" area. Geographic barriers, highways, shopping patterns, state borders, and cultural habits are but a few of the things influencing the boundaries of these areas.

To prevent unfair competition, the laws and court precedents of most states provide business owners with a right to protect their trade areas from competition by departing employees or sellers as long as the protective measures taken are reasonable. The difficulty encountered with these laws, though, is in determining where a majority of a business's clientele reside. The methods used to define a veterinary practice's trade area follow.

GEOGRAPHIC LIMITATIONS

Courts determine the reasonableness of geographic restraints on a case-by-case basis, just as they do when judging the length for time limitations. Since in most small animal practices small percentages of clients live 10 to 75 miles away (or in urban areas, 30 to 60 minutes from the practice), only a portion instead of all of a practice's clientele is protectable. Generally, courts enforce geographic restraints that protect 80% to 85% of the practice's clientele.[12] Although the use of the word "radius" implies air miles, it is wise to use the words "air-mile radius" in covenants to avoid confusion.

For example, in Cockerill v. Wilson, the Illinois Court of Appeals found a 20-mile geographic restraint judicious because 90% of the practice's clients lived within that radius.[12,42] Although the Illinois Supreme Court reversed the appellate decision on other grounds, it upheld the lower court's finding of reasonableness.

In a 1945 case, Brecher v. Brown,[43] the Iowa Supreme Court held that a 25-mile geographical restraint in a mixed animal practice was overreaching, as only one of the employer's clients lived outside of that radius. The Supreme Court ruled that the restricted area was greater than necessary to protect the employer.

In 1976, the New Hampshire Supreme Court addressed geographic restraints in Moore v. Dover Veterinary Hospital, Inc.[35] The plaintiff, Moore, sought a declaratory judgment to render a restrictive covenant entered into with his employer unenforceable. Under the agreement, Moore had promised not to compete within a 20-mile radius of an AAHA small animal hospital. The Supreme Court upheld the restrictive covenant and stated that the enforceability of restrictive covenants hinges on whether space and time restraints are reasonable. The reasonableness of geographic restraints is determined by the employer's normal marketplace. Evidence showed that the 20-mile radius represented an approximate measure of the employer's market.

Finally, in Cukjati v. Burkett, Burkett entered into an employment contract with Cukjati, the owner of two veterinary facilities.[44] The contract contained a restrictive covenant prohibiting Burkett from practicing veterinary medicine within a 12-mile radius of either veterinary clinic for 3 years postemployment. After voluntarily terminating employment, Burkett took a job at another veterinary clinic within the restricted area. Burkett sought declaratory relief, arguing that the restrictive covenant was invalid. Cukjati countersued. The trial court entered summary judgement in favor of Burkett; Cukjati appealed.

The Texas Court of Appeals affirmed the lower court opinion for several reasons, one of which was that the territorial restriction was unreasonable. Burkett produced uncontroverted evidence demonstrating that most of the pet owners in the area traveled only a few miles to receive veterinary medical care. Consequently, the Court ruled that the 12-mile restriction was unreasonable.

SCIENTIFIC ANALYSES VS. STANDARD NORMS

Traditionally, employers have determined reasonable geographic distances by relying on standard norms similar to those presented in Table 9.3. These guidelines generally take into account practice type, population densities, and community size, which courts recognize affect geographical limitations.[12] Although such boundaries can be realistic in some cases, they may be nothing more than speculation in others.

Small animal practices provide services to clients from relatively smaller "catchment" areas than do equine or food animal practices. According to a 1989 *JAVMA* article, 75% of urban small animal practitioners' clients live within 8 miles of the practices they patronize. The same percentage of small animal clients in rural areas live within 19 miles of their practices. Equine practitioners' clients live within an average radius of 27 miles from their veterinarians. Food animal practitioners' clients live an average of 23 miles from the practices.[45] Finally, ambulatory practices, which service animals at the owners' premises, serve larger areas than do hospitals, and thus have larger geographic scopes.[12] Although these may have been realistic guidelines for the 1980s, and still are considered the norm today, increasingly dense populations of people and veterinary practices make these less reliable figures as the turn of the century approaches.

A more recent study of 37,000 pet owners and 535 veterinary practices involving the demographics of small animal practice showed the following:

- 27% of pet owners lived less than 2 miles from the veterinary practice they frequented,

- 38% lived between 2 and 5 miles from the practice (total of 65% living less than 5 miles from the practice),

- 20% lived between 6 and 10 miles away, and

- 15% lived 10 or more miles from the practice.[46]

In that study, the national mean distance was 5.3 miles. Owners who lived more than two miles from the practice said that friends and relatives influenced their decision. Older pet owners were more concerned with location than younger ones.

Standard norms are beneficial, especially to employees who need guidelines during contract negotiations to help them determine whether covenant restrictions are fair. However, standard norms are general guidelines and often are overly broad, leaving employers vulnerable to challenges or causing undue hardship to employees and the public. Employers and employees are urged to use compasses to plot boundaries in advance of signing contracts with noncompete agreements to help determine the reasonableness of the distances. The failure to do this often results in the absence of a geographic reality check and, thus, the inclusion of unreasonable and unenforceable distances in employment contracts.

Examples of the standard norms found within the industry can be seen in Table 9.3.

THE SCIENTIFIC APPROACH TO DETERMINING TRADE AREAS

Although standard norms are used more commonly than scientific analyses when setting restrictive covenant boundaries, they are not nearly as reliable. In fact, as the numbers of private practitioners and veterinary practices have increased in the past decade, as human populations per veterinarian have decreased (from 6,000 people per DVM to 3,000 per DVM in some regions of the country), and as computer tracking systems of clients have improved, the old "standard norm"

Table 9.3. Guidelines for Standard Norms*

Small animal practices	High-rise, densely populated urban areas	1-2 miles or by streets
	Densely populated urban setting	2-3 miles or zip codes
	Suburbia	3-6 miles
	Exurbia**	5-12 miles
	Rural areas	10-20 miles
Feline practices	Dense urban	2-5 miles
	Suburbia	8-12 miles
Large animal practices	States with reasonably dense animal populations	10-25 miles
	States with sparse animal/human populations	15-50 miles
	Dairy practices - could be limited by distance or to	
	specific producers who are clients	10-25 miles
Equine practices	Depends on density of equine population and the	
	type of practice, with differences among pleasure,	
	racetrack, and broodmare practices	10-35 miles
Specialty practices	Including surgery, ophthalmology, dermatology, etc.,	
	depends on population densities and numbers of	
	competing specialists in same specialty	10-50 miles
Emergency practices	Dense urban	15-25 miles
	Suburban to exurban areas	20-35 miles

* Note: These numbers were derived upon review of more than 550 veterinary employment contracts and the geography of over 200 restrictive covenants.

** *Exurbia* is defined as distant suburbs not immediately connected to a major urban area.

method seems to make less and less sense. Furthermore, this approach does not take into consideration the presence of natural and manmade barriers.

When utilizing the scientific approach, it is suggested that employers start with detailed maps of the area to determine the presence of naturally occurring geographic borders like freeways, mountain ranges, highways, and bodies of water. When that has been completed, random samples of 1% of their practices' active clients should be plotted on detailed maps of their trade areas. Active clients are those seen by the practice in the past two years.

Once the maps of client addresses are plotted, employers calculate the radii (or determine the actual geographic boundaries) in which 80% to 85% of the clients reside. Although this can be time consuming, it is worthwhile because it produces scientifically based decisions, establishing trade areas that are more likely to be defended and upheld if challenged. Additionally, completing such an analysis generally proves to be a valuable marketing exercise for practice owners. Once they know which sections of their trade areas are the strongest, they can develop marketing plans to develop those areas where their client numbers are weak.

GEOGRAPHIC LIMITATIONS: NATURAL AND MANMADE BARRIERS

Most practices draft geographic limitations by calculating radii. When mapping out the boundaries of trade areas, though, it is critical to consider natural and manmade barriers in order to draft reasonable covenants. The only way to do this effectively is to purchase detailed maps of the trade area and use a compass or connect lines involving natural street borders on the map to plot the boundaries. Using this technique, employees, employers, sellers, buyers, and courts can get a feel for the geography and locate other practices that compete within their trade areas.

For example, practices adjacent to large bodies of water usually have major highways running parallel to the water. These circumstances affect radii calculations. One practice near the New Jersey shore with a satellite practice 7 miles south of its main hospital has the Atlantic Ocean 1½ miles to the east and the Garden State Parkway 2½ miles to the west. As a result of a careful analysis of a random 1% of the practice's clientele, it was determined that 80% of the clients reside within a rectangle 15 miles north of the central practice and 8 miles south of the satellite practice, and 1½ miles to the east and 2½ miles to the west. Thus, a 15-mile radius in all directions of the practice would have been overly broad and unreasonable, whereas a rectangular catchment area appears reasonable and defensible.

To assure reasonably accurate geographic boundaries, it is recommended that the scientific approach be used while taking barriers into consideration. In urban or densely populated suburban areas, zip code analyses of 100% of the client residences often help locate accurate boundaries for 80% to 85% of the clients.

A list of criteria to be considered when evaluating natural boundaries includes the following:

- rivers and the locations of bridges across them
- oceans, lakes, parks, and mountain ranges
- freeways and the location of access points traversing them
- traffic patterns and bottlenecks that prevent residents from traveling in certain directions during rush hours
- borders between states that alter legal, cultural, and business practices
- locations of jobs for the general work force in given areas
- shopping patterns
- ethnic boundaries beyond which most residents do not shop for services

GEOGRAPHIC LIMITATIONS: SATELLITE CLINICS

Some employers own one or more satellite clinics in addition to a central hospital. Restrictive covenants that prohibit employees from working within "x" miles of any and all locations the employer owns either before and/or after they start their jobs are likely to be held to be unreasonably restrictive. After all, how can clients form bonded relationships with all of the doctors at all of the hospitals, especially when some doctors only work at certain practices within the group a few shifts or days per year?

For example, in Stringer v. Herron, the South Carolina Court of Appeals invalidated a restrictive covenant which placed a 15-mile restraint from any of three hospitals operated by the employer.[47] Veterinarians Stringer and Herron entered into an employment contract with a restrictive covenant. The covenant prohibited Herron from practicing veterinary medicine for three years from termination of employment within 15 miles of any of the three veterinary practices owned by Stringer. After three years, Herron voluntarily terminated his employment. Shortly thereafter, Herron began a mobile veterinary practice which provided services to clients who lived within the prohibited boundaries. Stringer brought suit to enforce the restrictive covenant agreement. The Circuit Court of Anderson County granted an injunction, enjoining Herron from practicing within the restricted area. The Appellate Court reversed the lower court opinion.

At issue was whether the geographic limit was reasonable. The Court stated that a geographic limitation will be upheld only if it covers an area necessary to protect the employer.

The Court noted that 96% of Stringer's clients lived within 15 miles of the practices. However, since 84% of Stringer's clients lived within 10 miles of one of the practices, the geographic boundaries were overly broad. The Court held that the restrictive covenant was unreasonable and, therefore, unenforceable.

There is no question that competition from any new veterinary practice can negatively impact the success of a multipractice owner's satellite clinic. It could be argued, though, that employees who work only a few days each year at a particular satellite clinic have no bigger advantage in the community than outsiders who choose to establish practices in that vicinity. Of course, former employees should not be able to use consistent exposure to clients or confidential information acquired during the course of employment to gain an unfair business advantage over their employers.

A CONTRACT CLAUSE FOR SATELLITE CLINICS

The following clause is suggested to provide employees with some latitude while preventing unreasonable competition near their employers' satellite clinics:

The terms of this restrictive covenant apply equally to any satellite or ancillary (small?, mixed?, equine?) animal veterinary facility(ies) that Employer currently owns or acquires in the future at which Employee works greater than 1 full day per week for 6 or more months of any contract year or greater than 10 full days per quarter, the total of which constitutes more than 40 days per contract year.

GEOGRAPHIC LIMITATIONS: ZONE OF COMMONALITY

A doctrine affecting restrictive covenants conceived and advanced by Owen McCafferty, CPA, North Olmsted, Ohio, is entitled the "zone" or "doctrine of catchment commonality." An illustration of this doctrine would be as follows. Dr. A's trade or catchment area consists of a radius of four miles, so that a departing Dr. B must move at least eight miles in any direction to avoid sharing a portion of the trade area which is common to both practices. The theory behind this is that if the trade radius of Dr. A's practice is four miles, it is likely that the trade area for Dr. B's practice will be four miles, too. Consequently, Dr. B needs to relocate at least eight miles away so as not to share any of the catchment area which would be common to both practices.

Although this seems logical, the authors' opinion is that relying on such large radii often provides employers with greater protection than is reasonably needed. For example, if the bulk of Dr. A's clients reside to the northwest, west, and southwest of the practice, and Dr. B moves to a practice location a tenth of a mile outside the eastern boundary of the noncompete clause, a relatively small portion of Dr. B's clientele will reside within the zone that overlaps with Dr. A's trade area (see Figure 9.1).

Conversely, if the majority of Dr. A's clients reside to the east of the hospital, and Dr. B moves to a practice a tenth of a mile outside the eastern border, Drs. A and B are likely to share a significant volume of the same clients (Figure 9.2).

As a result of these types of variations in trade areas, there may be times when restrictive covenant radii will need to extend beyond the point where 80% to 85% of a practice's clientele reside in order to provide the practice owner with reasonable protection. In such situations, it may be appropriate to extend the distances to 1.5 to 1.75 times the actual radius within which 80% to 85% of the practice's clients reside (Figure 9.3). Under circumstances such as this, though, extending the entire 360°E radius to 1.5 to 1.75 times the distance within which 80% to 85% of the clients live will probably cause unreasonable restraints of trade. What makes sense, instead, is extending the restrictive covenant in the direction of the dense population of clientele to a longer distance than to that of the sparse population (Figures 9.4 and 9.5).

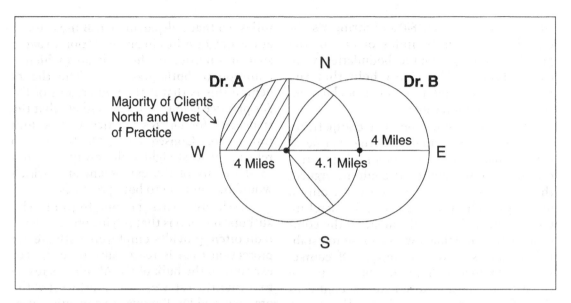

Figure 9.1. The total distance from Dr. A's practice to the border is equal to the radius within which 80% to 85% of Dr. A's clients reside. If Dr. B leaves Dr. A's practice and opens a facility 4.1 miles from Dr. A, just outside the 4-mile restrictive covenant zone, the two parties will share nearly 1/3 of the same trade area. Since most of Dr. A's clients live north and west of the practice, though, the effect on Dr. A's practice should be limited.

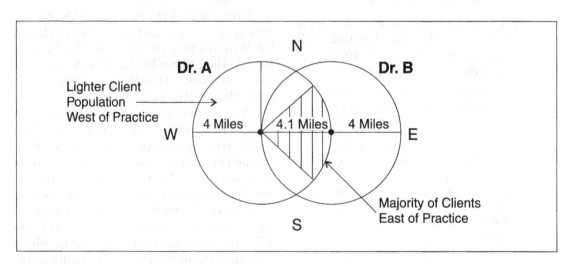

Figure 9.2. Same scenario as Figure 9.1, but since the majority of Dr. A's clients live east of the practice, competition from Dr. B for the overlapping trade area could be significant.

Zones of Commonality— Some Final Thoughts

As can be seen from the previous diagrams, zones of catchment commonality can significantly impact competition within specific sectors of some practice trade areas. Nonetheless, it is only reasonable that practice owners wishing to extend their boundaries based on this rationale be

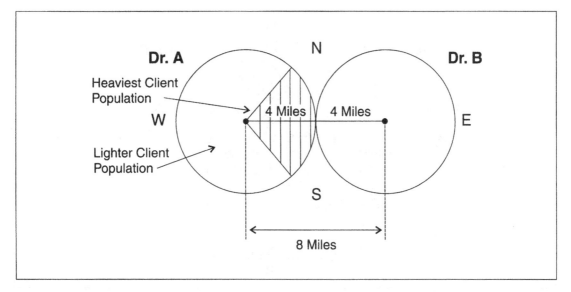

Figure 9.3. The total distance from Dr. A's practice is 2 times the radius. However, even though most clients are in the direction of Dr. B's clients, that practice now is farther away and less likely to impact Dr. A's practice.

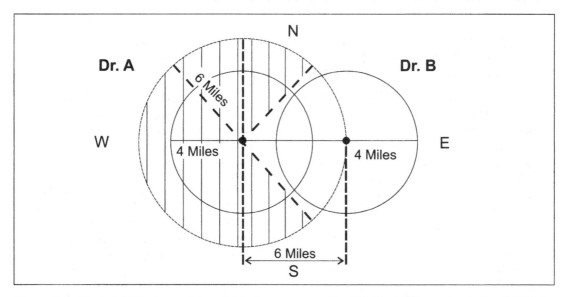

Figure 9.4. The total distance of the restrictive covenant (6 miles) is 1.5 times the radius in which 80% to 85% of clients reside. Thus, a complete circle of 6 miles is greater protection to the north, south and west than Dr. A needs.

required to determine client densities in the various quadrants of their trade areas based upon the scientific analysis of client addresses. Only by assuming this addi- tional burden are businesses justified in extending their restrictive covenant bound- aries beyond the standard 80% to 85% pro- tection areas.

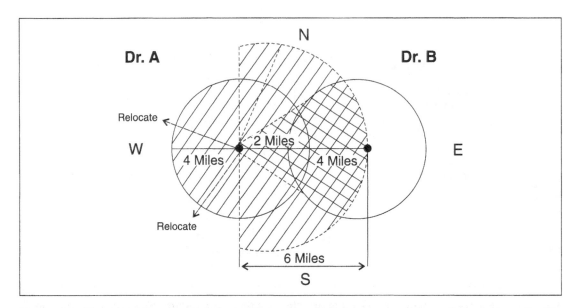

Figure 9.5. The restrictive covenant is 4 miles to the northwest, west and southwest where Dr. A's clientele is sparsely populated, and a half-circle radius of 6 miles to the northeast, east and southeast where Dr. A's clients are concentrated. This gives ample protection to Dr. A, forcing Dr. B to go more than 6 miles to the east if she wants to work in that direction.

A CLAUSE FOR ACTIVITY RESTRICTIONS AND TIME/GEOGRAPHIC LIMITATIONS

The following contract clause addresses activity restrictions as well as time and geographic limitations:

As a material inducement to Employee to enter into this agreement, Employee shall be provided with professional education, experience, and training and the compensation and benefits heretofore agreed upon. Employee agrees that during the period of this agreement and for a period of (one?, two?, three?) years after the termination or expiration of this contract, Employee will not render, offer to render, or attempt to render; serve as an independent contractor for; own, manage, operate, or control; be employed by, participate in, or have an interest in, or be connected in any manner with the ownership, management, operation, or control of any business or profession, including that of a mobile practice, engaged in (small animal?, emergency?, mixed animal?, equine?, food animal?) veterinary services simi-lar in scope to those provided by the Employer within a (three?, five?, ten?) air-mile radius of the Employer's practice location. (Note: in some cases it may be essential to use streets, freeways, rivers, mountains or other natural business barriers as boundaries rather than mileage radii. Also, if employees are engaged in mixed animal practice, it may be necessary to use two different radii: a longer radius for large animal ambulatory clientele, and a shorter radius for small animal clients.)

During the term of such restrictive covenant, Employee may be employed as (1) a government employee, as long as the work performed for a governmental employer does not compete with the services offered by the Employer in this Agreement; (2) a relief veterinarian for veterinary practices within the previous boundaries as long as such employment is not greater than 6 consecutive days per month at any one practice, does not exceed 10 days during any 3-month quarter of a calendar year, and is not a consistent day of the week for greater than 3 consecutive weeks; (3) a veteri-

narian at a humane society or govern-
mentally supported low-cost spay and
neuter facility (note: assuming
Employer does not operate such a facil-
ity); or (4) a clinician at a night-
time/weekend emergency clinic that
routinely is open for business when the
Employer in this Agreement is closed.

THE ISSUE OF CONSIDERATION

Consideration, a necessary element for all contracts, is the cause, motive, or impelling influence that induces contracting parties to enter into agreements. For example, if a contract states: "To induce Employee to enter into an employment contract, Employer agrees to pay Employee compensation and provide benefits, professional education, and training," the consideration is the employee's work in exchange for compensation, benefits, professional education, and training.

Like all contracts, restrictive covenants must be supported by consideration. With the sale of a business interest in a partnership or stock in a corporation, the consideration is the exchange of money for the sale and transfer of the practice's goodwill. Most courts do not question the existence of consideration for restrictive covenants in such contracts.[12]

In contrast, courts pay greater attention to the consideration issue in employment contracts. Because of the unequal bargaining power between employers and employees, courts look to the circumstances surrounding the negotiation process to ensure that the restrictive covenant was part of a bargain for exchange. Moreover, if employers and employees enter into restrictive covenants weeks, months, or years after the commencement of employment, additional consideration must be provided to employees for the covenant to be held valid.[12]

The Restatement (Second) of Contracts states that in an ongoing transaction or relationship, a promise not to compete may be made before the termination of the relation-

ship and still be ancillary as long as it is supported by consideration and meets other requirements for enforceability.[48] For example, if parties enter into an oral agreement which includes a restrictive covenant and later put the employment agreement in writing, the written covenant is supported by the original consideration associated with the hiring of the party at the time of the oral agreement. However, if a covenant is added to an already established contract, additional consideration is needed for the covenant to be enforceable.

In *Stevenson v. Parsons*, the employee signed a restrictive covenant after the commencement of employment without receiving additional consideration.[49] The Trial Court entered a summary judgement for the employee stating that, as a matter of law, the covenant was void for lack of consideration. The North Carolina Court of Appeals reversed the Trial Court opinion and sent the case back for a trial, holding that a genuine issue of fact did exist. The Appellate Court ruled that if the facts presented at trial showed that the promise not to compete was agreed upon before employment commenced and in exchange for being hired, then the covenant was valid.

Courts usually will not assess the adequacy of consideration in most routine contract disputes. However, since restrictive covenants can be oppressive and the bargaining power between employers and employees often unequal, courts are more willing to analyze the adequacy of consideration in restrictive covenants in employment agreements.[12]

In *Hopper v. All Pet Animal Clinic, Inc.*, the parties entered into an oral employment agreement and mentioned a restrictive covenant, but did not specify its terms.[37] A written agreement was established about 10 months later, and the terms of the restrictive covenant were addressed. Six months after implementing the written agreement, both parties agreed upon an addendum. The addendum stated that Hopper would provide professional services to a newly acquired animal hospital, Alpine Animal Hospital, in addition to All Pet Animal Clinic. The addendum also included a $550 per month raise in Hopper's salary; the restrictive covenant remained the same.

The trial court held and the Supreme Court of Wyoming affirmed that since the oral agreement never addressed a specific geographic radius or time frame in which Hopper was prohibited from practicing veterinary medicine, the restrictive covenant was not ancillary to the employment agreement. Since no additional consideration was given, the covenant failed for lack of consideration. But the courts ruled that the addendum providing the salary increase was separate consideration. Thus, the restrictive covenant was enforced.

In *Kramer* v. *Robec, Inc.*, Kramer worked for Robec as an at-will employee, meaning that termination of employment by the employer could occur at any time.[50] During the employment period, Robec made Kramer an offer: In exchange for $1,000 and changing Kramer's employment status to a guaranteed 2½ years, terminable only for good cause, with 180 days notice of severance by either employer or employee, Kramer would enter into a covenant not to compete. Kramer signed the agreement. Later, Kramer left Robec to work for a competitor. At issue was whether Kramer was bound by the covenant.

The District Court for the Eastern District of Pennsylvania held that, although the agreement was entered into after Kramer began work, the additional consideration of change of employment status and $1,000 was adequate to make the covenant valid. The Court noted, however, that the $1,000 alone would not have been adequate consideration. Thus, if Robec had not changed the employment status, the covenant would not have been enforceable under the circumstances of this case. The court did not reach any decision regarding whether the change to new employment status from at-will to

an agreed-upon term alone would constitute adequate consideration.

In a 1995 case entitled *Admiral Services, Inc.* v. *John Drebit*,[51] the court shed some light on whether a change in employment status alone constitutes the "fundamental change in employment" needed to be deemed adequate consideration. After finding a "raise in the employee's salary, an additional paid holiday, a cash bonus, a longevity bonus plan, and the use of a bigger company truck," to be a "corresponding benefit" which suffices as adequate consideration, the court went on to add that "continued employment is not sufficient consideration for a covenant not to compete which the employee signed after the inception of employment, where the employer makes no promise of continued employment for a definite term."

This does seem to suggest that a situation such as in *Kramer* v. *Robec, Inc.*, where an employee's status is changed from at-will to some significant guaranteed time, would be considered a fundamental change in employment, since it does change the nature of the at-will employment entirely. However, an insignificant change in employment from, e.g., at will to 15 days would not constitute a change in the terms of employment fundamental enough to satisfy the consideration requirement.

When analyzing case law concerning this issue, it is important to recognize that the term *continued employment* lends itself easily to confusion and error; thus, the intent or precedent as an authority for a legal opinion can be misconstrued. In Pennsylvania, for example, continued employment, as in continuing with the status quo, does not amount to adequate consideration— only continued employment where the employment status has been fundamentally changed does. This becomes problematic when cases in Pennsylvania or elsewhere refer to opinions from previous legal cases involving "continued employment" without actually ascertaining which type of "continued employment" situations occurred in those earlier cases.

To add to the confusion, although courts always examine the adequacy of consideration when determining the enforceability of restrictive covenants, ultimately it is up to each individual state and court to determine what is adequate. In *Kida* v. *Chesterfield Veterinary Clinic, Inc.*, for example, the Circuit Court of Chesterfield County, Virginia held that an additional $1,000 in salary was adequate consideration.[52]

In another case, *Loescher* v. *Policky*, the Supreme Court of South Dakota ruled that an employer's compliance with contract terms and willingness to extend the contract indefinitely was adequate consideration. Loescher practiced veterinary medicine for Policky.[53] Both parties agreed to the terms of a contract, which included a restrictive covenant. Policky complied with the contract and agreed to continue it indefinitely. After two years, however, Loescher voluntarily terminated employment and, a week later, began practicing veterinary medicine within the restricted area and time. The trial court held that the agreement was enforceable. Loescher appealed on several grounds, including inadequacy of consideration. The South Dakota Supreme Court upheld the lower court opinion and stated that the employer's compliance with the contract terms and willingness to continue the contract for an indefinite period provided adequate and valuable consideration.

Clearly, courts have been inconsistent when determining the adequacy of continued employment as consideration; thus, there is no set rule of law defining adequate consideration as it pertains to this issue.

SOLICITING CLIENTS BEFORE AND AFTER TERMINATION OF EMPLOYMENT

Employers and associates who enter into restrictive covenant agreements must con-

sider what behaviors are allowable when employment ends. For example, is it acceptable for departing associates to inform clients about their new job location "just down the road" while they still are working for their employers? What information can associates who have departed expect their former employers to pass on to clients who question their whereabouts? Is it appropriate and legal for associates to recruit fellow employees to come with them to their new places of employment? If the restrictive covenant prohibits employment or ownership of a practice within a given radius, and a departed employee moves outside the radius to establish a new practice, can that party solicit business from animal owners who live inside the restricted trade area but who were not clients of the former employer? What constitutes the solicitation of a previous client or a fellow staff member, and what is a "previous client?"

The answers to these questions are contingent upon the language of restrictive covenant agreements. Most noncompete provisions in veterinary contracts contain only time restraints and geographic limits. These agreements do not prohibit employees from discussing new jobs with clients and staff, nor do they prohibit employees from recruiting clients or staff to join them at their new places of employment. The omission of such provisions in employment agreements can create major conflicts and bad will between employers and employees.

DEFINING SOLICITATION AND ADVERTISING

Employers and employees often have remarkably different ideas as to what *solicitation* means. Since this is an area where disputes frequently occur, contracts would best specify the type of conduct that constitutes solicitation. The AVMA Principles of Veterinary Medical Ethics defines solicitation as "advertising intentionally directed to specific individuals."

Webster's Dictionary defines *advertise* as "to tell about a service as through newspapers, handbills, radio, and television so as to make people want to buy it." The AVMA Principles of Veterinary Medical Ethics defines advertising as "newspaper and periodical announcements and listings; professional cards; office and other signs; letterheads; telephone and other directory listings; and any other form of communication designed to inform the public about the availability, nature or prices of products or services." Thus, any form of advertising aimed at specific animal owners within the restricted trade area would be disallowed should advertising be prohibited in a restrictive covenant.

Soliciting and advertising would include uttering comments across the exam table or at the farm informing existing clients of one's pending departure and encouraging them to call for appointments. Other forms of soliciting and advertising would be handing out business cards, sending announcements through the mail, or making phone calls informing individual animal owners within the restricted area of one's availability at a new place of employment. Soliciting and advertising should not, however, be construed so broadly as to encompass general press releases announcing employment or the purchase or starting of a practice in the same business community. Basic information aimed at the animal-owning public at large and placed in the Yellow Pages, newspaper, or radio ads is allowable.

According to Jerrold Tannenbaum's *Veterinary Ethics* book, the official codes of ethics of several professions view solicitation as inherently coercive and therefore prohibited conduct.[54] Tannenbaum quotes the 1983 American Bar Association rules of professional conduct where it says,

...a person who is solicited often feels overwhelmed by the situation giving rise to the need for legal services, and may have an impaired capacity for reason, judgment, and protective self-interest. Furthermore, the lawyer seeking the retainer is faced with a conflict stemming from the lawyer's own interest, which may color the advice and representation offered the vulnerable prospect.

This discussion seems equally relevant to solicitous comments by veterinarians because it puts clients in the awkward position of having their loyalty tested. Encouraging clients to choose between a veterinary practice that may have served them well for years and an associate veterinarian at a new place of business who most recently treated their animals creates some ill will. If departing doctors think all their clients "love them so dearly" that they would gladly follow them elsewhere, they are in for a rude awakening. Sooner or later clients who were solicited behind closed doors will inform the solicitor's employer of the circumstances, resulting in an embarrassing and adversarial situation.

It is for this reason that many employers prefer to terminate the contracts of their associate veterinarians or practice managers on the spot at the end of a work shift rather than allow the situation to linger. Many such prudent employers provide their departing employees with one to four weeks of "guilt" money, also known as "in lieu of notice pay," rather than allow them to work through the end of their contracts, during which time they might intentionally or unintentionally solicit clients and staff members to follow them.

A Definition of Solicitation

Clearly, contracts that include antisolicitation clauses should define the prohibited conduct. Such a definition could read as follows:

For the purpose of this agreement, "solicitation" means all advertising directed intentionally to specific individuals. This includes any type of in-person communication with existing clients within the restricted trade area, where such discussion is designed to

inform such people about the availability, nature, and/or prices of veterinary products or services and attract those clients to seek the services of the departing or departed Employee at the Employee's future place of veterinary employment. Solicitation does not include general press releases, advertising to the public at large, or professional listings in telephone books.

AMBULATORY PRACTICE CONSIDERATIONS

Unique problems occur with respect to prohibitions restricting departing ambulatory veterinarians from competing with their former employers or co-owners. As discussed previously in this chapter, most noncompete clauses prohibit former employees or practice sellers from owning, managing, operating, or controlling; being employed by, participating in, or having an interest in; or being connected in any manner with the ownership, management, operation, or control of any business or profession engaged in the provision of veterinary services similar in scope to those provided by the employer. This makes sense because practice owners or purchasers who have invested heavily in the creation and maintenance of the goodwill that attracted their clients in the first place have a right to protect their investments.

One must ask, though, whether this type of carte blanche prohibition is fair to the animal owners who live within the proscribed areas who never have or have not recently been clients of the practice. As long as former employees or practice sellers fulfill their contractual obligations to establish places of business outside the restricted zone, it seems unreasonable to prohibit them from offering their services to animal owners who have rarely or never been clients at the veterinary practices at which they previously worked. If these clients are solicited to leave the restricted trade area and travel to a neutral location outside the

boundary, former employers have nothing to lose, and the public and departed employees have everything to gain. Furthermore, if that represents fairness and reasonableness, then why not extend the privilege to travel back into the restricted zone to these same ambulatory clinicians and allow them to provide veterinary services for animal owners who never were serviced by the former employers in the first place?

The authors have found that in some settings a provision like this works extremely well, while in others it creates a nightmare. For example, in cases where ambulatory clinicians treat one owner's herds of dairy cattle and swine, or flocks of sheep or poultry, few problems and no competition occur with prior employers. Equine practices, though, present different problems. Many horses are housed at stables where there are up to 50 different horse owners but only one person requesting the veterinary care for these horses, i.e., the stable manager or trainer. Confusion and opportunities for covenant violations arise when veterinarians treat horses whose owners never had utilized their previous employers' services, but they are prohibited from soliciting and/or treating upon request the horse(s) in adjoining stalls because they had been patients of the prior employer.

The philosophical question is, should restrictive covenants that preclude working for or owning practices within the restricted zone also prohibit departed employees from fulfilling the veterinary needs of people inside the restricted zone who never or rarely have been clients? The answer seems to lie with allowing this type of solicitation in some types of practices but prohibiting it in others, recognizing that a need to share medical records ultimately may be required to settle disputes. Alternatively, legal disputes concerning such issues could involve mediation and settlements whereby the interests of all parties, i.e., the employer, the employee, and the public, are fulfilled in a reasonable manner. The authors have been retained in a dozen or more such disputes where creativity and rational communications have prevented expensive legal actions. In many of these cases, even the friendships of the parties were preserved.

Answering Questions about Staff Departures

When clients question the whereabouts of departed associates, employers and staff are obligated to answer truthfully. Antisolicitation clauses govern the behavior of employees, not clients. Thus, clients who question the whereabouts of departing employees, staff, or employers are entitled to honest answers. Furthermore, employers who provide clients with deceptive answers are violating the Principles of Veterinary Medical Ethics.[14]

Employers should be able to prohibit departing employees from soliciting clients and instructing them to transfer their animals' care and patient records. Conversely, clients can ask, and should not be discouraged from asking, why their doctors no longer will be available and where they are going. Similarly, veterinarians who have signed restrictive covenants should not approach clients and solicit their business at new places of employment.

Aside from the ethical considerations, employers also may have medical obligations to patients who require ongoing care. This is particularly true in situations where patients have been receiving care from specialists and need continuing supervision from those same or equally qualified specialists. Failing to inform the owners of such patients of the departing specialist's new location during a time when no equally qualified specialist has been hired could result in the filing of a legal action for professional negligence or unprofessional conduct. This would be based upon a breach of the duty to offer a referral when the animal's condition merits it or a failure to offer a referral to a client who requests one.

To minimize legal, ethical, and public relations risks, employers should consider reviewing the medical status of those patients afflicted with complex, ongoing ailments. If they conclude that their staff is not sufficiently trained and experienced to provide competent, contemporary veterinary services to those patients, employers should allow departing veterinarians to continue serving patients needing ongoing treatments of diagnosed problems at their new locales, even though this violates the antisolicitation language in their restrictive covenants.

Lastly, some antisolicitation clauses also prohibit employees from recruiting staff to join them at their new places of employment. Depending on the attitude of employers on this issue, they may wish to include such provisions in their contracts, especially if their staff members have received bonuses or extensive training and/or continuing education in recent months or years. Refer to Table 9.4 for an overview of the authors' data concerning antisolicitation clauses.

Table 9.4. Percentage of Contracts with Antisolicitation Clauses[1]

Restrictive Covenants	Percentage
Client antisolicitation clauses	48
Employee antisolicitation clauses	20

A CLAUSE FOR CLIENT ANTISOLICITATION

The following clause addresses antisolicitation issues regarding employers' clients:

During the 60 days preceding the expiration or termination of this contract and for (one?, two?) years after its expiration or termination, Employee agrees not to solicit (as that word is defined in this Agreement) business of a nature similar to that of the Employer from any of Employer's past or present clients or give any person, firm, or corporation the right to do so. For the purpose of this section, clients shall be defined as any person or entity who, directly or indirectly, through one or more intermediaries, owns the animal or controls the medical decision making for an animal that received veterinary care from the Employer's business within the two years immediately preceding Employee's departure.

The goal of this clause is to be restrictive, yet reasonable. Because of this, only the solicitation of existing clients, not the public at large nor owners of animals who are not active patients of the employer, is prohibited. If the former employer (or owner who has sold the practice) has had no prior business relationship with animal owners residing in the restricted trade area, it seems unreasonable to prohibit a departed veterinary associate from soliciting clients who are not currently clients of that employer.

EMPLOYEE ANTISOLICITATION CLAUSES

Just as the solicitation of clients by departing veterinary associates poses risks to employers, so does the solicitation of employees. In fact, in some cases the loss of key employees is more damaging than the solicitation and departure of clients.

Long-term prohibitions against the solicitation of employees pose serious obstacles to job mobility for existing employees who, in most cases, are not involved in the contractual relationships between employers and associate veterinarians. On the other hand, the raiding of experienced staff members by departing veterinary associates or office managers is unfair to the employers who have invested heavily in their compensation, training, and fringe benefits. Because of these clashes, clauses prohibiting the solicitation of employees typically are limited to one year.

An antisolicitation clause for employers' employees follows:

During the 60 days preceding the expiration or termination of this contract and for one year after its expiration or termination, the Employee agrees not to solicit (as defined in this Agreement), recruit, or encourage any employee employed by Employer to work for, participate in, or assist with the formation or operation of any business that com- *petes or intends to compete with the Employer or to do any act that is disloyal to the Employer or inconsistent with the Employer's interests or any provision of this Agreement.*

UNENFORCEABILITY OF COVENANTS DUE TO MATERIAL BREACHES

A material breach of a contract is a violation of contract terms that is so substantial it invalidates the contract. If employers materially breach contracts containing restrictive covenants, courts may determine that the covenants should not be enforced. The rationale for this is that employers who materially breach their contractual obligations should not be allowed to force employees to honor their obligations.

In *Laconia Clinic, Inc.* v. *Cullen,* the Supreme Court of New Hampshire affirmed a lower court ruling excusing the employee from honoring a restrictive covenant because of the employer's material breach.[55] The employer had mismanaged funds, causing the employee financial hardship; this was affirmed as a material breach. The Court stated, "It has been generally held that a restrictive clause in an employment contract preventing future competition by the employee may not be enforced where there has been a breach by the employer of his own obligations under the contract."

According to a "Legal Brief" article published in *JAVMA,* other examples of material breaches are when employers demand that employees work substantially different numbers of hours than those stated in the contract, when employers mislead employees about their job duties, or when employers are dishonest about the nature of their practices.[56]

Examples of issues raised on one or more occasion wherein one of the authors was asked to serve as an expert witness include: poor financial and personnel management; allegations of cruelty to animals on the part of practice owners; controlled substances storage and record-keeping violations; persistent employee safety and overtime violations leading to penalties to employers by state labor commissioners and OSHA administrators; material misrepresentations of fact regarding earning power anticipated under percentage-based compensation contracts; repeated late payments of commissions on previous months' income generation figures; hospital equipment, instruments, supplies, and drug inventories inadequate to practice veterinary medicine within the standard of care; corroborated claims of sexual harassment or sexual misconduct by a practice owner; inadequate and inaccurate medical record keeping, in violation of regulations set forth by state boards of examiners; the persistent requirement by employers that employees use outdated drugs and vaccines in spite of complaints by employees; and chronic support staff turnover or shortages. How many of these must exist or how serious the mismanagement must be before an employer will elect to settle out of court or before the court elects not to enforce a noncompete agreement depends on the facts presented in each case.

WAIVERS PROVIDED BY GENEROUS EMPLOYERS

Occasionally, employers include provisions in their restrictive covenants stipulating that under specific circumstances, their restrictive covenants will not be enforced against former employees. One such section of a contract reads as follows:

The only exception to the enforceability of this covenant is termination by Employer without cause. For the purpose of this agreement, the term cause shall be defined as the inability of Employee to meet professional practice standards commensurate with Employee's education and experience or the inability of Employee to successfully relate to the clients and/or other employed staff members. Cause does not include dismissal of Employee from the staff for economic reasons or

because of natural disasters such as flood or fire.[57]

When the covenant in this contract was challenged in court by an employee who resigned after working for her employers for six years, evidence of this additional generosity and reasonableness was introduced into the trial to enhance the employer's position. The viewpoint of the employers and their expert witness was that a six-mile, one-year covenant not to compete was reasonable for an employee who had worked at the practice six years. The court must have looked favorably on the overall fairness of the terms, enhanced by the reasonableness of the above clause, because it found for the employers and dismissed all claims raised by the employee.

Another contract providing waiver language that could preclude enforcement of a noncompete clause included the following statement:

The foregoing (restrictive covenant language) notwithstanding, in the event that the Employer unilaterally terminates the Employee's employment during the term of this Agreement for reasons other than those stated in the Agreement (for cause), the two year noncompetition prohibition of this paragraph will not apply.[1]

Clauses such as these are rare. When present, they reflect a genuine attitude of reasonableness, good faith, and fair dealing that sets them apart from usual contracts. The authors found that the veterinarians who included these clauses in their contracts managed state-of-the-art practices and had considerable self-confidence. They stated that if they elected to lay off associates they had hired because of economic downturns or for personal rather than performance reasons, they were not concerned about competition from such terminated employees.

Perhaps it is naive on the part of employers to offer former employees such generous reasons for not enforcing their noncompete agreements. However, employees who see clauses like these in contract offers should consider this a good omen with respect to the quality of the practice and judgment of the employers.

LIQUIDATED DAMAGES

When a breach of contract has occurred and been proved, the nonbreaching party is entitled to some form of remedy. This usually involves requiring the breaching party to pay the damages incurred by the nonbreacher. Unfortunately, a breach and the resulting damages can take months or years to determine and thousands of dollars in legal and expert witness fees to prove.

Because of this, many employers attempt to predetermine an amount of money that would be required to offset their losses if an employee violated his or her agreed-upon covenant. With preset damages, if employees compete in violation of restrictive covenant clauses, they are liable to employers for the preset amount. Establishing this predetermined figure relieves the courts of the difficult task of calculating damages as the result of unfair competition and speeds the resolution of disputes.

At issue is what constitutes "reasonable estimations of anticipated damages." Most courts will not enforce liquidated damages clauses if they are so disproportionate to the actual damages incurred as deemed to be punitive in nature. Conversely, if the dollar amount is unrealistically low, some employees will breach the agreement and simply pay the liquidated damages, in effect buying themselves out of their contracts. What is reasonable, then, is a wide-open question which requires careful thought and reasonable calculations before inclusion in any employment contract. In the authors' opinion, liquidated damages should be high enough to allow employers to advertise for, interview, select, hire, and train replacement veterinarians to fill the shoes of the person who departed and breached the restrictive covenant. This can vary considerably from associate to associate depending upon experience, years of employment, medical competence, bedside manner, and communication skills. Using these guidelines, liquidated damages in Table 9.5 could be argued to be reasonable:

The departure of experienced clinicians can cause more damage than departing new graduates, and departing specialists can cause more damage than generalists. With respect to generalists, losses are related to the difficulties locating and the lead time required to hire experienced clinicians; costs incurred advertising for applicants and interviewing and selecting prospects; time and money involved in training replacement

Table 9.5. Reasonable Liquidated Damages

Description of Employed Veterinarian	Amount of Damages
1. Recent graduate completing 1st year of training and employment	One year's salary
2. Recent graduate completing greater than 1 year of employment	Most recent year's salary plus 10% for each year of employment beyond one year, to a maximum of 150% of the most recent year's salary
3. General practitioner with greater than 2 years of experience when initially hired	115% of first year's salary
4. Experienced clinician who remains employed longer than 2 years	115% of most recent year's salary plus 15% for each year of employment beyond the first year, to a maximum of 175% of most recent year's salary
5. Board-eligible or board-certified specialist completing first year of employment	150% of first year's salary
6. Board-eligible or board-certified specialist with more than 2 years of employment at the practice	200% of most recent year's salary

veterinarians to become competent and efficient doctors; and the time required to bond clients to the new doctors.

With respect to departing specialists who violate their restrictive covenants, even greater losses can occur. First of all, because of the scarcity of residency programs, lag times of one to two years to fill specialty positions are not unusual, during which time employers can incur considerable lost income. Secondly, specialists need to bond with only 50 to 100 referring veterinary practices to be able to make a good living in a local veterinary community, whereas generalists require 1,000 to 2,500 individual animal owners in their practice to ensure adequate personal income. Thus, specialists can develop competing practices more easily than generalists.

Lastly, employers often need to purchase tens of thousands of dollars of equipment, make major investments in staff training, provide paid or unpaid time off for board-eligible specialists to study for boards, and hire replacements or forego income during the time these people are off work studying. It is because of these issues that liquidated damages must be much higher for specialists than they are for generalists.

The authors analyzed the inclusion of liquidated damages clauses in their study of several hundred veterinary employment contracts. Twenty-nine percent of the employment contracts contained liquidated damages clauses, consisting of a wide variety of terms. The following are samples of amounts and payment time frames from several of the liquidated damages clauses that were reviewed:[1]

1. The Associate shall pay the lump sum of $75,000 in liquidated damages.

2. For a period of two years after termination of this Agreement, Employee shall pay to the Corporation as liquidated damages, and not as penalty, 90% of all fees received by Employee from any client who was a client of the Corporation during the previous 36 months.

3. Reimbursement for breach of this restrictive covenant will be in the amount equal to fifty percent (50%) of one year's gross production of the Employee, calculated on the twelve (12) months previous production of the Employee prior to termination of the Employment Agreement. Fifty percent (50%) of this amount will be due immediately, with the balance to be paid over five (5) years.

4. The Employee shall pay the Employer the sum of $20,000 in liquidated damages if such violation occurs during the first year after this Agreement. The amount of liquidated damages for which Employee shall be liable shall be increased by ten percent (10%) for each year after the first year.

Final Thoughts about Liquidated Damages

In summary, because employers will be required to live with the damage amounts they establish in their restrictive covenants, they are advised to ensure that the amount specified is a reasonable estimate of anticipated damages. Excessively high estimates or unrealistically low ones will create bonanzas that benefit their employees rather than themselves. In such cases, employers will find that they would have been better off omitting such clauses than including unfounded or unscientific ones.

A CONTRACT CLAUSE FOR LIQUIDATED DAMAGES

Suggested contract language for liquidated damages reads as follows:

If Employee violates any of the terms of the restrictive covenant, the Employer shall be entitled to any and all remedies at law and equity, which remedies may be cumulative, and shall include, but not be limited to, the right of injunction or the right to seek damages. Alternatively, because the Employee's services are of a special and unusual character which have a unique value to the Employer, the loss of which cannot ade-

quately be compensated by damages in an action at law and, if used in competition with the Employer would cause serious harm to Employer, and because actual damages may be difficult to determine without protracted litigation, in the event of repeated violations by the Employee of any part of this restrictive covenant, the Employee shall pay the Employer the sum of (one year's salary?, $60,000?, 125% of employee's current year's salary?) in liquidated damages if such violation occurs during the first year of this agreement. The amount of liquidated damages for which Employee shall be liable shall be increased by (10%?, 15%?) for each year after the first year of employment up to a maximum of (150%?, 175%?) of Employee's current year salary.

IMPROPERLY DRAFTED RESTRICTIVE COVENANTS

In the past, courts that found restrictive covenants to be unreasonable often held the entire covenant invalid. The majority of jurisdictions no longer reach such harsh conclusions today; instead, they usually invalidate only the unreasonable portions.[12] Courts accomplish partial enforcement by applying either the blue pencil doctrine or engaging in judicial rewriting.[58]

Blue Pencil Doctrine

The blue pencil doctrine, employed by some state courts, stipulates that if courts can render unreasonable restraints reasonable by excising (blue penciling out) the oppressive components of the covenants, they should do so and enforce the remainder. Courts only can blue pencil specific clauses if the contract remains grammatically correct, the remaining language is reasonable, and the contract needs no rewriting.[12]

Rewriting Restrictive Covenants

Another more common remedy courts utilize when faced with unreasonable

restrictive covenants is rewriting.[59] Jurisdictions that utilize this remedy take overly broad agreements and transform them to provide reasonable protection for employers without excessively restricting employees.

The Supreme Court of Iowa decided to follow this modern trend and overruled its longstanding landmark case, *Brecher* v. *Brown*.[60] In that 1945 case, both parties were mixed animal practitioners who entered into an employment agreement that included a restrictive covenant. The restrictive covenant clause prohibited Brown from practicing veterinary medicine within 25 miles of Brecher's practice for an indefinite period of time. Less than a year into the agreement, Brown terminated employment and soon thereafter opened and operated a veterinary hospital about 100 feet from Brecher's veterinary practice. The trial court did not enforce the restrictive covenant, and Brecher appealed.

The Court stated that restrictive covenants were reasonable if they protected the employer without causing undue hardship to employees and the public. The Court then held that the 25-mile geographical restraint in this mixed animal practice was overreaching, as only one of the employer's clients lived outside of that radius. Consequently, the Supreme Court ruled that the restricted area was broader than necessary to protect the employer and, therefore, unenforceable.

Moreover, the 1945 Supreme Court stated that since they were not at liberty to rewrite or modify the contract, it would be rejected or upheld as written. It went on to say that employers "desiring the maximum protection have no doubt a difficult task. When they fail, it is commonly because, like the dog in the fable, they grasp too much and so lose all."[61]

In 1971, the Iowa Supreme Court decided to follow the modern trend and overrule *Brecher* v. *Brown* so that its courts could rewrite overly broad covenants. In *Ehlers* v. *Iowa Warehouse Co.*, the Court expressly rejected the "all or nothing rule" and adopted rewriting.[59]'

Similarly, in *Raimonde* v. *Van Vlerah*, the Ohio Supreme Court adopted the rewriting doctrine.[62] Van Vlerah entered into an employment contract with Raimonde. The contract included a restrictive covenant which restricted Van Vlerah from practicing veterinary medicine within 30 miles of the city of Defiance, Ohio for a period of 3 years from termination of employment. After eight months of practicing, Van Vlerah terminated employment and subsequently began practicing veterinary medicine within the restricted area.

The trial court upheld the restrictive covenant but reduced the geographic limitation from 30 miles to 18 miles. The Court of Appeals reversed the trial court decision, stating that the contract was unreasonable and that the trial court did not have the power to rewrite it. The Supreme Court disagreed. It stated that the trial court could modify the noncompete clause so as to protect the employer's business interests reasonably.

A problem arises, though, in that this may encourage employers to draft overly broad restraints knowing that most employees cannot afford the legal fees and economic risks required to challenge such clauses. In the few cases where they are challenged, employers can rely on courts simply to rewrite rather than invalidate their overly protective agreements.[12]

To address this issue and minimize the drafting of overly broad clauses, courts can (1) modify clauses only if good-faith bargaining is evident, (2) rewrite clauses so that they are below minimum standards of reasonableness, or (3) invalidate overly broad covenants.[2] Employers need to know which of these remedies the courts in their jurisdiction employ before they draft restrictive covenants that are unreasonably protective. Such practices may lead to costly litigation; result in courts invalidating their covenants, giving employers no protection in the process; create adverse relations among job

applicants and employers; and drive away potential employees.[63]

A "Savings" Clause for an Improperly Drafted Restrictive Covenant

Knowing that it is impossible to anticipate every contract dispute or how each court will decide such disputes, attorneys routinely include "savings" clauses in contracts that prevent courts from voiding the contract rather than rewriting it. Such clauses are particularly useful with restrictive covenants. A savings clause for what might turn out to be an improperly drafted restrictive covenant reads as follows:

> *In the event that any of the provisions of the restrictive covenant shall be held to be invalid or unenforceable, the remaining provisions shall nevertheless continue to be valid and enforceable as though the invalid or unenforceable parts had not been included herein. In the event that any provision of the time period and/or areas of restriction shall be declared by a court of competent jurisdiction to exceed the maximum time period or areas as such court deems reasonable and enforceable, the time period and/or areas of restriction shall be deemed to become and thereafter be the maximum time period and/or areas that the court deems reasonable and enforceable.*

Conclusion

Both employers and employees invest in their professional success by committing to one another. For employers, this commitment means providing employees contact with clientele, experienced staff, agreed-upon compensation, fringe benefits, in some cases trade secrets, and training. Employers are entitled to protect these assets. For employees, this commitment means promising that as part of their bargained-for exchange of time and effort in return for money, fringe benefits, and experience, they will not compete upon leaving. When covenants not to compete are drafted as reasonable documents, each party can respect the rights of the other without the emotional and financial expenses associated with legal challenges. When they are blatantly unreasonable, employees often refuse to accept the job or sign the contract under duress and, instead, engage in legally, emotionally, and financially draining battles at the time they consider resigning, after submitting their resignation, or at the time they are terminated.

Employers and employees must determine whether their state permits restrictive covenants (Appendix III). If such agreements are recognized, an understanding of the principles governing restrictive covenants is necessary. Finally, to minimize disputes and assure that their contracts are properly drafted for each state, it is essential that parties retain local legal counsel to review their restrictive covenant clauses before signing any agreements.

REFERENCES

1. Wilson J, Nemoy J: Retrospective study of 200 veterinary employment contracts. Yardley, PA, 1987-1997.
2. Wilson JF: *Law and Ethics of the Veterinary Profession*. Priority Press, Ltd, PO Box 306, Yardley, PA 19067, ph 215-321-9488, 1988, pp 176-184.
3. 15 USC 1.
4. *Standard Oil Co* v *United States*, 221 US 1 (1911).
5. *Board of Trade* v *United States*, 246 US 231, 238 (1918).
6. *Arizona* v *Maricopa County Medical Society*, 457 US 332 (1982).
7. Van Cise JG, Lifland WT, Sorkin LT: *Understanding the Antitrust Laws*, ed 9. New York, Practicing Law Institute, 1986, pp 26, 31, 33-34, 42, 45.
8. Hills CA: *Antitrust Adviser*, ed 3. Colorado Springs, CO, Shepard's McGraw-Hill, pp 7,8, 1985.
9. Florida Statutes § 542.33, Colorado Statutes § 8-2-113, Calif Bus and Prof Code § 16601.
10. 421 US 773 (1975).
11. *Williams* v *St. Joseph Hospital*, 629 F.2d 448, 7th Cir (1980).
12. *Bishop* v *Lakeland Animal Hospital PC* (1994) 644 NE.2d 33 (Ill App 2 Dist 1994).
13. Grossman M, Scoggins G: The legal implications of covenants not to compete in veterinary contracts. *Nebr Law Rev* 71:826-878, 1992.
14. Restatement, Torts §757.
15. Principles of veterinary medical ethics options and reports of the judicial council. *American Veterinary Medical Association Membership Directory and Resource Manual*. Schaumburg, IL, American Veterinary Medical Assoc, 1997, pp 43-47.
16. Restatement, Second, Contracts §188.
17. *Durio* v *Johnson*, 358 P.2d 703-705 (NM 1961).
18. *Restrictive Covenant Survey*. The Health Care Group, Plymouth, PA, 1996, pp 1-69.
19. California Business and Professions Code §16600.
20. Montana Code Annotated §28-2-703, 704, 705.
21. 15 OS 1991, §217, 218, 219.
22. NCDD §9-08-06.
23. Alabama Code 1975 §8-1-1.
24. *Friddle* v *Raymond*, 575 So.2d 1038 (AL 1991).
25. WIST §103.465. *See also, Restrictive Covenant Survey*. The Health Care Group, Plymouth, PA, p 68, 1996.
26. SDCL 1990 §§ 53-9-8/-9/-10/-11. *See also, Restrictive Covenant Survey*. The Health Care Group, Plymouth, PA, p 59, 1996.

27. FS §542.33(2)(a).

28. *City of Coral Springs v Florida Nat'l Properties, Inc,* 340 So.2d 1271, 1272 (Fla 4th DCA 1976).

29. Samuels LK: Florida's Amended Noncompetition Statute: A Reasonable Approach. *Fla Bar J* (July/Aug):60-63, 1991.

30. *Tench v Weaer,* 374 P.2d 27-30 (Wyo 1962).

31. *Spring Harbor Veterinary Assoc v Schackter,* 287 NW.2d 517 (Wis 1980) (unpublished limited precedent opinion).

32. GA ST 13-8-2.1. *See also, Restrictive Covenant Survey.* The Health Care Group, Plymouth, PA, p 59, 1996.

33. *Chaichimansour v Pets are People Too,* 485 SE.2d 248 (Ga 1997).

34. *Lassen v Benton,* 346 P. 2d 137 (Ariz 1959); reaffirmed in *Lassen v Benton,* 347 P. 2d 1012 (Ariz 1959)

35. *Moore v Dover Veterinary Hospital, Inc,* 367 A.2d 1044-1049 (NH 1976).

36. Fish v Collins, 9 Va Cir 64 Lexis 54 1987.

37. *Hopper v All Pet Animal Clinic, Inc,* 861 P.2d 531 (Wyo 1993).

38. *Phoenix Orthopaedic Surgeons, Ltd v Richard Peairs and Jane Doe Peairs,* 164 Ariz 54, 790 P.2d 752 (1990).

39. *Griffen v Hunt,* 268 P.2d 874 (OK 1954)

40. *Boggs v Couturier* 321 NW.2d 794 (Mich App 1982).

41. *Marysville Animal Care Center, Inc v Andreas,* 1991 Ohio App LEXIS 4470 (on-line only).

42. *Cockerill v Wilson,* 281 NE.2d 648-651 (Ill 1972). *See also, Cockerill v Wilson,* 265 NE.2d 514 (Ill App).

43. *Brecher v Brown,* 17 NW.2d 377-380 (Iowa 1945).

44. *Cukjati v Burkett,* 772 SW.2d 215 (Tex App Dallas 1989).

45. Wise JK: Size and practice density of local veterinary service areas, 1988. *JAVMA* 195(2):251-252, 1989.

46. Meyers WS: Who are your clients? *Vet Econ* 38(5):46-53, 1997.

47. *Stringer v Herron,* 424 SE.2d 547 (SC App 1992).

48. Restatement, Second, Contracts § 187.

49. *Stevenson v Parsons,* 384 SE.2d 291-298 (NC App 1989).

50. *Kramer v Robec, Inc,* 824 F Supp 508-513 (ED Penn 1992).

51. *Admiral Services v John Drebit,* US Dist Ct (East Dist PA), 1995 US Dist LEXIS 3897.

52. *Kida v Chesterfield Veterinary Clinic, Inc,* 519 SW.2d 511 (Va Cir 1990).

53. *Loescher v Policky,* 173 NW.2d 50 (SD 1969).

54. Tannenbaum J: *Veterinary Ethics.* Baltimore, Williams and Wilkins, 1989, p 170.

55. *Laconia Clinic, Inc v Cullen,* 408 A.2d 412-414 (NH 1979).

56. Hannah H: Covenants not to compete-ten questions. *JAVMA* 200-201:38-39, 1992.

57. Endnote Text

58. Hannah H: Restrictive covenants: recent cases, court modification, and statutory provisions. *JAVMA* 208(11):1825-1826, 1996.

59. *Ehlers v Iowa Warehouse Co,* 188 NW.2d 368 (Iowa 1971).

60. *Brecher v Brown,* 235 Iowa 17 NW.2d 377 (Iowa 1945).

61. *Id.* (citing *Samuel Stores, Inc v Abrams,* 108 A 541 (Conn 1919)).

62. *Raimonde v Van Vlerah* 325 NE.2d 544 (Ohio 1975).

63. Hannah H: Court modifications of covenants against competition. *JAVMA* 201-203:399-401, 1992.

Chapter 10

INDEPENDENT CONTRACTORS

By Jeffrey D. Nemoy, DVM and James F. Wilson, DVM, JD

For years veterinary practice owners have attempted to save taxes and reduce payroll administrative work by paying veterinarians, practice managers, veterinary technicians, and groomers as independent contractors rather than as employees. At the same time, numerous relief veterinarians have chosen to be self-employed business people rather than employees so that they can deduct routine business expenses and make pension contributions.

Unfortunately, many veterinarians and other health care professionals, accountants, and general practitioner attorneys are unfamiliar with the countless mutable rules regarding the creation of independent contractor relationships. This chapter presents the most current guidelines for developing independent contractor status; however, final materials and contract language should be reviewed by local legal counsel before documents are signed to be sure no significant changes in the tax codes or legal precedents have occurred.

There has been much confusion over what constitutes a relief doctor, a relief technician, or a consultant and whether such people legally can be considered independent contractors. Many practice owners have errantly classified relief workers as independent contractors, paying them flat hourly, daily, weekly, or monthly stipends

unchallenged by the Internal Revenue Service, a worker's compensation office, or a state taxing agency. Anecdotal reports received by the authors indicate that California veterinarians have faced more challenges regarding independent contractor classifications than practice owners in other states. This appears to be related to the fact that the California Employment Development Department (managing state governmentally regulated unemployment insurance) has aggressively reviewed such relationships in order to bolster income for its department.

The veterinary profession can be grateful for the efforts put forth by the San Diego and California VMA's Committees on Independent Contractors and the Veterinary Independent Contractor Association cited frequently herein. Over the years, these organizations have invested considerable time, energy, and financial resources developing guidelines for the profession.

In an effort to clear up much of the confusion surrounding this subject, this chapter will review the legal issues pertaining to the independent contractor relationship with discussion of

- the advantages and disadvantages of establishing independent contractor relationships with workers,

- the criteria which determine whether relief veterinarians are independent contractors or employees and addressing exceptions to the criteria,

- IRS rulings that have determined whether workers were properly classified as independent contractors,

- the steps necessary to create independent contractor relationships,

- the risks of misclassifying workers who do not qualify for independent contractor status,

- many of the issues inherent in independent contractors contracts,

- ancillary legal concerns, and

- various tax forms required by the independent contractor relationship.

Additional resources to assist practice owners and workers with business management issues concerning independent contractor relationships are given at chapter's end.

An Overview

Independent contractors (also called *contractors*) are workers contracted by veterinary practice owners (called *clients* here) to perform certain jobs, independent of control by such clients.[1] Conversely, employees are contracted by practice owners to perform specified job tasks but are subject to the authority and control of their employers.[2] It is the delegation of control to the practice owner (establishing an employee:employer relationship) vs. the retention of control by the independent contractor (establishing a contractor:client relationship) that spells the difference between these two entities.

Harold Hannah, LL.B., the author of the "Legal Brief" column for *JAVMA* for many years, stated that

a regularly employed veterinarian receiving a stipulated salary from the employer and not engaging in practice outside of the employment is an employee, but those veterinarians...[who make] themselves available to any practice requiring their services and who simply take over while the employing veterinarian is away, are independent contractors.[1]

Establishing independent contractor status is important for tax purposes, as large tax penalties can be incurred if workers and employers file taxes incorrectly. Workers who behave like employees but file taxes according to independent contractor status risk losing their retirement plans and tax deductions.[2] Employers who do not file taxes and who misclassify employees as independent contractors may have to pay all past due employment taxes plus interest and penalty charges.[3] Thus, a thorough understanding of the independent contractor:veterinary practice relationship and strict adherence to the applicable principles and laws are essential.

Relief Veterinarians vs. Independent Contractors

Relief veterinarians and independent contractors are not the same entity. Many professionals equate relief veterinarians with independent contractors without understanding the legal criteria required to differentiate independent contractors from employees. Examples of relief veterinarians who probably qualify as employees rather than as independent contractors include

- general practitioners who work the same day, hours, or days of the week for the owner of one or more veterinary practices and use the staff, fee schedules, and billing procedures of the practice owners—even if they work for more than one practice

- general practitioners who work specified shifts at emergency clinics on a part-time but consistent basis

- general practitioners who work as employees in one practice but fill in occasionally for a few days at a time at only one other practice

- veterinarians who work as relief veterinarians but who have no formal contract with their clients identifying them as independent contractors

Examples of veterinarians who probably can meet the difficult independent contractor criteria include

- specialists who work as mobile surgeons, ultrasonographers, endoscopists, and telephone or on-premise consultants for other practitioners, who withdraw after having completed their surgical procedures or consultations, leaving the postoperative or postvisit care to the veterinary practice for which they worked

- veterinarians who are called to perform surgeries on specific patients at emergency clinics but who do not develop veterinarian-client-patient relationships with the owners of such animals

- large animal practitioners who perform embryo transfers, surgeries, cardiology consultations, endoscopic examinations, or alternative medicine treatments for other large animal practitioners without establishing veterinarian-client-patient relationships with the animals' owners or the owners' agents

- veterinarians who work short periods of time at multiple veterinary practices, filling in for absent practice owners or associates in those practices who are on vacation, maternity or family leave, attending continuing education seminars, or ill

Confusion often reigns over who is a relief veterinarian and who is an independent contractor. Typically, veterinarians who function as independent contractors are called relief veterinarians. But some veterinarians who work as part-time employees also are referred to as relief veterinarians even though they do not qualify as true independent contractors. Thus, two relief veterinarians can have the same title, but one is an independent contractor and the other an employee.[4] The remainder of this chapter delineates the two.

ADVANTAGES AND DISADVANTAGES OF THE INDEPENDENT CONTRACTOR: VETERINARY PRACTICE RELATIONSHIP

THE INDEPENDENT CONTRACTOR'S PERSPECTIVE

Because they are self-employed, independent contractors have great flexibility when practicing veterinary medicine. They establish the fees for their time, maintain their own work schedules, determine how much vacation they will take and when to take it, and decide which continuing education seminars to attend. These workers deduct business expenses, establish and maintain retirement plans, and choose the types and numbers of practices for which they work. They control professional decision making, such as diagnosing and treating diseases, performing surgeries, and prescribing medications. Independent contractors can hire other relief veterinarians and veterinary assistants to help them accomplish their jobs. Finally, they can pursue dual careers or other degrees while practicing veterinary medicine.[2,5]

Although working independently has many advantages, it also entails more risks. Contractors may lose money. Their salaries may vary from job to job, month to month, season to season, and year to year. They must pay business taxes and expenses and fund their own fringe benefits.

In reality this means that because they are required to pay the employer's 7.65%

share of FICA and Medicare, as well as their own 7.65%, they must charge 7.65% more than the accepted daily stipend paid to employed associates. Additionally, they should understand that to duplicate the workers' compensation insurance provided by employers via their own workers' comp coverage or disability income insurance, 4% to 8% must be added to the daily salary paid employed veterinarians to handle these potential job-related disabilities. Lastly, to provide allowances for vacations and sick leave, cover the costs of health insurance, provide for continuing education expenses, and pay for association dues, professional liability insurance, and licensing fees, they need to add another 10% to 12% to the daily amount received by employed veterinarians.

When these numbers are cumulated, it becomes obvious that to do as well financially as their employed counterparts, independent contractors must charge fees for their time that are 22% to 27% higher than the daily salaries received by employed veterinarians — without any allowance for contributions to self-funded pension plans. Moreover, depending on the state in which they work, they may be ineligible for workers' compensation, unemployment insurance, and state disability insurance, and they are not covered under equal employment opportunity laws.[2,5]

THE VETERINARY PRACTICE'S PERSPECTIVE

Veterinary practices benefit financially by using independent contractors. They do not pay any federal or state income, payroll, Medicare, or FICA taxes on income earned by independent contractors.[3] They have no responsibility to provide fringe benefits, such as health, disability, and professional liability insurance; vacation, continuing education, and sick leave; moving allowances; discounted pet care; fees for association memberships, licenses, and DEA registrations or contributions to pension plans.[2] The aggregate cost of these taxes and

benefits can amount to 25% to 32% of an employee's daily pay; i.e., associates earning $200 per day can cost employers $250 to $266 per day.[6] In practices where owners are contributing the maximum amount allowed by the IRS to their associate veterinarians' pension plans, aggregate costs can reach as high as 47% of salaried associates.

Using independent contractors rather than employees provides other advantages for veterinary practices. Practices are able to contract with independent contractors for short time periods, and tax filing requirements are minimal. Furthermore, practice owners are not liable for damages to third parties caused by independent contractors except, as discussed later in the chapter, where they knew or should have known of the incompetence of the independent contractors or in cases where there were inherent dangers in the work required.[2,7] Inherent dangers are more likely to occur with subcontractors in the building and construction trades than in veterinary medicine.

Mistakenly classifying employees as independent contractors can result in disciplinary actions by the IRS and state taxing agencies including forced payment of back taxes plus interest and penalties.[3] The worst case scenarios occur when veterinarians who are misclassified fail to file and pay their estimated FICA, Medicare, and state and federal withholding taxes. In the event they skip town or are unable to pay these taxes, the owners of the veterinary practice with which they contracted are liable for payment of all back taxes plus interest and penalties.[3]

Practices that make classification errors also become vulnerable to costly veterinary malpractice and civil suits. Additionally, employers may be underinsured because they were under the impression that their workers were personally liable for their own mistakes, negligence, and legal fees, only to discover after the fact that their contractors were misclassified and had no personal or professional insurance coverage. In such cases, plaintiffs in lawsuits will most certainly sue the veterinary practices for which the independent contractors worked, in hopes of recovering something. In these circumstances the misclassifications could result in the loss of considerable time and expense defending such suits in addition to liability for the acts of any misclassified independent contractors.

Workers who think that they are incorrectly classified as independent contractors can sue practices for denying them certain employee benefits like unemployment insurance or disability or workers' compensation insurance.[4] Should misclassified contractors who carry no workers' compensation insurance on themselves be injured during the "course of employment," one of the biggest risks for the veterinary practices that hired them is that their injured associates will sue for medical expenses and lost wages incurred during their terms as misclassified contractors. This is discussed in more detail later in the chapter.

For practice owners, a final disadvantage of retaining independent contractors is loss of control. Veterinary practices cannot direct, supervise, or instruct independent contractors as to how they are to complete their work. They cannot decide how independent contractors diagnose and treat diseases, perform surgeries, prescribe medications, or organize and complete their surgical and treatment procedures. They can establish fee schedules for their veterinary practices; however, they cannot require that their independent contractors comply with such schedules. Also, due to contractual obligations, independent contractors cannot be terminated until the work for which they have been contracted has been completed.[2] The primary things over which practice owners do have control is that they can set standards of conduct for medical, surgical, and anesthetic competence, punctuality, and communication with staff and clients by which contractors are expected to comply.

INDEPENDENT CONTRACTOR OR EMPLOYEE: MAKING THE DETERMINATION

THE IRS'S TWENTY COMMON LEGAL FACTORS

Because of losses in tax revenue and difficulties determining if people classified as independent contractors were in fact employees, in 1986 the IRS developed a 20-factor list to help determine whether workers are independent contractors or employees. The factors focus on whether independent contractors retain control over their work. The more factors with which workers comply, the more likely they will be considered independent contractors. Status does not hinge on one factor, nor must every requirement be met;[2,8] however, one issue can be determinative if it indicates that the veterinary practice controls the worker.[4] The 20 factors are as follows:[2,9,10]

1. Independent contractors are not required to follow instructions about how to accomplish a job.

2. Independent contractors ordinarily do not receive training by the veterinary practice and typically use their own methods to accomplish the work.

3. The veterinary practice's success or continuation should not depend on the services performed by the independent contractor; therefore, contracting with independent contractors is nonessential to the veterinary practice's survival.

4. Independent contractors furnish results. If services must be rendered by the independent contractor personally, then veterinary practices are interested not only in results, but also in control. They may hire others to provide the actual work.

5. Independent contractors have the sole discretion to hire, direct, and pay assistants.

6. Relationships between independent contractors and veterinary practices should

be for limited time periods. The work can be short or long term, but it takes place at irregular intervals.

7. Independent contractors establish and control their own work hours.

8. Independent contractors do not work full time for one practice. They have the right to pursue other job opportunities.

9. Independent contractors control where they work. If they work at veterinary practice sites, they do so independently, without supervision and direction from the practices.

10. Independent contractors retain the right to control the order in which the work is accomplished.

11. Independent contractors are not required to provide oral or written reports to veterinary practices regarding the progress of their work. State practice acts and regulations often mandate, however, that all attending veterinarians keep written medical records.

12. Independent contractors are paid by the job and not by time, such as by the hour, week, or month. Relief veterinarians typically charge per day for that day's services, although they also may charge a percentage of income produced.

13. Independent contractors are responsible for their own business expenses, such as legal, accounting, health insurance, DEA registration, association dues, travel, and continuing education expenses.

14. Independent contractors furnish their own tools, a requirement that surgeons often can meet more easily than other specialists.

15. Independent contractors strengthen their status by making investments in the facilities within or equipment with which they work, i.e., renting office space or upgrading or purchasing additional diagnostic instruments and equipment or computer hardware and bookkeeping, accounting, word processing, and referral software programs.

16. Independent contractors realize profits or suffer losses as a result of contracting for and providing their services.

17. Independent contractors have the right to work for more than one veterinary practice at a time and are more likely to be classified as independent contractors if they do so.

18. Independent contractors offer their services to the general public via listings in telephone directories or by advertising in veterinary association newsletters, with placement services, on web sites, and in veterinary journals.

19. Independent contractors who perform their responsibilities according to their contracts with practices cannot be discharged.

20. Independent contractors are responsible for completing their work and performing their jobs in a satisfactory manner.

In summation, veterinarians who perform work under their own supervision are considered independent contractors. They control their professional decisions, such as how to diagnose and treat diseases, perform surgeries, prescribe medications and, using their clients' fee schedules as guides, assess fees for services rendered to clients whose animals are under their care. They control their personal and business finances, standards of professional ethics, and practice philosophies.[2] The Code of Federal Regulations states:

Generally, physicians, lawyers, dentists, veterinarians...and others who follow an independent trade, business, or profession, in which they offer their services to the public, are not employees.[11]

On the other hand, veterinarians who are supervised, directed, and controlled with respect to their services are considered employees. Once the veterinary practices have the right to control workers, regardless of whether they exercise the right, the relationship becomes more like that of an employer/employee.[2] For more information regarding the 20 common law factors, see Revenue Ruling 87-41.

NEW IRS GUIDELINES

In 1995, the IRS expanded upon the 20-factor test because employers and workers were having difficulties applying it.[12] The new guidelines, which further elucidate application of the 20 factors,[13] also focus on control and are categorized in three general areas: behavioral control, financial control, and the relationship between employers and workers.[14]

Behavioral Control[13,14]

The considerations under behavioral control examine the extent to which the business (client) has the right to direct or control a worker's (contractor's) performance, focusing most specifically on the area of worker's instructions and training.

- The more the business's instructions are targeted to how jobs get done, rather than the end results, the more likely that workers are employees.

- The imposition of instructions mandated by government regulations or industry standards is irrelevant.

- When instructions come from businesses' customers, they may or may not be relevant. However, when businesses adopt their customers' instructions as if they were their own and pass them on to their workers, this is evidence that the workers are employees.

- When businesses instructions are not mandatory but merely suggestions, workers are more likely independent contractors.

- Workers are more likely to be classified as employees if businesses require them to wear uniforms or other identification or to place the businesses' names on their vehicles. An exception exists if workers' occupations require identification with the businesses for security purposes, such as entry to customers' homes.

- Highly trained professionals, such as doctors, lawyers, accountants, engineers, and computer specialists, often require little or no training or instruction on how to perform their services. For such workers, considerations involving behavioral control are less relevant than businesses' financial control and the nature of the parties' relationship.

- Employment relationships may exist even though jobs are performed with minimal direction and control by employers. Jobs such as a store clerks or gas station attendants may require little instruction. The key factor to consider is whether the businesses retain the right to direct work, regardless of whether they actually exercise that right.

- Workers who receive periodic or ongoing training about procedures to be followed and methods to be used at work are more likely to be employees. However, certain types of training are irrelevant to the employee-independent contractor inquiry. These include: (1) orientation to matters such as business policies, new product lines, or applicable statutes or government regulations; and (2) training for unpaid volunteer programs.

Financial Control[13,14]

The factors in this group examine whether clients (veterinary practices) have the right to direct or control the economic aspects of their contractors' activities:

- The central question is whether businesses have the right to direct and control business-related means and details of their workers' performance, not whether their workers are economically dependent on or independent of the business.

- Workers who make significant investments to perform services for others are likely to be independent contractors, although such investments are not required. While there are no precise dollar amounts defining "significant" investments, the investments must have substance. As long as workers pay fair market/rental value for the subject of their investments, workers' relationships to sellers/lessors are irrelevant.

- The more workers bear the costs of business expenses such as rent, utilities, equipment, training, advertising, wages, licenses, supplies, insurance, and travel, the more likely they are independent contractors.

- The more unreimbursed expenses workers have, the more likely they are independent contractors. However, relatively minor expenses incurred by workers, or more significant expenses that are customarily borne by employees in particular lines of business, such as tools for auto mechanics and carpenters, generally do not indicate that workers are independent contractors.

- Workers who advertise, maintain visible business locations, and are available to work for relevant markets ordinarily are independent contractors.

- Compensation on an hourly, daily, weekly, or similar guaranteed basis is evidence that workers are employees. Compensation in the form of flat fees is evidence that workers are independent contractors – especially if workers incur the expenses of performing the services. Nevertheless, in some lines of business, such as the practice of law, it is typical to pay independent contractors on an hourly basis.

- Probably the strongest evidence that workers are independent contractors is that workers may realize profits or incur losses by making decisions that affect their bottom lines, not just the employers' bottom lines. However, a worker's ability to receive more money by working more hours or less money by working fewer hours is consistent with employee status and is not the type of discretion contemplated by this factor.

The Relationship Between Employer and Worker [13,14]

The factors under this heading revolve around how the parties perceive their relationship.

- Written contracts designating workers as independent contractors are evidence of the parties' intent. Although such designations can be dispositive in close cases, they usually do not determine worker status by themselves. Generally, the substance of the contracts, such as methods of compensation, expenses that workers will incur, and the rights and obligations of the parties with respect to how the work will be done, is primarily relevant.

- Filing W-2 tax forms usually indicates the parties' belief that workers are employees. However, workers have been held to be independent contractors even when W-2 forms were filed.

- Workers who create corporations or other business entities through which they perform services usually are viewed as employees of their corporations or businesses, not of the businesses that engaged the workers' corporations or other businesses.

- Providing workers with employee benefits, such as paid vacation, paid sick days, health insurance, life insurance, disability insurance, or pensions, is evidence that workers are employees. The evidence is strongest when workers are provided with benefits under tax-qualified retirement plans, Internal Revenue Code section 403(b) annuities, or cafeteria plans, which federal statutes specify may be provided only to employees.

- Excluding workers from benefit plans because businesses do not consider them to be employees is evidence of independent contractor status. But if the workers are excluded for other reasons, such as their work locations or business units, the exclusion is irrelevant.

- While state laws often define "employees" for purposes such as workers' compensation and unemployment insurance, these definitions are irrelevant to the IRS definition.

- Under the IRS's former 20-factor test, the right that employers had to discharge workers at any time without penalty, and workers' right to quit at any time without penalties were seen as evidence that workers were employees. But because of developments in contract and employment law, this is no longer true. Now a worker's ability or inability to quit at any time without penalty is relevant. Moreover, while the right of businesses to freely discharge workers is by itself no longer evidence of independent contractor status, a business's ability to refuse payment for a worker's unsatisfactory work is.

- Businesses that hire workers with the expectation that the relationships will continue indefinitely is evidence that workers are employees. When businesses hire workers for specific periods or projects, it is evidence that workers are independent contractors. However, relationships that are long-term, but not indefinite, are a neutral fact.

- Temporary relationships also constitute neutral facts. To determine whether temporary workers are employees hired on seasonal bases, for certain projects, or on an "as needed" basis, or whether they are, instead, independent contractors, the IRS will examine the services performed by the workers. If those services are a key aspect of the company's regular business, the workers are more likely employees.

The IRS's new guidelines make clear that all of the above factors must be considered, viewing the relationship as a whole. The presence of one or two factors does not override all the other considerations.

STATE LAWS

State agencies may use other criteria in addition to the IRS 20 common law factors when challenging independent contractor status. For example, the Employment Development Department (EDD), a California agency that administers unemployment benefits, disability benefits, and state income taxes, uses 14 criteria. Eight are from the IRS 20 common law factors, and 6 are unique. The EDD's focus is similar to that of the IRS, determining whether the businesses or workers retain control.[15] The six unique criteria are as follows:

- Are the workers skilled?

- Do the workers have a specific business or occupation?

- Are the workers supervised?

- Are independent contractors typically used in the industry?

- Do both parties intend to establish the independent contractor relationship?

- Is the party who hired the worker a business or individual?[4]

Unlike their federal counterpart, some states require that all workers be covered by workers' compensation and/or unemployment insurance. Thus, even if the IRS considers workers to be independent contractors, such workers may need to carry and pay for their own workers' compensation and/or unemployment insurance to comply with state laws. To learn more about relevant state laws, contact state employment boards, boards of revenue, and labor boards.[5]

Exceptions to the IRS Rules

IRS Safe Harbor Rules

Section 530 of the Revenue Act of 1978 gives businesses another way to classify workers as independent contractors. Businesses that mistakenly classify workers as independent contractors and meet section 530 requirements may nonetheless treat workers as independent contractors and be exempt from federal employment taxes.[16]

Section 530 was designed to protect businesses, and not workers, from employment tax liabilities. Thus, the IRS may audit the misclassified workers and disqualify their retirement plans and, at the same time, protect the businesses for whom they work from undesirable tax consequences. However, Section 530 does not apply to local or state government classifications. Consequently, workers occasionally may be classified as independent contractors under federal law and as employees under state law.[2]

Section 530 contains three requirements, *all* of which must be met for businesses to qualify their workers as independent contractors and, thus, avoid tax liability for errant decisions regarding independent contractor classifications:[17]

1. The business had a reasonable basis for treating workers as independent contractors. This can be substantiated by relying on one of the following:

   - court cases regarding federal taxes;
   - IRS rulings issued to the business;
   - past IRS audits of the business which did not reclassify similar workers from independent contractors to employees; professional norms, treating similar workers as independent contractors; or

   - some other reasonable basis, such as advice from attorneys or certified public accountants.

2. The business and any predecessor business have treated similar workers as independent contractors since 1978.

3. The business and any predecessor business have treated workers as independent contractors and filed Form 1099-MISC for each worker who exceeded earnings of $600 per year in all filing periods after 1978.

For more information regarding eligibility, refer to the Revenue Act of 1978, section 530 and attorneys who specialize in labor or tax law.

Supplement to IRS Safe Harbor Rules

IRS Revenue Procedure 85-18 further protects employers who misclassify employees as independent contractors and do not meet the Safe Harbor Rules. It states:

> A taxpayer who fails to meet any of the three 'safe havens' may nevertheless be entitled to relief if the taxpayer can demonstrate, in some other manner, a reasonable basis for not treating the individual as an employee. In H.R. Rep. No. 95-1748...it is indicated that 'reasonable basis' should be construed liberally in favor of the taxpayer.[18]

For more information regarding eligibility, refer to the Revenue Procedure 85-18 and an attorney specializing in labor or tax laws.

Good Faith Belief

Employers who do not qualify for the Safe Harbor and supplemental rules but who honestly mistake employees as independent contractors may owe only employment back taxes and no penalties.[4] Pursuant to the Internal Revenue Code section 3509, honest employers are fined less than businesses who misclassify purposefully.[19]

In *Diaz* v. *U.S.*, the employer classified workers who conformed to some of the 20 common law factors as independent contractors. The IRS reclassified the workers as employees. As a result of the misclassification, the IRS sought back taxes and penalties. The court held that in order for the IRS to impose penalties, it had the burden of showing that the employer acted with willful neglect. Because the employer had a good faith belief that his employees were independent contractors, no penalties were imposed.[20]

IRS RULINGS

The IRS makes private rulings for taxpayers who need assistance in determining whether workers are employees or independent contractors. The rulings are published, but information concerning the parties involved is confidential. The following rulings illustrate how the IRS uses its guidelines.

VETERINARIANS

An owner and operator of a veterinary clinic engaged a veterinarian to render professional services. The veterinarian performed services either at the clinic or from the owner's ambulatory vehicle. The owner set appointments for the veterinarian, set fees, and collected the fees. The clinic owner supervised and corrected the veterinarian's services, and hired, paid, and controlled the support staff.

RULING: The veterinarian is an employee.[21]

VETERINARIANS

An animal hospital retained a veterinarian to provide professional services. The hospital instructed and supervised the veterinarian to some degree. The veterinarian was subject to a restrictive covenant upon resignation. Initially the hospital paid the veterinarian a salary and then later paid the doctor based on a percentage of gross receipts. The hospital supplied all necessary equipment.

RULING: The veterinarian is an employee.[22]

PHYSICIANS

A hospital contracted with a radiologist, psychiatrist, physiologist, pathologist, and several emergency room physicians. The doctors were not subject to hospital rules applicable to employees. The doctors created their own schedules and were permitted to hire and pay assistants. The doctors were not eligible for employment benefits and supplied their own malpractice insurance.

RULING: The physicians are independent contractors.[23]

PHYSICIANS

Doctors worked for a corporation that provided emergency medical care. The corporation determined the doctors' schedules and required them to work a minimum number of hours. The corporation provided the facility, equipment, supplies, support staff, and administrative services. The doctors were paid hourly and had no financial interest in the corporation. Contracts between both parties stated that the doctors were independent contractors.

RULING: The physicians are employees.[24]

PHYSICIANS

A doctor was associated with a firm which provided anesthesiology services to a hospital. The contract between the firm and the doctor indicated that the firm billed and collected the doctor's fees, deducted the doctor's business expenses, and paid the doctor an annual salary. The firm did not guarantee minimum compensation or provide benefits. The services provided to the hospital were rendered by the doctor personally. The doctor was not restricted from practicing outside the firm.

RULING: The physician is an independent contractor.[25]

DENTISTS

A dental partnership contracted with dentists. The dental practice provided the facilities, equipment, and support staff. The dentists set their own schedules and fees. They directed the assistants and had complete control over the care provided their patients. The fees collected were paid to the dental practice, which in turn provided the dentists with 45% of the profits and utilized the remaining 55% for business expenses.

RULING: The dentists are independent contractors.[26]

DENTISTS

Dentists worked for a dental practice. The dentists received a percentage of fees collected for rendering professional services. The practice did not train or instruct the dentists but did evaluate their procedures and recommend changes. The practice provided office space, equipment, and support staff for a fee. Both parties could terminate the relationship at will.

RULING: The dentists are employees.[27]

VETERINARIAN'S ASSISTANTS

A veterinary practice hired a veterinary assistant to clean and assist with examinations and treatment of animals. The assistant received instructions, supervision, and review by the practice. The assistant assumed no risk of loss, had no investment in the veterinary practice, and did not offer services to the general public.

RULING: The assistant is an employee.[28]

SMALL ANIMAL GROOMERS

A dog groomer was paid based on the number of dogs groomed and was supplied with the equipment necessary to perform the job. The groomer and the hirer could terminate employment at will.

RULING: The groomer is an employee.[29]

SMALL ANIMAL GROOMERS

Dog and cat groomers received fees directly from customers and split the fees equally with the hirer. The groomers set their own hours but had to report daily to the hirer. The hirer provided towels and shampoos for the groomers, and the groomers furnished their own clippers and scissors.

RULING: The groomers are employees.[30]

DOG OBEDIENCE TRAINERS

A dog trainer was retained by an organization to teach dog obedience classes. The trainer determined class schedules and supplied all the materials. The organization furnished the classroom. The trainer was paid on a commission. The relationship could be terminated by either party at any time.

RULING: The dog trainer is an independent contractor.[31]

HORSE TRAINERS

A horse trainer was hired to break quarter horses to ride for sale and show. The trainer was paid a fixed amount and supplied none of the necessary equipment. Either party could terminate employment at will.

RULING: The trainer is an employee.[32]

HOW TO ESTABLISH INDEPENDENT CONTRACTOR STATUS

By adhering to state and federal guidelines and following the steps in this section, workers and veterinary practices can establish independent contractor:veterinary practice relationships. The responsibilities of independent contractors and veterinary practices are listed below. The more steps both parties follow, the more likely an independent contractor relationship is established.

STEPS FOR INDEPENDENT CONTRACTORS

1. Establish independent contractor contracts with veterinary practices and abide by them. Contracts may show the intent of the parties, but they are considered meaningless if independent contractors and veterinary practices do not adhere to them.[33]

2. Charge for professional services on a per-job basis rather than by the hour or week.[2] Billing statements submitted by independent contractors should include the business name, address, phone number, a brief description of the job performed, beginning and ending dates, the amount due, and a social security or employer identification number.[34] Keep copies of all billing statements.

3. Pay the required estimated state and federal taxes on a quarterly basis.[35] Contact a tax attorney or certified public accountant to be certain tax payments and forms are submitted properly.

4. Apply for an employer's identification number (EIN). This is the taxpayer identification number used by independent contractors who pay wages to employees or file for certain retirement plans. Otherwise, use a social security number as the business taxpayer identification number.[5] The EIN application, Form SS-4 (Figure 10.1) is obtained by calling 1-800-TAX-FORM or by downloading it from the Internet by accessing the IRS web site at http://www.irs.ustreas.gov.

5. Obtain copies of IRS Form 1099-MISC (Figure10.2) from all contracting veterinary practices. Veterinary practices are required to submit this form to the IRS for independent contractors paid more than $600 per year.[3] Do not fill out a W-4 form and do not accept a W-2 form from the veterinary practices.

6. Purchase health, disability, professional liability insurance, and workers' compensation insurance.[35,36] Do not accept any coverage for these benefits from clients.

7. Procure a DEA registration number and, if necessary, a state pharmacy license. Call the relevant state veterinary board to determine if a state pharmacy license is required.[5]

8. Obtain city and state business licenses.[5]

9. Obtain a USDA accreditation certificate authorizing the signing of health certificates for animals transported interstate or across international boundaries.[5]

10. Set up an office in home or elsewhere. Establish a business telephone line and a business checking account.[5]

11. Purchase homeowner's, renter's, and/or personal articles insurance covering the general liability of the business and for professional instruments and equipment.[5]

12. Create professional letterhead for stationery and business cards.[35]

13. Advertise in veterinary journals, state and local veterinary association newsletters, and veterinary-related web sites, and become listed on the AVMA relief veterinarians' list.[37]

14. Lease facility and on-site equipment from each veterinary practice at which one contracts for a flat daily rate, such as $10 per day.[38] Document the lease by including lease payments on billing statements and including such payments in contracts.[35]

15. Keep records of business expenses such as office supplies, veterinary equipment, transportation mileage, and auto costs. Contact tax attorneys or certified public accountants about eligible tax deductions and proper filing forms.

16. File for business names so that clients can write checks to those names. Even

though independent contractors are not required to have business names, this step further substantiates their independent contractor status.[4]

See Table 10.1 for an independent contractor's checklist.

Steps for Veterinary Practices

1. Establish contracts with independent contractors and abide by them.

2. Submit Form 1099-MISC (Figure 10.2) to the IRS no later than February 28 when contracting with independent contractors whose services exceed $600 annually. Keep one copy on file and send a copy to independent contractors after the jobs are completed or no later than January 31. Veterinary practices are not required to file 1099-MISC forms for independent contractors who are incorporated.[4] Forms are obtained by calling 1-800-TAX-FORM or by downloading them from the Internet by accessing the IRS web site.

3. Send one 1096 transmittal form (Figure 10.3) with all the 1099-MISC forms submitted to the IRS no later than February 28.[39] Forms are obtained by calling 1-800-TAX-FORM or by downloading them from the IRS web site.

4. Create a vendor file for independent contractors (Table 10.2). This file is kept with other vendor files, such as plumbers, electricians, x-ray processor maintenance firms, and oxygen supply and janitorial service companies rather than with the practice's employee files. Since materials contained in these files can be reviewed by the IRS or state auditing agencies, keep only those documents that substantiate the independent contractor relationship, such as the independent contractor's contract; Form 1099-MISC; the Independent Contractor Information Sheet (Figure 10.4); billing

Table 10.1. Checklist for an Independent Contractor's Portfolio

✓ independent contractor's contract

✓ billing statements

✓ proof of quarterly taxes paid

✓ employer identification number or social security number

✓ copies of 1099-MISC forms

✓ certificates for health, disability, professional liability coverage, workers' compensation, automobile, and homeowner's or renter's insurance

✓ DEA registration number

✓ pharmacy license where required

✓ city and state business license

✓ USDA accreditation certificates

✓ business telephone statements

✓ business checking account statements

✓ professional letterhead, business cards, and copies of advertisements

✓ records of business expenses

✓ certificate of business name

Table 10.2. Checklist for a Veterinary Practice's Vendor File

✓ independent contractor's contract

✓ Form 1099-MISC

✓ a copy of the 1096 transmittal form

✓ independent contractor information sheet

✓ billing statements

✓ copies of independent contractors' business licenses

✓ copies of independent contractors' health, disability, professional liability, workers' compensation, and auto insurance policies

✓ any other documents that substantiate the independent contractor's status such as business advertisements, business cards, and letters on their stationery

statements; copy of the contractors' business licenses; statements verifying the existence of the contractors' insurance policies and quarterly estimated tax filings; business advertisements; and business cards.[15]

5. Require billing statements before payment.[4]

6. Pay independent contractors from the business account used for other contractors rather than from the employee payroll account.[4] Pay independent contractors on the same day as other vendors rather than on a standard employee payday. Write checks to the business name rather than the name of the veterinarian whenever possible, even though independent contractors are not required to have business names.[4]

7. Lease the facility and the on-site equipment to independent contractors for a flat daily rate, such as $10 per day. Document the lease by incorporating lease terms in the independent contractor's contract. Roger Tenney, owner and manager of Veterinary Relief Services and creator of the Veterinary Independent Contractor's Association, stated that

> the lease-per-day rate is intended to create a paper trail on behalf of the hospital if a relief doctor's status is

challenged by a regulatory or insurance agency. Subsequently, hospitals should lessen their chances of receiving negative determinations and misclassifications in an audit utilizing relief doctors who either supply their own equipment or lease the on-site equipment per day.[38]

8. Make staff meetings optional and without pay.[4]

9. Call state unemployment and workers' compensation departments to determine whether the state has more stringent requirements than the IRS.

INDEPENDENT CONTRACTOR'S CONTRACTS

Independent contractor contracts evince the intent of both parties to create an independent contractor relationship. Evidence of this intent is clear when contract terms (1) meet federal and state requirements of control and (2) clarify the responsibilities for both the independent contractors and the veterinary practices. Moreover, both parties must abide by the contract terms.[40]

Extensive, detailed contracts that focus on control are most likely to substantiate workers as independent contractors; however, lengthy contracts sometimes intimidate veterinary practice owners who are undereducated regarding this topic or independent contractors who abhor record keeping and the potential for conflicts with clients.[41] Contracts must be sufficient to substantiate workers as independent contractors but straightforward and coherent enough to encourage these working relationships.

Contracts designating workers as independent contractors are not absolute proof of independent contractor status.[42] These contracts cannot negate the existence of employer-employee relationships when the parties fail to meet the criteria discussed earlier in the chapter. As stated in the Code of Federal Regulations:

> If the relationship of employer and employee exists, the designation or description of the relationship by the parties as anything other than that of employer and employee is immaterial. Thus, if such relationship exists, it is of no consequence that the employee is designated...as an independent contractor or the like.[43]

A sample independent contractor contract[44] addressing the issues included in this chapter can be purchased though the publisher of this book, or an affiliate thereof, but must be reviewed by local legal counsel to address individual state idiosyncracies before final adoption.

Contract Terms: Federal and State Requirements of Control

IRS and state laws determine whether workers are independent contractors or employees.[4] Since control is the most important factor in determining independent contractor status, the terms of the contract must focus on that. For example, contracts should include statements claiming that workers are independent contractors and have complete control over services rendered; fees charged; diagnostic procedures performed; and the selection of medical, surgical, and dental procedures. Furthermore, it should state that independent contractors control their own finances including paying required federal and state taxes and business expenses.[44]

The contract terms should include provisions stating that independent contractors have the right to hire and control other veterinarians and veterinary assistants. There should be stipulations regarding the independent contractors' rights and responsibilities to compensate such people, withhold required payroll taxes, provide mandated worker's compensation and unemployment insurance for them, and cover all other business expenses related to their employment.[44]

Contract terms should not contain clauses that restrict independent contractors from working for other veterinary practices in the community, as that would restrict their right to control their businesses. One certified public accountant knowledgeable about veterinary independent contractor issues was so bold as to state, "If the practice owner establishes a requirement that the person providing the service sign a covenant not to compete, the independence test is completely flunked."[45] Other references support that position.[4] No legal cases have been found to substantiate such a definitive position and, as discussed previously, the IRS considers at least 20 factors before upholding or denying the existence of an independent contractor relationship. Nonetheless, restrictive covenants in independent contractors' contracts certainly raise red flags regarding the independence of the contractor and the independent contractor relationship.

Careful draftsmanship in independent contractor contracts is essential if practice owners are to protect their businesses against unfair competition by independent contractors without fueling the legal challenges to the independent relationship of the parties. This entails customizing the confidentiality and nonsolicitation clauses found in Chapter 9 to protect a practice's medical records and client list from competition by a contractor without jeopardizing the tax status of the contractor. A limited application of a restrictive covenant in these contracts can prohibit independent contractors from using confidential information gleaned from the practices without barring the contractors from working for other practices in the local trade or catchment area.

Finally, contracts should stipulate that veterinary practices cannot discharge workers at will. Independent contractors are not employees and, thus, both parties are under contractual obligations until the terms of the contract are completed. Contracts are terminated only upon completion, mutual written consent, or when material breaches or valid excuses by either party exist, such as death, illness, or a disability. [44]

CONTRACT TERMS: BOTH PARTIES' RESPONSIBILITIES

Contract terms should address the responsibilities of both independent contractors and practice owners. Verbal agreements alone are insufficient when misunderstandings arise. Moreover, in the event of litigation over contract disputes, the written terms enable courts to enforce the intended agreements. [5]

Responsibilities of independent contractors include (1) abiding by the laws and professional standards established by state licensing boards and maintaining good standing with such boards, (2) possessing licenses to practice in relevant states, and (3) honoring the ethical norms established by the American Veterinary Medical Association. [44]

Contracts also should define the bilateral financial responsibilities of the parties. First, they should state a flat fee per project payable by veterinary practices upon satisfactory completion of the contractors' work. Next, they should state the daily facility and on-site equipment leasing fee due from independent contractors. [44]

Finally, contracts should state commencement and termination dates and include cancellation policies stipulating that practices that do not cancel scheduled work within defined time periods before contracted work dates will be required to pay specified amounts to independent contractors. [44]

ANCILLARY LEGAL CONCERNS

INDEPENDENT CONTRACTORS AND PART-TIME EMPLOYEES

Veterinarians can work as part-time employees for one practice and as independent contractors for others. Workers who are employees and independent contractors for the same veterinary practice within the same tax year, however, are considered employees by the IRS. [5] A past chairperson of the San Diego County Veterinary Medical Association Investigative Committee on Independent Contractor Relationships stated, "never should one's employment status be changed within the same tax year by the same hiring firm." [35]

Veterinarians who function as part-time employees and independent contractors should consult labor or tax attorneys to address the complications of such relationships. For example, part-time veterinarians who sign contracts with restrictive covenants may jeopardize their ability to offer services as independent contractors to other practices in the restricted area. [5]

In *Fish* v. *Collins*, both Fish and Collins were veterinarians who worked with large animals. They entered into an employment contract which included a restrictive covenant. At the end of the one-year term, employment was terminated. Collins began practicing as an independent contractor for other practices within the restricted territory and time. By engaging in an independent contractor relationship, he maintained that he was not in violation of the contract.

In reviewing the issues, the court said, "Not only is the proscribing language of the covenant sufficiently clear and inclusive to cover that modality,...to hold otherwise would...allow the defendant to circumvent the covenant and accomplish indirectly what he could not accomplish directly." Thus, the Circuit Court of Frederick County, Virginia upheld the restrictive covenant against working as an independent contractor as well as working as an employee of another practice.[46]

Tax Audits

Since the federal government has been balancing the need to rebuild the country's infrastructure and pay off its enormous national debt with financing programs that benefit society, it has been forced to explore avenues to increase revenue.[47] By eliminating tax loopholes, such as reclassifying workers as employees who are mistakenly classified as independent contractors, the government collects more revenue through more reportable income and required tax payments, fewer tax deductions, and collection of back taxes, interest, and penalties for misclassifications. The IRS estimates that over $1.5 billion per year is lost as a result of misclassifications.[48]

During a tax audit, the IRS may examine all independent contractor relationships of a business, regardless of the reason the IRS initially decided to conduct the audit. The IRS generally assumes that an employer/employee relationship exists unless it is shown to be otherwise. Thus, veterinary practices have the burden of proving that their relief veterinarians are independent contractors. Similarly, state auditing agencies place the burden on veterinary practices to prove that relief veterinarians are independent contractors.[4,15]

Situations that prompt the IRS and state agencies to challenge independent contractor working relationships include:

- veterinary practices paying unincorporated independent contractors over $600 annually and not submitting 1099-MISC forms;

- independent contractors not filing estimated quarterly taxes;

- contractors claiming disability, unemployment, or workers' compensation in states that do not cover them; and

- either party submitting Form SS-8 for determination of a worker's employment status.[41]

If the IRS audits a practice and disagrees with an independent contractor classification, it will send the practice a letter within 30 days of the completion of the audit stating its position. Once the letter is received, the practice has 30 days to respond. The Tax Court does not have jurisdiction over employment tax issues and, thus, the practice must pay the required back taxes, interest, and penalties for the workers while simultaneously filing suit in a United States District Court for a refund. The practice bears the legal burden of proof to show the independent contractor status of the workers at issue. When seeking representation for legal challenges, labor lawyers or tax attorneys with experience in IRS and state audits should be consulted.[2]

Liability for Actions of Independent Contractors

As a general rule, employers are liable to third parties injured by the negligent acts of employees. Conversely, veterinary practices generally are not liable for injuries suffered by third parties injured as the result of the negligence of their independent contractors.[2] Nonetheless, they can become liable for injuries caused or incurred by independent contractors under the following circumstances:

- The work exposes the independent contractors to unreasonable risks of harming others.

- The work requires the independent contractors to harm others.

- Veterinary practices are negligent in selecting, evaluating, and retaining their independent contractors.

- Practices knowingly contract with incompetent independent contractors — and continue to renew their contracts.

- Practices exert sufficient control over their independent contractors or their work so that courts conclude such parties were actually employees.

- Independent contractors injure third parties while performing nondelegable duties or ultrahazardous activities.[4]

- Independent contractors assume such relationships with veterinary practices at the insistence of practice owners, fail to obtain their own worker's compensation coverage, and are injured on the job. Practices can be held liable for medical expenses and loss of income based on the premise that these parties were employees, not independent contractors, and the practices errantly classified them as contractors to save money.

FORMS FOR ESTABLISHING INDEPENDENT CONTRACTOR STATUS

The forms presented in this section will help independent contractors and veterinary practices establish independent contractor status. As discussed previously, original forms are obtained by calling 1-800-TAX-FORM. Individuals with computers and Internet access can download forms from the IRS website at http://www.irs.ustreas.gov. Attorneys or certified public accountants should be consulted as needed to assist in completing the forms.

FORM SS-4 APPLICATION FOR EMPLOYER IDENTIFICATION NUMBER

The employer identification number (EIN) is the taxpayer's identification number. It is used by independent contractors and veterinary practices that pay wages to employees or have certain retirement plans. If no such criteria exist, the use of a social security number as the business taxpayer identification number suffices. The EIN application, Form SS-4 (Figure 10.1) discusses in further detail who should file this form, and when and where to do it.

FORM 1099-MISC

Veterinary practices must submit Form 1099-MISC (Figure 10.2) to the IRS no later than February 28 for each independent contractor it pays more than $600 annually. One copy of this form is kept in the independent contractor's file at the veterinary practice and another is sent to the person after completion of a job or by January 31 of each calendar year. Veterinary practices are not required to file 1099-MISC forms for independent contractors who are incorporated.[4]

TRANSMITTAL FORM 1096

Veterinary practices send one 1096 transmittal form (Figure 10.3) with the 1099-MISC forms to the IRS no later than February 28.[4]

INDEPENDENT CONTRACTOR INFORMATION SHEET

The Independent Contractor Information sheet in Figure 10.4 lists general information about independent contractors.[15] This document can help substantiate independent contractor status to auditing agencies that question the relationship. Independent contractors should keep this

Form **SS-4**
(Rev. February 1998)
Department of the Treasury
Internal Revenue Service

Application for Employer Identification Number

(For use by employers, corporations, partnerships, trusts, estates, churches, government agencies, certain individuals, and others. See instructions.)

▶ Keep a copy for your records.

EIN

OMB No. 1545-0003

Please type or print clearly.

1 Name of applicant (legal name) (see instructions)

2 Trade name of business (if different from name on line 1)

3 Executor, trustee, "care of" name

4a Mailing address (street address) (room, apt., or suite no.)

5a Business address (if different from address on lines 4a and 4b)

4b City, state, and ZIP code

5b City, state, and ZIP code

6 County and state where principal business is located

7 Name of principal officer, general partner, grantor, owner, or trustor—SSN or ITIN may be required (see instructions) ▶

8a Type of entity (Check only one box.) (see instructions)
Caution: *If applicant is a limited liability company, see the instructions for line 8a.*

☐ Sole proprietor (SSN) _____
☐ Partnership   ☐ Personal service corp.
☐ REMIC   ☐ National Guard
☐ State/local government   ☐ Farmers' cooperative
☐ Church or church-controlled organization
☐ Other nonprofit organization (specify) ▶ _____
☐ Other (specify) ▶

☐ Estate (SSN of decedent) _____
☐ Plan administrator (SSN) _____
☐ Other corporation (specify) ▶ _____
☐ Trust
☐ Federal government/military
(enter GEN if applicable) _____

8b If a corporation, name the state or foreign country (if applicable) where incorporated

State

Foreign country

9 Reason for applying (Check only one box.) (see instructions)
☐ Started new business (specify type) ▶_____
☐ Hired employees (Check the box and see line 12.)
☐ Created a pension plan (specify type) ▶

☐ Banking purpose (specify purpose) ▶ _____
☐ Changed type of organization (specify new type) ▶ _____
☐ Purchased going business
☐ Created a trust (specify type) ▶ _____
☐ Other (specify) ▶

10 Date business started or acquired (month, day, year) (see instructions)

11 Closing month of accounting year (see instructions)

12 First date wages or annuities were paid or will be paid (month, day, year). **Note:** *If applicant is a withholding agent, enter date income will first be paid to nonresident alien. (month, day, year)* . . . . ▶

13 Highest number of employees expected in the next 12 months. **Note:** *If the applicant does not expect to have any employees during the period, enter -0-. (see instructions)* . . . . ▶

Nonagricultural	Agricultural	Household

14 Principal activity (see instructions) ▶

15 Is the principal business activity manufacturing? . . . . ☐ Yes   ☐ No
If "Yes," principal product and raw material used ▶

16 To whom are most of the products or services sold? Please check one box.   ☐ Business (wholesale)
☐ Public (retail)   ☐ Other (specify) ▶   ☐ N/A

17a Has the applicant ever applied for an employer identification number for this or any other business? . . . . ☐ Yes   ☐ No
Note: *If "Yes," please complete lines 17b and 17c.*

17b If you checked "Yes" on line 17a, give applicant's legal name and trade name shown on prior application, if different from line 1 or 2 above.
Legal name ▶   Trade name ▶

17c Approximate date when and city and state where the application was filed. Enter previous employer identification number if known.
Approximate date when filed (mo., day, year) | City and state where filed | Previous EIN

Under penalties of perjury, I declare that I have examined this application, and to the best of my knowledge and belief, it is true, correct, and complete.

Business telephone number (include area code)

Fax telephone number (include area code)

Name and title (Please type or print clearly.) ▶

Signature ▶   Date ▶

Note: *Do not write below this line. For official use only.*

Please leave blank ▶	Geo.	Ind.	Class	Size	Reason for applying

For Paperwork Reduction Act Notice, see page 4.   Cat. No. 16055N   Form **SS-4** (Rev. 2-98)

Figure 10.1. Form SS-4

9595	☐ VOID	☐ CORRECTED			
PAYER'S name, street address, city, state, ZIP code, and telephone no.		**1** Rents $	OMB No. 1545-0115		
		2 Royalties $	19**99**	**Miscellaneous Income**	
		3 Other income $	Form **1099-MISC**		
PAYER'S Federal identification number	RECIPIENT'S identification number	**4** Federal income tax withheld $	**5** Fishing boat proceeds $	**Copy A For**	
RECIPIENT'S name		**6** Medical and health care payments $	**7** Nonemployee compensation $	**Internal Revenue Service Center**	
Street address (including apt. no.)		**8** Substitute payments in lieu of dividends or interest $	**9** Payer made direct sales of $5,000 or more of consumer products to a buyer (recipient) for resale ▶ ☐	**File with Form 1096.** For Privacy Act and Paperwork Reduction Act Notice and	
City, state, and ZIP code		**10** Crop insurance proceeds $	**11** State income tax withheld $	instructions for completing this form, see the	
Account number (optional)	2nd TIN Not. ☐	**12** State/Payer's state number	**13** $	**1999 Instructions for Forms 1099, 1098, 5498, and W-2G.**	

Form **1099-MISC** Cat. No. 14425J Department of the Treasury - Internal Revenue Service
Do NOT Cut or Separate Forms on This Page — Do NOT Cut or Separate Forms on This Page

Figure 10.2. Form 1099-MISC

document in their portfolios, and veterinary practices should store it in their vendor files.

FORM SS-8 DETERMINATION OF EMPLOYEE WORK STATUS FOR PURPOSES OF FEDERAL EMPLOYMENT TAXES AND INCOME WITHHOLDINGS

Employers and workers have the option of filing a Form SS-8 (Figure 10.5) with the IRS to obtain a private ruling on whether workers are employees or independent contractors.[49] The form lists a series of questions which are based on the 20 common law factors. Most attorneys and certified public accountants do not suggest submitting the form. If the IRS makes a private ruling and determines that independent contractors are employees, the ruling becomes retroactive and back taxes can be imposed. The form is useful as a worksheet, though, to further guide employers and workers in assessing independent contractor working relationships.[4,5]

ADDITIONAL RESOURCES

Relief veterinarians and practice owners who want to learn more about business management and legal issues concerning the independent contractor:veterinary practice relationship can contact the associations and consultants listed here. These resources can help both parties address concerns such as the desirable characteristics of relief veterinarians and veterinary practices, necessary steps when interviewing relief veterinarians or veterinary practices, and what to look for in referral agencies that match relief veterinarians and veterinary practices.

ASSOCIATIONS

American Veterinary Medical Association
National Relief Veterinarian List
1931 North Meacham Road, Suite 100
Schaumburg, IL 60173
800-248-2862
FAX 847-925-1329

Veterinary Independent Contractors
Association

DO NOT STAPLE   6969

Form **1096**	Annual Summary and Transmittal of	OMB No. 1545-0108
Department of the Treasury Internal Revenue Service	U.S. Information Returns	19**99**

ATTACH IRS LABEL HERE

⌈ FILER'S name

Street address (including room or suite number)

City, state, and ZIP code ⌋

If you are not using a preprinted label, enter in box 1 or 2 below the identification number you used as the filer on the information returns being transmitted. Do not fill in both boxes 1 and 2.

Name of person to contact if the IRS needs more information

Telephone number
(   )

For Official Use Only

1 Employer identification number	2 Social security number	3 Total number of forms	4 Federal income tax withheld $	5 Total amount reported with this Form 1096 $

Enter an "X" in only one box below to indicate the type of form being filed.   If this is your FINAL return, enter an "X" here ▶ ☐

W-2G 32	1098 81	1098-E 84	1098-T 83	1099-A 80	1099-B 79	1099-C 85	1099-DIV 91	1099-G 86	1099-INT 92	1099-LTC 93	1099-MISC 95	1099-MSA 94	1099-OID 96
☐	☐	☐	☐	☐	☐	☐	☐	☐	☐	☐	☐	☐	☐

1099-PATR 97	1099-R 98	1099-S 75	5498 28	5498-MSA 27
☐	☐	☐	☐	☐

Please return this entire page to the Internal Revenue Service. Photocopies are NOT acceptable.

Under penalties of perjury, I declare that I have examined this return and accompanying documents, and, to the best of my knowledge and belief, they are true, correct, and complete.

Signature ▶   Title ▶   Date ▶

Instructions

Purpose of form. Use this form to transmit paper Forms 1099, 1098, 5498, and W-2G to the Internal Revenue Service. *(See Where To File on the back.)* DO NOT USE FORM 1096 TO TRANSMIT MAGNETIC MEDIA. See **Form 4804,** Transmittal of Information Returns Reported Magnetically/Electronically.

Use of preprinted label. If you received a preprinted label from the IRS with Package 1099, place the label in the name and address area of this form inside the brackets. Make any necessary changes to your name and address on the label. However, do not use the label if the taxpayer identification number (TIN) shown is incorrect. **Do not prepare your own label. Use only the IRS-prepared label that came with your Package 1099.**

If you are not using a preprinted label, enter the filer's name, address (including room, suite, or other unit number), and TIN in the spaces provided on the form.

Filer. The name, address, and TIN of the filer on this form must be the same as those you enter in the upper left area of Form 1099, 1098, 5498, or W-2G. A filer includes a payer, a recipient of mortgage interest payments (including points) or student loan interest, an educational institution, a broker, a barter exchange, a creditor, a person reporting real estate transactions, a trustee or issuer of any individual retirement arrangement or a medical savings account (MSA) (including a Medicare+Choice MSA), and a lender who acquires an interest in secured property or who has reason to know that the property has been abandoned.

Transmitting to the IRS. Send the forms in a flat mailing (not folded). Group the forms by form number and transmit each group with a **separate** Form 1096. For example, if you must file both Forms 1098 and 1099-A, complete one Form 1096 to transmit your Forms 1098 and another Form 1096 to transmit your Forms 1099-A. You need not submit original and corrected returns separately. **Do not** send a form (1099, 5498, etc.) containing summary (subtotal) information with Form 1096. Summary information for the group of forms being sent is entered only in boxes 3, 4, and 5 of Form 1096.

Box 1 or 2. Complete only if you are not using a preprinted IRS label. Individuals not in a trade or business must enter their social security number in box 2; sole proprietors and all others must enter their employer identification number in box 1. However, sole proprietors who do not have an employer identification number must enter their social security number in box 2.

Box 3. Enter the number of forms you are transmitting with this Form 1096. Do not include blank or voided forms or the Form 1096 in your total. Enter the number of correctly completed forms, not the number of pages, being transmitted. For example, if you send one page of three-to-a-page Forms 5498 with a Form 1096 and you have correctly completed two Forms 5498 on that page, enter "2" in box 3 of Form 1096.

Box 4. Enter the total Federal income tax withheld shown on the forms being transmitted with this Form 1096.

For more information and the Privacy Act and Paperwork Reduction Act Notice, see the 1999 Instructions for Forms 1099, 1098, 5498, and W-2G.

Cat. No. 14400O   Form **1096** (1999)

Figure 10.3. Form 1096

INDEPENDENT CONTRACTOR

Name

| Telephone number | Fax number |

E-mail

Business name

Business address

| Social Security # | Employer Identification # |

PROFESSIONAL DEGREE

Degree (DVM or VMD)

University

Date received

LICENSES

State veterinary license #

USDA accreditation #

DEA #

State pharmacy license #

Business license #

Motor vehicle operator's license #

INSURANCE POLICIES (CARRIER/POLICY #/EXPIRATION DATE)

Health

Professional liability

Disability

Workers' compensation

General liability

Motor vehicle

INDEPENDENT CONTRACTOR'S EQUIPMENT

Home computer, stethoscope, ophthalmoscope, otoscope?

MISCELLANEOUS

Figure 10.4. Independent contractor information sheet

Form **SS-8**
(Rev. June 1997)
Department of the Treasury
Internal Revenue Service

Determination of Employee Work Status
for Purposes of Federal Employment Taxes
and Income Tax Withholding

OMB No. 1545-0004

Paperwork Reduction Act Notice

We ask for the information on this form to carry out the Internal Revenue laws of the United States. You are required to give us the information. We need it to ensure that you are complying with these laws and to allow us to figure and collect the right amount of tax.

You are not required to provide the information requested on a form that is subject to the Paperwork Reduction Act unless the form displays a valid OMB control number. Books or records relating to a form or its instructions must be retained as long as their contents may become material in the administration of any Internal Revenue law. Generally, tax returns and return information are confidential, as required by Code section 6103.

The time needed to complete and file this form will vary depending on individual circumstances. The estimated average time is: **Recordkeeping,** 34 hr., 55 min.; **Learning about the law or the form,** 12 min.; and **Preparing and sending the form to the IRS,** 46 min. If you have comments concerning the accuracy of these time estimates or suggestions for making this form simpler, we would be happy to hear from you. You can write to the Tax Forms Committee, Western Area Distribution Center, Rancho Cordova, CA 95743-0001. **DO NOT** send the tax form to this address. Instead, see **General Information** for where to file.

Purpose

Employers and workers file Form SS-8 to get a determination as to whether a worker is an employee for purposes of Federal employment taxes and income tax withholding.

General Information

Complete this form carefully. If the firm is completing the form, complete it for **ONE** individual who is representative of the class of workers whose status is in question. If you want a written determination for more than one class of workers, complete a separate Form SS-8 for one worker

from each class whose status is typical of that class. A written determination for any worker will apply to other workers of the same class if the facts are not materially different from those of the worker whose status was ruled upon.

Caution: *Form SS-8 is **not** a claim for refund of social security and Medicare taxes or Federal income tax withholding. Also, a determination that an individual is an employee does not necessarily reduce any current or prior tax liability. A worker must file his or her income tax return even if a determination has not been made by the due date of the return.*

Where to file.—In the list below, find the state where your legal residence, principal place of business, office, or agency is located. Send Form SS-8 to the address listed for your location.

Location:	Send to:
Alaska, Arizona, Arkansas, California, Colorado, Hawaii, Idaho, Illinois, Iowa, Kansas, Minnesota, Missouri, Montana, Nebraska, Nevada, New Mexico, North Dakota, Oklahoma, Oregon, South Dakota, Texas, Utah, Washington, Wisconsin, Wyoming	Internal Revenue Service SS-8 Determinations P.O. Box 1231, Stop 4106 AUSC Austin, TX 78767
Alabama, Connecticut, Delaware, District of Columbia, Florida, Georgia, Indiana, Kentucky, Louisiana, Maine, Maryland, Massachusetts, Michigan, Mississippi, New Hampshire, New Jersey, New York, North Carolina, Ohio, Pennsylvania, Rhode Island, South Carolina, Tennessee, Vermont, Virginia, West Virginia, All other locations not listed	Internal Revenue Service SS-8 Determinations Two Lakemont Road Newport, VT 05855-1555
American Samoa, Guam, Puerto Rico, U.S. Virgin Islands	Internal Revenue Service Mercantile Plaza 2 Avenue Ponce de Leon San Juan, Puerto Rico 00918

Name of firm (or person) for whom the worker performed services

Name of worker

Address of firm (include street address, apt. or suite no., city, state, and ZIP code)

Address of worker (include street address, apt. or suite no., city, state, and ZIP code)

Trade name

Telephone number (include area code)
( )

Worker's social security number

Telephone number (include area code)
( )

Firm's employer identification number

Check type of firm for which the work relationship is in question:
☐ **Individual** ☐ **Partnership** ☐ **Corporation** ☐ **Other** (specify) ▶ ....

Important Information Needed To Process Your Request

This form is being completed by: ☐ Firm ☐ Worker

If this form is being completed by the worker, the IRS **must** have your permission to disclose your name to the firm.

Do you object to disclosing your name and the information on this form to the firm? . . . . . . ☐ Yes ☐ No

If you answer "Yes," the IRS cannot act on your request. **Do not complete the rest of this form unless the IRS asks for it.**

Under section 6110 of the Internal Revenue Code, the information on this form and related file documents will be open to the public if any ruling or determination is made. However, names, addresses, and taxpayer identification numbers will be removed before the information is made public.

Is there any other information you want removed? . . . . ☐ Yes ☐ No

If you check "Yes," we cannot process your request unless you submit a copy of this form and copies of all supporting documents showing, in brackets, the information you want removed. Attach a separate statement showing which specific exemption of section 6110(c) applies to each bracketed part.

Cat. No. 16106T

Form **SS-8** (Rev. 6-97)

Figure 10.5. Form SS-8

Form SS-8 (Rev. 6-97)   Page **2**

This form is designed to cover many work activities, so some of the questions may not apply to you. **You must answer ALL items or mark them "Unknown" or "Does not apply."** *If you need more space, attach another sheet.*

Total number of workers in this class. (Attach names and addresses. If more than 10 workers, list only 10.) ▶ _____

This information is about services performed by the worker from _____ to _____
                                                                                                (month, day, year)   (month, day, year)

Is the worker still performing services for the firm? . . . . ☐ **Yes** ☐ **No**

● If "No," what was the date of termination? ▶ _____
                                                                            (month, day, year)

1a Describe the firm's business ....

 b Describe the work done by the worker ....
....

2a If the work is done under a written agreement between the firm and the worker, attach a copy.

 b If the agreement is not in writing, describe the terms and conditions of the work arrangement ....
....
....

 c If the actual working arrangement differs in any way from the agreement, explain the differences and why they occur ....
....
....

3a Is the worker given training by the firm? . . . . ☐ **Yes** ☐ **No**
 ● If "Yes," what kind? ....
 ● How often? ....

 b Is the worker given instructions in the way the work is to be done (exclusive of actual training in 3a)? . ☐ **Yes** ☐ **No**
 ● If "Yes," give specific examples ....

 c Attach samples of any written instructions or procedures.

 d Does the firm have the right to change the methods used by the worker or direct that person on how to
 do the work? . . . . ☐ **Yes** ☐ **No**
 ● Explain your answer ....
....

 e Does the operation of the firm's business require that the worker be supervised or controlled in the
 performance of the service? . . . . ☐ **Yes** ☐ **No**
 ● Explain your answer ....
....

4a The firm engages the worker:
 ☐ To perform and complete a particular job only
 ☐ To work at a job for an indefinite period of time
 ☐ Other (explain) ....

 b Is the worker required to follow a routine or a schedule established by the firm? . . . . ☐ **Yes** ☐ **No**
 ● If "Yes," what is the routine or schedule? ....
....

 c Does the worker report to the firm or its representative?. . . . . ☐ **Yes** ☐ **No**
 ● If "Yes," how often? ....
 ● For what purpose? ....
 ● In what manner (in person, in writing, by telephone, etc.)? ....
 ● Attach copies of any report forms used in reporting to the firm.

 d Does the worker furnish a time record to the firm? . . . . ☐ **Yes** ☐ **No**
 ● If "Yes," attach copies of time records.

5a State the kind and value of tools, equipment, supplies, and materials furnished by:
 ● The firm ....
....

 ● The worker ....
....

 b What expenses are incurred by the worker in the performance of services for the firm? ....
....

 c Does the firm reimburse the worker for any expenses? . . . . ☐ **Yes** ☐ **No**
 ● If "Yes," specify the reimbursed expenses ....

Figure 10.5. Form SS-8 (cont.)

6a Will the worker perform the services personally? . . . . □ Yes □ No
  b Does the worker have helpers? . . . . □ Yes □ No
   • If "Yes," who hires the helpers? □ Firm □ Worker
   • If the helpers are hired by the worker, is the firm's approval necessary? . . . . □ Yes □ No
   • Who pays the helpers?   □ Firm □ Worker
   • If the worker pays the helpers, does the firm repay the worker? . . . . □ Yes □ No
   • Are social security and Medicare taxes and Federal income tax withheld from the helpers' pay? . . □ Yes □ No
   • If "Yes," who reports and pays these taxes?   □ Firm   □ Worker
   • Who reports the helpers' earnings to the Internal Revenue Service? □ Firm □ Worker
   • What services do the helpers perform? ....
7 At what location are the services performed? □ Firm's □ Worker's □ Other (specify) ....
8a Type of pay worker receives:
   □ Salary   □ Commission □ Hourly wage   □ Piecework □ Lump sum   □ Other (specify) ....
  b Does the firm guarantee a minimum amount of pay to the worker? . . . . □ Yes □ No
  c Does the firm allow the worker a drawing account or advances against pay? . . . . □ Yes □ No
   • If "Yes," is the worker paid such advances on a regular basis? . . . . □ Yes □ No
  d How does the worker repay such advances? ....
9a Is the worker eligible for a pension, bonus, paid vacations, sick pay, etc.? . . . . □ Yes □ No
   • If "Yes," specify ....
  b Does the firm carry worker's compensation insurance on the worker? . . . . □ Yes □ No
  c Does the firm withhold social security and Medicare taxes from amounts paid the worker? . . . . . □ Yes □ No
  d Does the firm withhold Federal income tax from amounts paid the worker? . . . . □ Yes □ No
  e How does the firm report the worker's earnings to the Internal Revenue Service?
   □ Form W-2 □ Form 1099-MISC □ Does not report □ Other (specify) ....
   • Attach a copy.
  f Does the firm bond the worker? . . . . □ Yes □ No
10a Approximately how many hours a day does the worker perform services for the firm? ....
  b Does the firm set hours of work for the worker? . . . . □ Yes □ No
   • If "Yes," what are the worker's set hours? _____ a.m./p.m. to _____ a.m./p.m. (Circle whether a.m. or p.m.)
  c Does the worker perform similar services for others? . . . . □ Yes □ No □ Unknown
   • If "Yes," are these services performed on a daily basis for other firms? . . . . □ Yes □ No □ Unknown
   • Percentage of time spent in performing these services for:
     This firm .... % Other firms .... % □ Unknown
   • Does the firm have priority on the worker's time? . . . . □ Yes □ No
   • If "No," explain ....
  d Is the worker prohibited from competing with the firm either while performing services or during any later
     period? . . . . □ Yes □ No
11a Can the firm discharge the worker at any time without incurring a liability? . . . . □ Yes □ No
   • If "No," explain ....
  b Can the worker terminate the services at any time without incurring a liability? . . . . □ Yes □ No
   • If "No," explain ....
12a Does the worker perform services for the firm under:
     □ The firm's business name   □ The worker's own business name   □ Other (specify) ....
  b Does the worker advertise or maintain a business listing in the telephone directory, a trade
     journal, etc.? . . . . □ Yes □ No □ Unknown
   • If "Yes," specify ....
  c Does the worker represent himself or herself to the public as being in business to perform
     the same or similar services? . . . . □ Yes □ No □ Unknown
   • If "Yes," how? ....
  d Does the worker have his or her own shop or office? . . . . □ Yes □ No □ Unknown
   • If "Yes," where? ....
  e Does the firm represent the worker as an employee of the firm to its customers? . . . . □ Yes □ No
   • If "No," how is the worker represented? ....
  f How did the firm learn of the worker's services? ....
13 Is a license necessary for the work? . . . . □ Yes □ No □ Unknown
   • If "Yes," what kind of license is required? ....
   • Who issues the license? ....
   • Who pays the license fee?

Figure 10.5. Form SS-8 (cont.)

Form SS-8 (Rev. 6-97)   Page **4**

14 Does the worker have a financial investment in a business related to the services
performed? . . . . ☐ **Yes** ☐ **No** ☐ **Unknown**
  ● If "Yes," specify and give amount of the investment ....
15 Can the worker incur a loss in the performance of the service for the firm? . . . . ☐ **Yes** ☐ **No**
  ● If "Yes," how? ....
16a Has any other government agency ruled on the status of the firm's workers? . . . . ☐ **Yes** ☐ **No**
  ● If "Yes," attach a copy of the ruling.
  b Is the same issue being considered by any IRS office in connection with the audit of the worker's tax
return or the firm's tax return, or has it been considered recently? . . . . ☐ **Yes** ☐ **No**
  ● If "Yes," for which year(s)? ....
17 Does the worker assemble or process a product at home or away from the firm's place of business? ☐ **Yes** ☐ **No**
  ● If "Yes," who furnishes materials or goods used by the worker? ☐ Firm   ☐ Worker   ☐ Other
  ● Is the worker furnished a pattern or given instructions to follow in making the product? . . . . ☐ **Yes** ☐ **No**
  ● Is the worker required to return the finished product to the firm or to someone designated by the firm? ☐ **Yes** ☐ **No**
18 Attach a detailed explanation of any other reason why you believe the worker is an employee or an independent contractor.

Answer items 19a through o only if the worker is a salesperson or provides a service directly to customers.

19a Are leads to prospective customers furnished by the firm? . . . . ☐ **Yes** ☐ **No** ☐ **Does not apply**
  b Is the worker required to pursue or report on leads? . . . . ☐ **Yes** ☐ **No** ☐ **Does not apply**
  c Is the worker required to adhere to prices, terms, and conditions of sale established by the firm? . . ☐ **Yes** ☐ **No**
  d Are orders submitted to and subject to approval by the firm? . . . . ☐ **Yes** ☐ **No**
  e Is the worker expected to attend sales meetings? . . . . ☐ **Yes** ☐ **No**
  ● If "Yes," is the worker subject to any kind of penalty for failing to attend? . . . . ☐ **Yes** ☐ **No**
  f Does the firm assign a specific territory to the worker? . . . . ☐ **Yes** ☐ **No**
  g Whom does the customer pay?   ☐ Firm   ☐ Worker
  ● If worker, does the worker remit the total amount to the firm? . . . . ☐ **Yes** ☐ **No**
  h Does the worker sell a consumer product in a home or establishment other than a permanent retail
establishment? . . . . ☐ **Yes** ☐ **No**
  i List the products and/or services distributed by the worker, such as meat, vegetables, fruit, bakery products, beverages (other
than milk), or laundry or dry cleaning services. If more than one type of product and/or service is distributed, specify the
principal one ....
  j Did the firm or another person assign the route or territory and a list of customers to the worker? . . ☐ **Yes** ☐ **No**
  ● If "Yes," enter the name and job title of the person who made the assignment ....
  k Did the worker pay the firm or person for the privilege of serving customers on the route or in the territory? ☐ **Yes** ☐ **No**
  ● If "Yes," how much did the worker pay (not including any amount paid for a truck or racks, etc.)? $ ....
  ● What factors were considered in determining the value of the route or territory? ....
  l How are new customers obtained by the worker? Explain fully, showing whether the new customers called the firm for service,
were solicited by the worker, or both ....
  m Does the worker sell life insurance? . . . . ☐ **Yes** ☐ **No**
  ● If "Yes," is the selling of life insurance or annuity contracts for the firm the worker's entire business
activity? . . . . ☐ **Yes** ☐ **No**
  ● If "No," list the other business activities and the amount of time spent on them ....
  n Does the worker sell other types of insurance for the firm? . . . . ☐ **Yes** ☐ **No**
  ● If "Yes," state the percentage of the worker's total working time spent in selling other types of insurance............... %
  ● At the time the contract was entered into between the firm and the worker, was it their intention that the worker sell life
insurance for the firm: ☐ on a full-time basis   ☐ on a part-time basis
  ● State the manner in which the intention was expressed ....
  o Is the worker a traveling or city salesperson? . . . . ☐ **Yes** ☐ **No**
  ● If "Yes," from whom does the worker principally solicit orders for the firm? ....
  ● If the worker solicits orders from wholesalers, retailers, contractors, or operators of hotels, restaurants, or other similar
establishments, specify the percentage of the worker's time spent in the solicitation .... %
  ● Is the merchandise purchased by the customers for resale or for use in their business operations? If used by the customers
in their business operations, describe the merchandise and state whether it is equipment installed on their premises or a
consumable supply

Under penalties of perjury, I declare that I have examined this request, including accompanying documents, and to the best of my knowledge and belief, the facts
presented are true, correct, and complete.

Signature ▶   Title ▶   Date ▶

If the firm is completing this form, an officer or member of the firm must sign it. If the worker is completing this form, the worker must sign it. If the worker wants a
written determination about services performed for two or more firms, a separate form must be completed and signed for each firm. Additional copies of this form may
be obtained by calling 1-800-TAX-FORM (1-800-829-3676).

✪

Figure 10.5. Form SS-8 (cont.)

Vet Web - newsletter
1 Argonaut, Suite 250
Aliso Viejo, CA 92656
714-457-8810

San Diego County Veterinary Medical
Association
Committee on Independent Contractor
Issues
7590 El Cajon Boulevard, Suite H
La Mesa, CA 91941
619-466-3400

CONSULTANTS ON INDEPENDENT CONTRACTOR ISSUES

Lacroix, Charlotte DVM, JD
Priority Veterinary Legal Consultants
16 S. Main Street
Yardley, PA 19067
215-321-9488 PA
908-534-2065 NJ
E-mail clacroix@pvmc.net

Gatto, Lou CPA
528 Arizona Avenue #201
Santa Monica, CA 90401
310-393-2434

McCafferty, Owen and Heinke, Marsha,
CPAs
P.O. Box 819
North Olmsted, OH 44070-0819
440-779-1099
E-mail omccaffert@aol.com

Smith, Carin DVM
19691 Highway 209
Leavenworth, WA 98826
509-763-2052
E-mail info@smithvet.com

Bent Ericksen & Associates
3941 Prk Drive, Suite 20-317
El Dorado Hills, CA 95762
916-933-5117

Veterinary Referral Services
800-447-5607
FAX 714-457-8814
E-mail VetRelief@aol.com
http://www.vetrelief.com

FEDERAL AND STATE AGENCIES (NAMES VARY FROM STATE TO STATE)

Internal Revenue Service
800-TAX FORM (800-829-3676)
http://www.irs.usteas.gov

Taxpayer Hotline or Taxpayer Education
Workshop
800-829-1040

Superintendent of Documents
Government Printing Office
Washington, DC 20402
http://www.access.gpo.gov

State Department of Taxation and Revenue:
state taxes and business licenses

State Employment Division: unemployment insurance

State Department of Labor: workers' compensation

Veterinary Medical Boards: professional and
accreditation licenses – available under the
"Practice Act" section of the AVMA Directory

CONCLUSION

Veterinarians who function as independent contractors retain the right to control
the means by which their work is accomplished. When veterinary practices have the
right to control, independent contractors are
then employees and the practices are the
employers.[50] With this in mind, veterinary
practices and independent contractors
should periodically reevaluate their working
relationships to ensure that they are abiding
by federal and state laws.[4]

Both parties should seek the advice of
labor attorneys knowledgeable about IRS
and state agency rules. Such professionals
can clarify any issues about independent
contractor status, cite the newest federal
and state rulings, advise about liability
issues, and review the independent contractor's contract before final adoption.[4]

REFERENCES

1. Hannah H: Employed veterinarians as independent contractors-some legal considerations. *JAVMA* 191(5):502-503 (citing 41 American Jurisprudence 2d 737), 1987.

2. Leet J:*Is That Person an Employee or an Independent Contractor?* Sacramento, CA, McDonough, Holland & Allen Publishers, 1992.

3. Gregory D, Leder W: Employee or independent contractor? *Vizcaino* v *Microsoft Corporation. Lab Law J* 47(12):749-754, 1996.

4. California Chamber of Commerce: *Independent Contractors: A Manager's Guide and Audit Reference.* Sacramento, CA, California Chamber of Commerce Publishers, 1996.

5. Smith C: *The Relief Veterinarian's Manual.* Leavenworth, WA, Smith Veterinary Services, 1996.

6. Veterinary Independent Contractor Association. *Vet Web* 1(2):1, 1995.

7. Veterinary Independent Contractor Association. *Vet Web* 1(4):1-5, 1995.

8. Kahler S: Concerns facing the profession, who's the boss? Answer holds key to independent contractor question. *JAVMA* 201:1, 1992.

9. San Diego County Veterinary Medical Association Committee on Independent Contractor Relationships: *Investigation of the Independent Contractor Status of Relief Veterinarians.* San Diego, CA, pp 1-8, March 1991.

10. Internal Revenue Service, Ruling 87-41: 20 common law factors.

11. CFR §31.3401(c)-1(c).

12. Leet J: Personal communication, Sacramento, CA, 1997.

13. Bender TJ: IRS issues new guidelines to distinguish employees from independent contractors. *Penn Employ Law Lett* 6(9):5-7, 1996.

14. *Internal Revenue Service Publication 15-A. Employee or Independent Contractor?* pp 4-5, 1996.

15. San Diego County Veterinary Medical Association Committee on Independent Contractor Relationships: *Investigation of the Independent Contractor Status of Relief Veterinarians.* San Diego, CA, pp 1-11, April 1991.

16. *Internal Revenue Service Publication 1976. Independent Contractor or Employee?* 1996.

17. Federal safe harbor for certain workers, Revenue Act of 1978, section 530.

18. IRS, Rev Proc 85-18. Supplement to Safe Harbor rules. p17.

19. Internal Revenue Code 3509

20. *Diaz* v *U.S. 90-1* US Tax Cases, (CCH) pp 50, 209.

21. IRS ltr rul 8453021.

22. IRS ltr rul 8453021.

23. IRS ltr rul 7904005.

24. IRS ltr rul 8033043.

25. IRS ltr rul 8014023.

26. IRS ltr rul 7934083.

27. IRS ltr rul 8909011.

28. IRS ltr rul 8239056.

29. IRS ltr rul 8647017.

30. IRS ltr rul 8833021.

31. IRS ltr rul 8629033.

32. IRS ltr rul 8640043.

33. San Diego County Veterinary Medical Association Committee on Independent Contractor Relationships: *Investigation of the Independent Contractor Status of Relief Veterinarians.* San Diego, CA, pp 1-2, Aug 1991.

34. Smith C: *The Employer's Manual: A Guide to Hiring Part-Time and Relief Veterinarians*. Leavenworth, WA, Smith Veterinary Services, 1996.

35. Veterinary Independent Contractor Association. *Vet Web* 2(1):1-5 June 1996.

36. AVMA PLIT Representative: Personal communications, Chicago, IL, AVMA PLIT office, business insurance department, 1997.

37. Smith C: Good communication key to relationship with relief veterinarian. *DVM Mag*(10): 52, 1991.

38. Veterinary Referral Services System Program. Lease per day http//www.vetrelief.com. Click on Doctor's Business Services, then click on lease per day. June 1997.

39. Internal Revenue Service, Form 1096. Annual summary and transmittal of US information returns, instructions section.

40. Wilson S: Letter re: independent contractor agreement. Littler, Mendelson, Fastiff & Tichy, Professional Law Corp, 1991.

41. Veterinary Independent Contractor Association. *Vet Web* 2(2):1-4, 1996.

42. McCoy C, Bank D: Microsoft loses appeal in worker-benefits case. *Wall Street J*:A3-A6, July 25, 1997.

43. CFR §31.3401(c)-1(e).

44. Sample Independent Contractor's Contract, compilation of work done by Dr. Rochelle Brinton, past Chairperson of the San Diego County Veterinary Medical Association Investigative Committee on Independent Contractor Relationships, the San Diego County Veterinary Medical Association's employment tax law advisors, attorneys who provided the 1991 Guide to Hiring Independent Contractors prototype for the California Chamber of Commerce. Customized and contemporized by James F. Wilson, DVM, JD, and Charlotte Lacroix, DVM, JD. Contact Priority Veterinary Legal Consultants, 16 S. Main St., Yardley, PA 19067, phone 215-321-9488.

45. McCafferty O: Independent contractor vs. employee in a veterinary practice. *Vet Econ* 31(5):74-79, 1990.

46. *Fish* v *Collins*, 9 Va Cir. 64 Lexis 54 1987.

47. Frederick G: The IRS and independent contractors: How to organize your business to comply. *Prof Speak*:26-27, 1993.

48. Veterinary Independent Contractor Association. *Vet Web* 1(3):1-4, 1995.

49. IRS Form SS-8. Determination of Employee Work Status for Purposes of Federal Employment Taxes and Income Tax Withholding, 1997.

50. Metelka E: Independent Contractor or Employee? *Vet Econ* 35(11):12-14, 1994.

PRINCIPLES OF VETERINARY MEDICAL ETHICS

OF THE AMERICAN VETERINARY MEDICAL ASSOCIATION (AVMA)

*(**Bold print states the Principles,** standard print explains or clarifies the Principle to which it applies)*

I. INTRODUCTION

A. Veterinarians are members of a scholarly profession who have earned academic degrees from comprehensive universities or similar educational institutions. Veterinarians practice the profession of veterinary medicine in a variety of situations and circumstances.

B. Exemplary professional conduct upholds the dignity of the veterinary profession. All veterinarians are expected to adhere to a progressive code of ethical conduct known as the Principles of Veterinary Medical Ethics (the Principles). The basis of the Principles is the Golden Rule. Veterinarians should accept this rule as a guide to their general conduct, and abide by the Principles. They should conduct their professional and personal affairs in an ethical manner. Professional veterinary associations should adopt the Principles or a similar code as a guide for their activities.

C. Professional organizations should establish ethics, grievance, or peer review committees to address ethical issues. Local and state veterinary associations should also include discussions of ethical issues in their continuing education programs.

1. Complaints about behavior that may violate the Principles should be addressed in an appropriate and timely manner. Such questions should be considered initially by ethics, grievance, or peer review committees of local or state veterinary associations and, if necessary, state veterinary medical boards. Members of local and state committees are familiar with local customs and circumstances, and those committees are in the best position to confer with all parties involved.

2. All veterinarians in local or state associations and jurisdictions have a responsibility to regulate and guide the professional conduct of their members.

3. Colleges of veterinary medicine should stress the teaching of ethical and value issues as part of the professional veterinary curriculum for all veterinary students.

4. The National Board Examination Committee is encouraged to prepare and include questions regarding professional ethics in the National Board Examination.

D. The AVMA Judicial Council is charged to interpret the AVMA Constitution and Bylaws, the Principles of Veterinary Medical Ethics, and other rules of the Association. The Judicial Council should review the Principles periodically to insure that they remain complete and up to date.

II. PROFESSIONAL BEHAVIOR

A. **Veterinarians should first consider the needs of the patient: to relieve disease, suffering, or disability while minimizing pain or fear.**

B. **Veterinarians should obey all laws of the jurisdictions in which they reside and practice veterinary medicine. Veterinarians should be honest and fair in their relations with others, and they should not engage in fraud, misrepresentation, or deceit.**

1. Veterinarians should report illegal practices and activities to the proper authorities.

2. The AVMA Judicial Council may choose to report alleged infractions by nonmembers of the AVMA to the appropriate agencies.

3. Veterinarians should use only the title of the professional degree that was awarded by the school of veterinary medicine where the degree was earned. All veterinarians may use the courtesy titles *Doctor* or *Veterinarian*. Veterinarians who were

awarded a degree other than DVM or VMD should refer to the *AVMA Directory* for information on the appropriate titles and degrees.

C. **It is unethical for veterinarians to identify themselves as members of an AVMA recognized specialty organization if such certification has not been awarded.**

D. **It is unethical to place professional knowledge, credentials, or services at the disposal of any nonprofessional organization, group, or individual to promote or lend credibility to the illegal practice of veterinary medicine.**

E. **Veterinarians may choose whom they will serve. Once they have started patient care, veterinarians must not neglect their patients, and they must continue to provide professional services until they are relieved of their professional responsibilities.**

F. **In emergencies, veterinarians have an ethical responsibility to provide essential services for animals when it is necessary to save life or relieve suffering. Such emergency care may be limited to euthanasia to relieve suffering, or when the client rejects euthanasia, to stabilize the patient sufficiently to enable transportation to another veterinary hospital for definitive care.**

1. When veterinarians cannot be available to provide services, they should arrange with their colleagues to assure that emergency services are available, consistent with the needs of the locality.

2. Veterinarians who are not qualified to manage and treat certain emergencies should arrange to refer their clients to other veterinarians who can provide the appropriate emergency services.

G. **Regardless of practice ownership, the interests of the patient, client, and pub-**

lic require that all decisions that affect diagnosis, care, and treatment of patients are made by veterinarians.

H. Veterinarians should strive to enhance their image with respect to their colleagues, clients, other health professionals, and the general public. Veterinarians should be honest, fair, courteous, considerate, and compassionate. Veterinarians should present a professional appearance and follow acceptable professional procedures using current professional and scientific knowledge.

I. Veterinarians should not slander, or injure the professional standing or reputation of other veterinarians in a false or misleading manner.

J. Veterinarians should strive to improve their veterinary knowledge and skills, and they are encouraged to collaborate with other professionals in the quest for knowledge and professional development.

K. The responsibilities of the veterinary profession extend beyond individual patients and clients to society in general. Veterinarians are encouraged to make their knowledge available to their communities and to provide their services for activities that protect public health.

L. Veterinarians and their associates should protect the personal privacy of patients and clients. Veterinarians should not reveal confidences unless required to by law or unless it becomes necessary to protect the health and welfare of other individuals or animals.

M. Veterinarians who are impaired by alcohol or other substances should seek assistance from qualified organizations or individuals. Colleagues of impaired veterinarians should encourage those individuals to seek assistance and to overcome their disabilities.

III. THE VETERINARIAN-CLIENT-PATIENT RELATIONSHIP

A. The veterinarian-client-patient relationship (VCPR) is the basis for interaction among veterinarians, their clients, and their patients. A VCPR exists when all of the following conditions have been met:

1. The veterinarian has assumed responsibility for making clinical judgements regarding the health of the animal(s) and the need for medical treatment, and the client has agreed to follow the veterinarian's instructions.

2. The veterinarian has sufficient knowledge of the animal(s) to initiate at least a general or preliminary diagnosis of the medical condition of the animal(s). This means that the veterinarian has recently seen and is personally acquainted with the keeping and care of the animal(s) by virtue of an examination of the animal(s), or by medically appropriate and timely visits to the premises where the animal(s) are kept.

3. The veterinarian is readily available, or has arranged for emergency coverage, for follow-up evaluation in the event of adverse reactions or the failure of the treatment regimen.

B. When a VCPR exists, veterinarians must maintain medical records (See section VII).

C. Dispensing or prescribing a prescription product requires a VCPR

1. Veterinarians should honor a client's request for a prescription in lieu of dispensing.

2. Without a valid VCPR, veterinarians' merchandising or use of veterinary prescription drugs or their extra-label use of any pharmaceuti-

cal is unethical and is illegal under federal law.

D. Veterinarians may terminate a VCPR under certain conditions, and they have an ethical obligation to use courtesy and tact in doing so.

1. If there is no ongoing medical condition, veterinarians may terminate a VCPR by notifying the client that they no longer wish to serve that patient and client.

2. If there is an ongoing medical or surgical condition, the patient should be referred to another veterinarian for diagnosis, care, and treatment. The former attending veterinarian should continue to provide care, as needed, during the transition.

E. Clients may terminate the VCPR at any time.

IV. ATTENDING, CONSULTING AND REFERRING

A. An *attending veterinarian* is a veterinarian (or a group of veterinarians) who assumes responsibility for primary care of a patient. A VCPR is established.

1. Attending veterinarians are entitled to charge a fee for their professional services.

2. When appropriate, attending veterinarians are encouraged to seek assistance in the form of consultations and referrals. A decision to consult or refer is made jointly by the attending veterinarian and the client.

3. When a consultation occurs, the attending veterinarian continues to be primarily responsible for the case.

B. A *consulting veterinarian* is a veterinarian (or group of veterinarians) who agrees to advise an attending veterinarian on the care and management of a case. The VCPR remains the responsibility of the attending veterinarian.

1. Consulting veterinarians may or may not charge fees for service.

2. Consulting veterinarians should communicate their findings and opinions directly to the attending veterinarians.

3. Consulting veterinarians should revisit the patients or communicate with the clients in collaboration with the attending veterinarians.

4. Consultations usually involve the exchange of information or interpretation of test results. However, it may be appropriate or necessary for consultants to examine patients. When advanced or invasive techniques are required to gather information or substantiate diagnoses, attending veterinarians may refer the patients. A new VCPR is established with the veterinarian to whom a case is referred.

C. The *referral veterinarian or receiving veterinarian* is a veterinarian (or group of veterinarians) who agrees to provide requested veterinary services. A new VCPR is established. The referring and referral veterinarians must communicate.

1. Attending veterinarians should honor clients' requests for referral.

2. Referral veterinarians may choose to accept or decline clients and patients from attending veterinarians.

3. Patients are usually referred because of specific medical problems or services. Referral veterinarians should provide services or treatments relative to the referred conditions, and they should communicate with the referring veterinarians and clients if

other services or treatments are required.

D. **When a client seeks professional services or opinions from a different veterinarian without a referral, a new VCPR is established with the new attending veterinarian. When contacted, the veterinarian who was formerly involved in the diagnosis, care, and treatment of the patient should communicate with the new attending veterinarian as if the patient and client had been referred.**

1. With the client's consent, the new attending veterinarian should contact the former veterinarian to learn the original diagnosis, care, and treatment and clarify any issues before proceeding with a new treatment plan.

2. If there is evidence that the actions of the former attending veterinarian have clearly and significantly endangered the health or safety of the patient, the new attending veterinarian has a responsibility to report the matter to the appropriate authorities of the local and state association or professional regulatory agency.

V. INFLUENCES ON JUDGEMENT

A. **The choice of treatments or animal care should not be influenced by considerations other than the needs of the patient, the welfare of the client, and the safety of the public.**

B. **Veterinarians should not allow their medical judgement to be influenced by agreements by which they stand to profit through referring clients to other providers of services or products.**

C. **The medical judgements of veterinarians should not be influenced by contracts or agreements made by their associations or societies.**

VI. THERAPIES

A. **Attending veterinarians are responsible for choosing the treatment regimens for**

their patients. It is the attending veterinarian's responsibility to inform the client of the expected results and costs, and the related risks of each treatment regimen.

B. **It is unethical for veterinarians to prescribe or dispense prescription products in the absence of a VCPR.**

C. **It is unethical for veterinarians to promote, sell, prescribe, dispense, or use secret remedies or any other product for which they do not know the ingredient formula.**

D. **It is unethical for veterinarians to use or permit the use of their names, signatures, or professional status in connection with the resale of ethical products in a manner which violates those directions or conditions specified by the manufacturer to ensure the safe and efficacious use of the product.**

VII. MEDICAL RECORDS

A. **Veterinary medical records are an integral part of veterinary care.** The records must comply with the standards established by state and federal law.

B. **Medical Records are the property of the practice and the practice owner.** The original records must be retained by the practice for the period required by statute.

C. **Ethically, the information within veterinary medical records is considered privileged and confidential. It must not be released except by court order or consent of the owner of the patient.**

D. **Veterinarians are obligated to provide copies or summaries of medical records when requested by the client.** Veterinarians should secure a written release to document that request.

E. **Without the express permission of the practice owner, it is unethical for a veterinarian to remove, copy, or use the** medical records or any part of any record.

VIII. FEES AND REMUNERATION

A. Veterinarians are entitled to charge fees for their professional services.

B. In connection with consultations or referrals, it is unethical for veterinarians to enter into financial arrangements, such as fee splitting, which involve payment of a portion of a fee to a recommending veterinarian who has not rendered the professional services for which the fee was paid by the client.

C. Regardless of the fees that are charged or received, the quality of service must be maintained at the usual professional standard.

D. It is unethical for a group or association of veterinarians to take any action which coerces, pressures, or achieves agreement among veterinarians to conform to a fee schedule or fixed fees.

X. ADVERTISING

A. Without written permission from the AVMA Executive Board, no member or employee of the American Veterinary Medical Association (AVMA) shall use the AVMA name or logo in connection with the promotion or advertising of any commercial product or service.

B. Advertising by veterinarians is ethical when there are no false, deceptive, or misleading statements or claims. A false, deceptive, or misleading statement or claim is one which communicates false information or is intended, through a material omission, to leave a false impression.

C. Testimonials or endorsements are advertising, and they should comply with the guidelines for advertising. In addition, testimonials and endorsements of professional products or services by veteri-

narians are considered unethical unless they comply with the following:

1. The endorser must be a bonafide user of the product or service.

2. There must be adequate substantiation that the results obtained by the endorser are representative of what veterinarians may expect in actual conditions of use.

3. Any financial, business, or other relationship between the endorser and the seller of a product or service must be fully disclosed.

4. When reprints of scientific articles are used with advertising, the reprints must remain unchanged, and be presented in their entirety.

D. The principles that apply to advertising, testimonials, and endorsements also apply to veterinarians' communications with their clients.

E. Veterinarians may permit the use of their names by commercial enterprises (e.g. pet shops, kennels, farms, feedlots) so that the enterprises can advertise 'under veterinary supervision', only if they provide such supervision.

X. EUTHANASIA

Humane euthanasia of animals is an ethical veterinary procedure.

I. GLOSSARY

1. PHARMACEUTICAL PRODUCTS

Several of the following terms are used to describe veterinary pharmaceutical products. Some have legal status, others do not. Although not all of the terms are used in the Principles, we have listed them here for clarification of meaning and to avoid confusion.

A. *Ethical Product*: A product for which the manufacturer has voluntarily limited the sale to veterinarians as a marketing decision. Such products are often given a different product name and are packaged differently than products that are sold directly to consumers. "Ethical products" are sold only to veterinarians as a condition of sale that is specified in a sales agreement or on the product label.

B. *Legend Drug:* A synonymous term for a veterinary prescription drug. The name refers to the statement (legend) that is required on the label (see *veterinary prescription drug* below).

C. *Over the Counter (OTC) Drug:* Any drug that can be labeled with adequate direction to enable it to be used safely and properly by a consumer who is not a medical professional.

D. *Prescription Drug:* A drug that cannot be labeled with adequate direction to enable its safe and proper use by non-professionals.

E. *Veterinary Prescription Drug:* A drug that is restricted by federal law to use by or on the order of a licensed veterinarian, according to section 503(f) of the federal Food, Drug, and Cosmetic Act. The law requires that such drugs be labeled with the statement: " Caution, federal law restricts this drug to use by or on the order of a licensed veterinarian."

2. DISPENSING, PRESCRIBING, MARKETING AND MERCHANDISING

A. *Dispensing* is the direct distribution of products by veterinarians to clients for use on their animals.

B. *Prescribing* is the transmitting of an order authorizing a licensed pharmacist or equivalent to prepare and dispense specified pharmaceuticals to be used in or on animals in the dosage and in the manner directed by a veterinarian.

C. *Marketing* is promoting and encouraging animal owners to improve animal health and welfare by using veterinary care, services, and products.

D. *Merchandising* is the buying and selling of products or services.

3. ADVERTISING AND TESTIMONIALS

A. *Advertising* is defined as communication that is designed to inform the public about the availability, nature, or price of products or services or to influence clients to use certain products or services.

B. *Testimonials* or endorsements are statements that are intended to influence attitudes regarding the purchase or use of products or services.

4. FEE SPLITTING

The dividing of a professional fee for veterinary services with the recommending veterinarian (See Section VIII B).

07/99

MANDATORY CONTINUING EDUCATION FOR VETERINARIANS

AVMA Survey as of July, 1996

(Since requirements change intermittently, up-to-date information on individual states' CE requirements is available only from the State Board of Veterinary Examiners in each state or through the American Association of Veterinary State Boards, ph. 816-931-1504.)

State/Province Territory	Year Implemented	CE hours/ Renewal Period (yrs)	Comments
Alabama	1975	20/1	One hour credit for each hour of attendance at an in-depth seminar that is medical/scientific in nature; One hour credit for local or state monthly business meetings up to a maximum of five hours per year; up to a maximum of five hours from verifiable audio, video and computer revision per year.
Alaska	1983	15/1	No more than 1/3 total hours may be in nonscientific topics; would be able to accept computer on-line CE.
Alberta		20/2	Annual license renewal, but CE credits submitted every two years.
Arizona	1979	20/2	A maximum of two hours may be in practice management and no more than 5 hours may be noncontact education, of which 2 hours may be tapes.
Arkansas	1975	20/1	No more than 5 hours accepted in the areas of practice management, business seminars, veterinary computer education and veterinary videos; 10 hours must be in the area of veterinary medicine and surgery. Veterinarians may earn up to 4 hours of credit for visitation with a colleague (not associated with his/her practice) at the facility of the colleague. One hour of credit will be given for each local district meeting (not to exceed 4 hours without approval of board prior to license renewal).

State/Province Territory	Year Implemented	CE hours/ Renewal Period (yrs)	Comments
British Columbia		20/2	Accepts all veterinary medical associations and university CE; excludes business and practice management courses and self-study programs.
California	1998	36/2	The law mandating CE was passed in late summer of 1998. Regulations stipulating what type of CE is acceptable have not been drafted as of press time for this book.
Colorado	1975	32/2	No practice management accepted. No provision in statute to allow computer on-line CE; require direct contact with and/or immediate access to the presenter to clarify information presented or address further questions. CE planners should seek prior approval from the board.
Delaware	1990	24/2	CE must be medical/scientific in nature; up to 12 hours/2 years can be from *The Compendium*, etc. Should first check with the board to be sure it meets with their approval.
District of Columbia	1988	36/2	
Florida	1969	30/2	Two hours must be in the area of dispensing scheduled drugs. Would be able to accept computer on-line CE; CE planners must seek prior approval from the board.
Georgia	1991	30/2	Only accept seminars considered scientific in nature. VCE Programs must seek prior approval from the board. Will accept up to 3 hours of computer on-line CE in the biennial renewed period.
Idaho	1989	30/3	Annual license renewal, but CE credits submitted every 3 years. Maximum of 9 hours in the area of practice management allowed. No provision in statute to allow computer on-line CE. Previously accepted video/audio tape materials, but the board voted to change this, as they feel interaction with peers is as important as the actual material presented.
Illinois	1977	20/2	Can earn hours any time between Jan. 1st and Dec. 31st of the following year. CE must be relevant to practice of veterinary medicine/surgery, and requirement is strictly enforced. Certain practice management courses are accepted. Would accept computer CE with verification of attendance.
Iowa	1978	60/3	CE must be medial/scientific in nature. Up to 1/3 VCE requirement may be fulfilled via independent study.
Kansas	1969	20/1	Wellness, stress reduction, etc. presentations that can be shown to be of benefit to the art of veterinary medicine through the doctor/client relationship are accepted up to a maximum of 4 hours. Present statute allows up to a total of 4 hours via computer on-line CE.
Kentucky	1977	15/1	Not more than 5 hours allowed in the area of practice management, etc.

State/Province Territory	Year Implemented	CE hours/ Renewal Period (yrs)	Comments
Louisiana	1990	16/1	Not more than 4 hours of self-help allowed (videos, *Compendium*, computer, etc.) nor more than 4 hours in the area of practice management. Check with board to ensure that specific self-instructional material will be accepted. Must have 12 CE hours in areas related directly to the practice of veterinary medicine.
Maine	1991	12/1	Accepts CE in the areas of medicine, surgery, diagnostics, and other subjects pertinent to the practice of veterinary medicine; up to 3 hours can be in the areas of practice management.
Maryland	1961	12/1	No practice management.
Minnesota	1995	40/2	Thirty hours must be from interactive sources, such as lectures, including on-line computer CE or interactive TV. Will accept up to 10 hours of self, non-interactive study. A maximum of 10 hours/biennial cycle of practice management is accepted.
Mississippi	1976	10/1	Clock hours to be reported from August 1st to August 1st.
Montana	1975	20/2	Up to 5 hours can be in the area of practice management; no independent study courses are approved.
Nebraska	1971	32/2	CE must be scientific in nature and related to the practice of veterinary medicine. Programs must be sponsored by state, national or local association or a college. No practice management or home study.
Nevada	1985	20/2	CE must be scientific in nature, will accept computer on-line CE.
New Hampshire	1979	12/1	No practice management. The board will have to review information from computer on-line CE before deciding if it will be accepted. The board feels interaction with peers is as important as the meeting itself; however, board has approved *The Compendium* with certificate for up to 4 hours.
New Mexico	1979	15/1	No more than 2 hours from local meetings with speakers. No practice management. Allow 15 hours to be carried over to next year. Will accept computer on-line CE.
North Carolina	1974	20/1	Up to 3 hours allowed for video or computer based training.
North Dakota	1985	12/1	Practice management seminars are accepted. Will accept computer on-line CE if verification of participation is provided.
Nova Scotia	1996	10/2	Proof of hours to be indicated with annual renewal form.
Ohio	1976	30/2	No less than 20 hours shall be specific to veterinary medicine and/or surgery. Up to a maximum of 10 hours of practice management. Up to 10 hours of biennium hours of computer on-line CE accepted.
Oklahoma	1982	20/1	Up to a maximum of 5 hours can be granted for reading scientific articles, and/or participating in autotutorial programs, and/or writing a peer-review article or giving a presentation.

State/Province Territory	Year Implemented	CE hours/ Renewal Period (yrs)	Comments
Oregon	1981	10/1	May consist of 2 hours audiovisual, 2 hours subscription, 2 hours practice management, and 4 hours classroom or any combination thereof; however, not more than 2 hours practice management. In regard to computer on-line CE, the board will probably approve the same number of credits as given to journals: 1 credit per journal for a maximum of 2 credits. A full course may be approved if some method of testing is available, as in video courses.
Pennsylvania	1963	8/2	No practice management; CE should have prior approval from the board. Legislation proposed in 1999 to allow board to establish a higher number of hours. Proposal includes language stipulating that courses in veterinary law, ethics, practice management, animal abuse and/or welfare or active service on a veterinary association peer review committee shall be acceptable forms of continuing education but shall not comprise greater than one fourth of the profession's mandated CE.
Prince Edward Island		20/2	Must be at conferences/meetings sponsored by veterinary associations or with veterinarians as speakers.
Puerto Rico	1983	30/3	Ten of the 30 hours must be completed during the last year.
Quebec		20/2	Obligation is tied to professional inspection program, not license renewal. Council can suspend license and have member follow a course or a clinical supervision in an accredited clinic. Up to 8 hours can be in the area of self-study.
Saskatchewan	1968	10/1	CE hours not bankable; however, a deficiency in 1 year must be corrected in the next year or member will be subject to discipline. Applies to all licensure that allows practice activity.
South Carolina	1966	15/1	No more than 4 hours in practice management or building. Will not accept computer on-line CE. CE planners should seek Board approval.
South Dakota	1960	16/2	CE must be scientific in nature. No provision in statute to accept computer on-line CE at this time. CE planners should seek Board approval.
Tennessee	1969	20/1	CE requirement is per calendar year, not license renewal period. Up to a maximum of 5 hours of practice management. There is currently a 5-hour limit on "correspondence"/ computer on-line CE courses. CE planners should seek prior approval from the Board.
Texas	1994	15/1	Effective 1995: Veterinarians renewing licenses in 1995 will be required to sign affidavit that they have acquired 15 hours of CE in previous 12 months. Must be obtained during preceding calendar year. No more than 5 hours of practice management. There is presently a 5-hour limitation on "correspondence" courses, but there is the possibility that additional credit will be given to computer on-line CE if a sound, accountable system was in place to verify participation.

State/Province Territory	Year Implemented	CE hours/ Renewal Period (yrs)	Comments
Utah	1993	24/2	No more than 6 hours accepted in the areas of practice management. No more than 5 hours for being primary author of published peer review article and no more than 2 hours for being a secondary author. VCE programs must receive prior approval from the VMA. Will accept computer on-line CE for board-approved courses.
Virginia	1997	15/1	Beginning with 1997 license renewals
Washington	1980	30/3	Annual license renewal, but CE credits submitted every 3 years. Licensee responsible for maintaining records, certificates or other evidence of compliance. Will accept computer CE.
West Virginia	1992	16/2	Six hours must be classroom, 2 hours may be audiovisual.
Wyoming	1995	6/1	Must be medical/surgical in nature. No practice management.

STATE LAWS AND PRECEDENTS COVERING RESTRICTIVE COVENANTS

Analyzing the legal precedents regarding restrictive covenants in all 50 states and the District of Columbia is a monumental task, one that was beyond the capabilities of the authors. Thus, when researching this subject for this book, the most complete synopsis of the law concerning health care professionals was found in the Restrictive Covenant Survey assembled by The Health Care Group® of Plymouth Meeting, PA. This publication, updated every few years, contains a reasonably complete synopsis of state statutes addressing covenants not to compete. Where no statutory law exists, it provides opinions about the case law in those states and its application to the health care professions.[1]

As is always the case with the law, statutes and case law precedents change from time to time with minimal notice to those whose lives or contracts are governed by such law. The authors of this book have updated information regarding some of the states in The Health Care Group's survey but have not verified the accuracy of the materials for all states. It is, nonetheless, being reproduced here with the permission of the publisher with the caveat that anyone who wishes to obtain contemporary information should (1) contact The Health Care Group® and purchase its latest edition of the survey, or (2) engage the services of a local attorney to research the law in the state in which a noncompete clause is being challenged to see if precedents exist that change any of the summaries provided herein.

ALABAMA

The Alabama statute provides that "every contract by which anyone is restrained from exercising a lawful profession, trade or business of any kind ... [is to] that extent void."

(1) "Professionals are subject to general statutory prohibitions against covenants not to compete; (2) exceptions to general rule, including the exception for sale of goodwill of business, are not available to professionals."(§ 8-1-1 Code 1975) (Includes 8 case citations, 1 veterinary case.)

ALASKA

Alaska does not statutorily prohibit restrictive covenants. (Includes no case citations.)

ARIZONA

Arizona does not statutorily prohibit restrictive covenants. The courts will enforce reasonable restrictions if they are ancillary to employment agreements and not injurious to the public. (Includes 3 case citations - 1 veterinary case.)

ARKANSAS

Arkansas does not statutorily prohibit restrictive covenants. The courts will enforce reasonable restrictions. (Includes 4 case citations.)

CALIFORNIA

The California statute provides that, except as specified below, "every contract by which anyone is restrained from engaging in a lawful profession, trade, or business of any kind is to that extent void." Exceptions: (1) Any person who sells the goodwill of a business or any shareholder of a corporation selling or otherwise disposing of all his shares in said corporation, or any shareholder which sells all or substantially all of its operating assets together with the goodwill of the Corporation...may agree with the buyer to refrain from carrying on a similar business within a specified county or counties, city or cities, or a part thereof, in which the business ... has been carried on, so long as the buyer...carries on a like business therein; (2) "Any partner may, upon or in anticipation of a dissolution of the partnership, agree that he will not carry on a similar business within a specified county or counties, city or cities, or a part thereof, where the partnership business has been transacted, so long as any member of the partnership...carries on like business therein." (3) "Any member may, upon or in anticipation of a dissolution of...or a sale of his...interest in a (LLC), agree that (he) will not carry on a similar business within a specified county or counties, city or cities, or a part thereof, where the (LLC) business has been transacted, so long as (the LLC) carries on a like business therein." (West's Ann Bus & Prof Code §§ 16600, 16601, 16602, 16602.5) (Includes 8 citations.)

COLORADO

Colorado's statute provides that "Any covenant not to compete as a provision of an employment, partnership or corporate agreement between physicians which restricts the right of a physician to practice medicine...upon termination of the agreement shall be void; except that all other provisions which require payment of damages in an amount that is reasonably related to the injury suffered by reason of termination of the agreement shall be enforceable. Provisions which require the payment of damages upon termination of the agreement shall be enforceable. Provisions which require the payment of damages upon termination of the agreement may include, but not be limited to, damages related to competition." To date, including a trial in which the author was an expert witness, this has meant that restrictive covenants in veterinary employment contracts will be enforced if they are reasonable, producing a different legal result than occurs with physicians' contracts. (CRS 1989 § 8-2-113(3)) (Includes 7 case citations.)

CONNECTICUT

Connecticut does not statutorily prohibit restrictive covenants. The courts will enforce restrictive covenants if they are ancillary employment contracts and limited as to time and place. Restrictions must provide only fair protection of employers' interests and must not interfere with the interests of the public. (Included 2 case citations.)

DELAWARE

Delaware statute provides that, for agreements entered into after 7/13/81, "Any covenant not to compete as a provision of an employment, partnership or corporate agreement between or among physicians which restricts the right of a physician to practice

STATE LAWS AND PRECEDENTS COVERING RESTRICTIVE COVENANTS /397

medicine in a particular locale and/or for a definite period of time upon the <u>termination</u> of the principal agreement of which the said provision is a part, shall be void; except that all other provisions of such an agreement shall be enforceable at law including provisions which require the payment of damages in an amount that is reasonably related to the injury suffered by reason of termination of the principal agreement. Provisions which require the payment of damages upon termination of the principal agreement may include, but not be limited to, damages related to competition." (6 Del C § 2707, 1990) Like Colorado, this statute applies only to physicians, not veterinarians. (Includes 1 case citation.)

DISTRICT OF COLUMBIA

The District of Columbia does not statutorily prohibit restrictive covenants. Federal antitrust laws permit reasonable restrictive covenants. (Includes 1 case citation.)

FLORIDA

Prior to June 28, 1990, employees bound by noncompetition agreements in Florida rarely prevailed in their attempts to invalidate their agreements. This was because court precedents had nearly always allowed employers to successfully enjoin employees from direct, or even indirect competition. Effective June 28, 1990, the new statutory provision governing noncompete clauses was amended to preclude courts from enforcing restrictive covenants against employees, independent contractors or agents when the agreements are either (a) contrary to public health, safety or welfare, (b) unreasonable, or (c) not supported by a showing of irreparable injury. Presumptions of irreparable harm arise only when employers can establish that employee's used specific trade secrets or customer lists or direct solicitation of existing customers. In all other violations of noncompete agreements,

employers must prove irreparable harm before courts will provide injunctive relief.

This 1990 statutory change places Florida within the mainstream of the American system of justice by precluding employers from enforcing noncompetition agreements with impunity and for the sake of prohibiting fair competition. Nonetheless, the new law still provides reasonable protection for them to protect their legitimate business interests.

The Florida statute §542.33 provides that

- (1) Notwithstanding other provisions of this chapter to the contrary, each contract by which any person is restrained from exercising a lawful profession, trade or business of any kind, as provided by subsections (2) and (3) hereof, is to that extent *valid*, and all other contracts in restraint of trade are *void*. (As seen by the following two sections, only certain types of restrictive covenants are enforceable and, even then, only under specified circumstances.)

- (2)(a) "One who sells the goodwill of a business or any shareholder of any corporation selling or otherwise disposing of all of his shares in said corporation, may agree with the buyer, and one who is employed as an agent or employee may agree with his employer to refrain from carrying on or engaging in a similar business and from soliciting old customers of such employer within a reasonably limited time and area, and so long as such employer continues to carry on a like business therein. Said agreements may, in the discretion of the court, be enforced by injunction. However, the court shall not enter an injunction contrary to the public health, safety, or welfare, or in any case where the injunction enforces an unreasonable covenant not to compete, or where there is no showing of irreparable injury. However, use of specific trade secrets, customer lists, or direct solicitation of existing customers shall be presumed to be an irreparable injury and may be specifically enjoined. In the event the seller of the goodwill of a business, or a shareholder selling or otherwise disposing of all his shares in a corporation, breaches an agreement to refrain from carrying on or engaging in a similar business, irreparable injury shall be presumed. (West's FSA § 542.33 (2)-(3) 1993)

Two excellent law review articles that explain these most recent changes are helpful references for readers concerned with Florida law.[2,3] (Includes 3 citations since the above amendment became law, amid a total of 15.)

GEORGIA

The Georgia statute provides that "contracts that restrain in a reasonable manner any party thereto from exercising any trade, business, or employment are contracts in partial restraint of trade and shall not be considered against the policy of the law, and such partial restraints, so long as otherwise lawful, shall be enforceable for all purposes."[5] The statute provides specific types of contracts that would be considered to be reasonable: (1) contracts for the sale of a business; (2) employment contracts, in which the reasonable duration would be 2 years in the case of an agreement not to compete after termination and 3 years in the case of an agreement not to solicit customers or attempt to recruit other employees of the business after termination; (3) "any restriction that operates during the term of an employment agreement,...partnership agreement...shareholders' agreement, or other ongoing business agreement shall not be considered unreasonable because it lacks any specific limitation upon scope of activity, duration, or territory"... (GA Statutes 13-8-2.1) (Includes 18 case citations.)

HAWAII

Hawaii does not statutorily prohibit restrictive covenants. The courts will enforce

postemployment covenants if they are reasonable in scope, do not impose undue hardship on the employee, and do not substantially lessen competition. (No case citations.)

IDAHO

Idaho does not statutorily prohibit restrictive covenants, but the courts will only enforce them if they are reasonable and consistent with the interests of the public. (Includes 3 case citations.)

ILLINOIS

Illinois does not statutorily prohibit restrictive covenants, but enforcement depends on the circumstances of the employee's departure. If the employee is dismissed without good cause and in bad faith, the restrictive covenants will not be enforced. Also, courts will enforce covenants if there was consideration, the restraint is limited as to time and place and is no greater than required to protect the legitimate interests of the employer, and there is no undue harm to the employee or public injury. (Includes 22 case citations - 2 veterinary case.)

INDIANA

Indiana does not statutorily prohibit restrictive covenants. The courts will enforce them if they are reasonably necessary to protect the interests of employers, if they are not unreasonably restrictive of the employee, and they cause no injury to the public. (Includes 8 case citations.)

IOWA

Iowa does not statutorily prohibit restrictive covenants. The courts will enforce them in employment agreements if they are necessary for the protection of the legitimate interests of the employer, they are not unreasonably restrictive of the employee, and they are not prejudicial to public interests. (Includes 6 case citations.)

KANSAS

Kansas does not statutorily prohibit restrictive covenants. The courts will enforce them when they are ancillary to employment agreements freely entered into with full knowledge of the restriction, if the restraint is reasonable, and if it is not inimical to the public welfare. (Includes 3 case citations.)

KENTUCKY

Kentucky's statute provides that

(1) Agreements between health care providers that allow or encourage the enforcement of contractual provisions by which one health care provider agrees not to compete against another health care provider or group of health care providers for a period of time upon severance of any relationship between the health care providers are unethical.....(T)hese agreements serve to increase health care costs by creating a barrier which forces the patient to seek alternate care from another health care provider....(T)hese agreements are contrary to the public policy of this Commonwealth.

(2) Agreements between health care providers that allow or encourage the enforcement of contractual provisions by which one health care provider agrees not to compete against another health care provider or group of health care providers for a period of time upon severance of any relationship between the health care providers shall be void as against public policy and not enforceable if the period of time is for one year or longer. (KRS § 118 Chapter 311.000 Part 17) (No mention of whether veterinarians are included in the definition of "health care providers." Includes 5 case citations.)

LOUISIANA

The Louisiana's statute provides that "every contract or agreement, or provision thereof, by which anyone is restrained from exercising a lawful profession, trade, or business...shall be null and void." However, a shareholder of a corporation "who sells the goodwill of a business may agree with the buyer that the seller will refrain from carrying on or engaging in a similar business...or from soliciting customers of the business...within a specified parish or parishes...so long as the buyer...carries on a like business therein...not to exceed a period of 2 years from the date of sale." Furthermore, "any person, including a corporation and the individual shareholders of such corporation, who is employed...may agree with his employer to refrain from carrying on or engaging in a business similar to that of the employer and/or from soliciting customers of the employer within a specified parish or parishes...so long as the employer carries on a like business therein...not to exceed a period of 2 years from termination of employment." Also applies to independent contractors and partners upon dissolution of the partnership. (LSA R.S. 23 : 921). Includes no citations.)

MAINE

Maine does not statutorily prohibit restrictive covenants, but courts find them contrary to public policy and will enforce them only if reasonable and no broader than necessary to protect business interest. (Includes 1 case citation.)

MARYLAND

Maryland does not statutorily prohibit restrictive covenants. Courts will enforce them in employment contracts when they are applied to employees who provide unique services and to prevent misuse of trade secrets or client lists. Restrictions are found to be justified when at least part of the compensated services performed by an employee creates client and customer "goodwill" and clients are likely to follow the employee. (Includes 2 case citations.)

Massachusetts

The Massachusetts statute provides that "Any contract or agreement which creates or establishes the terms of a partnership, employment or any other form of professional relationship with a physician...which includes any restriction of the right of such physician to practice medicine in any geographic area for any period of time after the termination of such partnership, employment or professional relationship shall be void and unenforceable with respect to said restriction; provide, however, that nothing herein shall render void or unenforceable the remaining provisions of any such....agreement." (MGLA c. 112 § 12X) (Includes 2 case citations.)

Michigan

Michigan's statute provides that "an employer may obtain from an employee an agreement or covenant which protects an employer's reasonable competitive business interests and expressly prohibits an employee from engaging in employment or line of business after termination of employment if the agreement or covenant is reasonable as to its duration, geographical area, and the type of employment or line of business. To the extent any such agreement or covenant is found to be unreasonable in any respect, a court may limit the agreement to render it reasonable in light of the circumstances in which it was made and specifically enforce the agreement as limited." Applies to agreements entered into after March 29, 1985. (MCLA 445.774a) (Includes 6 case citations - 1 veterinary case.)

Minnesota

Minnesota does not statutorily prohibit restrictive covenants. Courts will enforce reasonable restrictions. (Includes 9 case citations.)

Mississippi

Mississippi does not statutorily prohibit restrictive covenants. (Includes 3 case citation.)

Missouri

Missouri does not statutorily prohibit restrictive covenants. (Includes 8 cases - 1 veterinary case.)

Montana

Montana's statute provides that "Any contract by which anyone is restrained from exercising a lawful profession, trade, or business of any kind..is to that extent void." Except: (1) One who sells the goodwill of a business may agree with the buyer to refrain from carrying on a similar business within the areas provided (below) so long as the buyer...carries on a like business therein." Permissible areas are city and/or county where principal office is located and/or a city in any county adjacent to the county where the principal office is located and/or any such adjacent county. (2) "Partners may, upon dissolution of the partnership, agree that one or more of them may not carry on a similar business (within area described above)."(MCA §§ 28-2-703/704/705) (Includes 2 case citations.)

Nebraska

Nebraska does not statutorily prohibit restrictive covenants. Courts will enforce a restrictive covenant if the restriction is reasonable, no greater than is necessary to protect the legitimate interests of the employer, not unduly harsh to the employee, and not injurious to the public. (Includes 3 case citations.)

Nevada

Nevada does not statutorily prohibit restrictive covenants. (Includes 3 case citations.)

New Hampshire

New Hampshire does not statutorily prohibit restrictive covenants. Courts will enforce reasonable restrictions if they are no greater than necessary to protect the legitimate interests of the employer, and create no undue hardship for the employee and no public injury. A 1997 case, *Concord Orthopedics Professional Association v. Forbes* added an interesting quirk to its interpretation of a two-year, 25-mile noncompete covenant for an orthopedic surgeon. While the court found the restriction reasonable as to time and distance, it drew a basic distinction between existing patients and new patients. In summary, the physician was allowed to treat new patients (those who weren't patients of his prior employer) within the protected radius and time frame. Thus, the departing orthopod could establish a practice within the 25-mile radius as long as he did not see any patients that had been patients of his prior employer. This is more lenient than the position taken by many other state courts but fits within New Hampshire's public policy encouraging free trade and discouraging covenants not to compete. (Includes 4 case citations - 1 veterinary case.)

New Jersey

New Jersey does not statutorily prohibit restrictive covenants, and courts enforce them as long as they are reasonable. (Includes 5 case citations.)

New Mexico

New Mexico does not statutorily prohibit restrictive covenants. (Includes 3 case citations.)

New York

New York does not statutorily prohibit restrictive covenants. (Includes 19 case citations.)

North Carolina

North Carolina does not statutorily prohibit restrictive covenants. Courts will enforce them if they are part of the written employment contract; restrictions are reasonable as to time, territory, and consideration thereof; and they create no injury to the public. (Includes 7 case citation - w veterinary case.)

North Dakota

The North Dakota statute provides that "Every contract by which anyone is restrained from exercising a lawful profession, trade or business of any kind is to that extent void, except: (1) One who sells the goodwill of a business may agree with the buyer to refrain from carrying on a similar business within a specified county, city, or part of either so long as the buyer...carries on a like business therein; (2) Partners, upon or in anticipation of a dissolution of the partnership, may agree that all or any number of them will not carry on a similar business within the same city where the partnership business has been transacted, or within a specified part thereof." (Includes 3 case citations.)

Ohio

Ohio does not statutorily prohibit restrictive covenants. Courts will enforce them if restraint is required to protect the employer, there is no undue hardship to employee, and they are not injurious to public. (Included 7 case citations - 1 veterinary case.)

Oklahoma

Oklahoma prohibits enforcement of all restrictive covenants except in the case of the sale of goodwill, wherein the buyer carries on the business, and in anticipation of or upon dissolution of a partnership, to restrict practice within the city or county (or part thereof) (only city or town or part thereof for partnership) where the business was transacted. (15 OS 1991 §§ 217/218/219) (Includes 5 case citations - 1 veterinary case.)

OREGON

Oregon's statute provides that "A noncompetition agreement entered into between an employer and employee is void and shall not be enforced by any court...unless the agreement is entered into upon the initial employment of the employee...or subsequent bona fide advancement of the employee with the employer." "A noncompetition agreement means an agreement, written or oral, express or implied ...under which the employee agrees that the employee either alone or as an employee of another person, shall not compete with the employer in providing products, processes or services, that are similar to the employer's...for a period of time or within a specified geographic area after termination of employment." This prohibition does not apply to bonus restriction agreements which are lawful. "Bonus restriction agreement means an agreement, written or oral, express or implied, under which: (1) Competition by the employee with the employer is limited or restrained after termination of employment, but the restraint is limited to a period of time, a geographic area and specified activities, all of which are reasonable (under the circumstances); (2) the services performed by the employee... include substantial involvement in the management of the business, personal contact with customers, knowledge of customer requirements...or knowledge of trade secrets or other proprietary information; and (3) penalty imposed on employee for competition is limited to forfeiture of profit sharing or other bonus compensation that has not yet been paid to the employee..." Exception for initial employment agreement applies only to agreements entered into after July 22, 1977. All other exceptions apply to agreements entered into after October 15, 1983. (ORS 653.295) (Includes 4 cases - 1 veterinary case.)

PENNSYLVANIA

Pennsylvania does not statutorily prohibit restrictive covenants. The courts will enforce reasonable covenants if they are part of the initial employment agreement or sale of business including goodwill. Restrictions must be reasonable as to time and territory. Needs of the community must take precedence over the rights of parties to covenant. A trial court decision in June of 1999 in which the author was an expert witness shortened a 3-year covenant to a year and a half but left a 10-mile radius intact in spite of clear and uncontroverted evidence that 10 miles was excessive. (Includes 11 case citations.)

RHODE ISLAND

Rhode Island does not statutorily prohibit restrictive covenants; however, courts do not favor them in employment agreements and carefully scrutinize them. (Includes 1 case citation.)

SOUTH CAROLINA

South Carolina does not statutorily prohibit restrictive covenants. Courts will enforce reasonable restrictions in employment agreements if they are necessary to protect the legitimate interests of the employer, they are not unduly burdensome to the employee, and there is no public injury. Courts will enforce nonsolicitation agreements and bonus restriction agreements. (Includes 1 case citation - 1 veterinary case.)

SOUTH DAKOTA

The South Dakota statute provides that "Every contract restraining exercise of a lawful profession, trade or business is void to that extent, except as provided: (1) one who sells the goodwill of a business may agree with the buyer to refrain from carrying on a similar business within a specified county, city or part thereof, so long as the buyer...carries on a like business therein. (2)

Partners may, upon or in anticipation of a dissolution of the partnership, agree that none of them will carry on a similar business within the same city or town where the partnership business has been transacted or within a specified part thereof. (3) An employee may agree at the time of his employment or at any time during his employment (not to compete) for any period not exceeding two years from the date of termination of the agreement and not to solicit existing customers...within a specified county, first or second class municipality or other specified area for any period not exceeding two years from the date of termination of the agreement, if the employer continues to carry on a like business therein." (SDCL 1990 §§ 53-9-8/-9/-10/-11) (Includes 1 case citation - 1 veterinary case.)

TENNESSEE

Tennessee does not statutorily prohibit restrictive covenants. The courts will enforce them if they are reasonable and given for consideration. (Includes 5 case citations.)

TEXAS

The Texas statute provides that "a covenant not to compete is enforceable if it is ancillary...to an otherwise enforceable agreement at the time the agreement is made to the extent that it contains reasonable limitations as to time, geographical area and scope of activity to be restrained (and) do(es) not impose a greater restraint than is necessary to protect the goodwill...." (Tx BUS & COM § 15.50) (1991)

"Procedures and Remedies in Actions to Enforce Covenants not to Compete." (Tx BUS & COM § 15.51) (Includes 11 case citations - 1 veterinary case.)

UTAH

Utah does not statutorily prohibit restrictive covenants. (Includes 1 case citation.)

VERMONT

Vermont does not statutorily prohibit restrictive covenants. (No case citations.)

VIRGINIA

Virginia does not statutorily prohibit restrictive covenants. The Code of Virginia does contain legal ethics opinions, though. These provide that (1) "it is not proper for a law firm, which is a professional corporation, to implement an unqualified deferred compensation plan which contains an agreement restricting employee attorneys from practicing within a 'reasonable radius' after voluntarily withdrawing from the firm...when the plan involves deferred compensation or interest earned on the investment of that attorney's deferred compensation." "It is not improper...if the benefits from such a plan come from funding by the employer corporation or partnership or third part." (LE Op. No. 880) (2) "...it is not improper for a professional corporation to enter into an agreement with attorneys of the corporation which states that the value of withdrawing attorney's stock would be reduced if he or she (a) withdraws in concert with other attorneys and/or (b) carried with him, her or them clients of the firm." (LE Op. No. 985) Disciplinary Rule 2-106(A) states that "a lawyer shall not be a party to a partnership or employment agreement that restricts the right of the lawyer to practice law after the termination of a relationship created by the agreement, except as a condition to payment of retirement benefits." (Includes 3 case citations.)

WASHINGTON

The Washington courts will uphold covenants not to compete if both the duration and geographic area are reasonable. (WA ST 19.86.030, 1991 Annotations) (Includes 5 case citations.)

West Virginia

West Virginia does not statutorily prohibit restrictive covenants. The courts will enforce reasonable restrictions. (Includes 4 case citations.)

Wisconsin

The Wisconsin statute provides that "A covenant...not to compete with his employer or principal...within a specified territory and during a specified time is lawful and enforceable only if the restrictions imposed are reasonably necessary for the protection of the employer or principal. Any such restrictive covenant imposing an unreasonable restraint is illegal, void and unenforceable even as to so much of the covenant or performance as would be a reasonable restraint." (WI ST 103.465) (Includes 5 case citations.)

Wyoming

Wyoming does not statutorily prohibit restrictive covenants. (Includes 3 case citations - 2 veterinary cases.)

References

1. *Restrictive Covenant Survey*, The Health Care Group®, 1997, Meetinghouse Business Center, 140 W. Germantown Pike, Suite 200, Plymouth Meeting , PA 19462, ph. 610-828-3888 (A phone call to this resource in July of 1999 indicated that a newer edition of this survey had not been researched nor published since 1997).

2. Samuels LK: Florida's amended noncompetition statute: A reasonable approach. Fla Bar J (July/Aug):60-64, 1991.

3. Coffey KB, Nealon TF: Noncompete agreements under Florida law: A retrospective and a requiem? *Fla State Univ Law Rev* 19:1105-1144, 1992.

Index

I

M

N

R

S

T